Computers in Health Care

Kathryn J. Hannah   Marion J. Ball
Series Editors

D1712964

Computers in Health Care

Series Editors:
Kathryn J. Hannah   Marion J. Ball

M.J. Ball   K.J. Hannah
S.K. Newbold   J.V. Douglas
Editors

Nursing Informatics

Where Caring and Technology Meet

Second Edition
Foreword by Salah H. Mandil

With 30 Illustrations

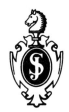

Springer-Verlag
New York Berlin Heidelberg London Paris
Tokyo Hong Kong Barcelona Budapest

Marion J. Ball
Vice President, Information
  Services
University of Maryland
Baltimore, Maryland 21201 USA
mjb@umabnet.ab.umd.edu

Kathryn J. Hannah
Professor, Department of Community
  Health Sciences
Faculty of Medicine, The University of
  Calgary
Calgary, Alberta T2N 4N1 Canada
khannah@acs.ucalgary.ca

Susan K. Newbold
Doctoral Student
University of Maryland
Baltimore, Maryland 21201 USA
snewbold@umabnet.ab.umd.edu

Judith V. Douglas
Director, Information Services
University of Maryland
Baltimore, Maryland 21201 USA
judy@umabnet.ab.umd.edu

Cover image courtesy of Dr. Richard Lichenstein, University of Maryland Medical System, Baltimore, Maryland. The health professionals simulate a mock cardiac arrest with a child mannequin, exemplifying the integration of caring and technology.

Library of Congress Cataloging-in-Publication Data
Nursing informatics : where caring and technology meet / M.J. Ball . . .
  [et al.], editors — 2nd ed.
      p.   cm. — (Computers in health care)
  Includes bibliographical references and index.
  ISBN 0-387-94476-1 (alk. paper)
    1. Nursing informatics.   2. Information storage and retrieval
systems—Nursing.   I. Ball, Marion J.   II. Series.   III. Series:
Computers in health care (New York, N.Y.).
    [DNLM: 1. Computers.   2. Information Systems.   3. Nursing.   WY
26.5 N974 1995]
RT50.5.N87   1995
610.73'0285—dc20
DNLM/DLC
for Library of Congress   95-6681

Printed on acid-free paper.

Production coordinated by Chernow Editorial Services, Inc., and managed by Natalie Johnson; manufacturing supervised by Jacqui Ashri.
Typeset by Impressions, a Division of Edwards Brothers, Inc., Madison, WI.
Printed and bound by R.R. Donnelley and Sons, Harrisonburg, VA.
Printed in the United States of America.

9 8 7 6 5 4 3 2 1

ISBN 0-387-94476-1 Springer-Verlag New York Berlin Heidelberg

To Dr. Gary D. Hales
1949–1995
Founding editor of Computers in Nursing
A pioneer and inspiration to us all

Foreword

There is something very special about nursing that seems to bond the members of this profession into some sort of a fellowship or order. This is apparent at the national level, in every country, as well as at the international level. In recent years, this cohesion has both contributed to, and benefited from, the efforts to introduce and use computing, networking, and communications support in nursing practice, administration, research, and education—so much so that nursing informatics has become a subject in its own right.

Unlike some professions, which initially resisted the introduction and uses of computing, nursing has been, from the outset, an active and lively component of health informatics—a term we use to refer generically to the uses of computing, networking, and communications in health-related fields such as medicine, nursing, pharmacy, and dentistry. As such, health informatics also encompasses health telematics.

The relatively high propulsion or drive of nursing informatics is mainly due to the fact that those working in nursing informatics are often practicing nurses and nursing educators, planners and managers, or individuals or groups with a strong interaction and synergism with those in nursing practice. On the other hand, a critical review of what has been written and published in nursing informatics has been predominantly focused on hospital-based nursing in industrially developed countries. But what about nursing beyond the hospital and nursing in developing communities and countries? Following some major international consultations, the nursing profession is adapting to meet the challenges of the shift from a cure orientation based on hospital medicine to a prevention orientation based on the practice of primary health care in the community. The nursing profession is adding to its computing uses those of modern tools of networking and communications techniques and educational technology. Thus, changes have already started, and the difference between the overall content of this book and that of its first edition bears witness to these significant changes.

The economic value of a good national healthcare system is still not well understood. Often, economic considerations conflict with the caring philosophy of the health profession, including nursing. In contrast, the economic value of the uses of informatics to support nursing practice is much less questioned than are those in other disciplines of health care. In recent years and in a variety of national situations, the increasing costs of health care have been directly attributed to the increasing uses of technology, particularly high technology, which is costly. This is largely true when taking health care as a whole, but in nursing, technology support will be found to be cost-effective.

Such a view of the value of technology support to health care appears fragmented and runs the risk of contrasting with the need to integrate further the various facets of healthcare services, or at least to suggest that such integration might have economic disadvantages. This is certainly not intended, and the points to underline here are, first, that integration remains an important objective aimed at improving the quality, efficacy, effectiveness, and economy of health care; and, second, that much experience, research, and development are still needed to learn how best to integrate the various components of the healthcare system. The methods of work and of national and international cooperation in nursing informatics do provide us with lessons in integration.

Nursing plays a major role in health care, a role that has progressively increased and will continue to increase, particularly insofar as primary health care is concerned. For example, it has been established that for certain categories of patients, "hospital care at home," which is primarily nursing care at home, achieves a faster and better recovery of the patient and is more economical. Another example is the increasing advocacy for the "named nurse" approach, whereby a specific qualified nurse, midwife, or health visitor is assigned to deliver nursing or midwifery care to a specific patient. The main arguments of the advocates of these relatively new notions in nursing include reliance on the increasing availability of informatics tools to support nursing.

The question of standards must also be stressed even at the risk of repeating the obvious. The problems here result from political and commercial differences, which combine to inflate technical differences and to reduce that essential requisite to standards setting—the will to compromise. International professional societies of medical imaging have set the example on how to overcome most of such problems and agree on working standards. It is also my opinion that the emerging collaboration, across national borders, and the rush of commercial interests in the various aspects of TeleMedicine could propel the relatively slow pace of achieving consensus in standards for certain aspects of health informatics. Those involved in nursing informatics can increase their significant contributions to health informatics by reaching, and demonstrating how to reach, agreements on the basics of informatics standards (e.g., minimum data sets) that are within reach.

Informatics tools in support of nursing may be a major contributor to the school of thought suggesting that some countries are gradually moving toward nurse-led national healthcare services.

SALAH H. MANDIL, PHD
Director-Advisor on Informatics
World Health Organisation
Geneva, Switzerland

Series Preface

This series is intended for students and practitioners of the health professions who are seeking to expand their knowledge of computers in health care. Our editors and authors, experts in their fields, offer their insights into innovations and trends. Each book is practical and easy to use.

Since the series began, in 1988, we have seen increasing acceptance of the term "informatics" and of the innovations it brings to health care. Today more than ever we are committed to making this series contribute to the field of healthcare informatics, the discipline "where caring and technology meet."

MARION J. BALL
KATHRYN J. HANNAH

Preface

This volume updates the successful first edition of Nursing Informatics: Where Caring and Technology Meet. Much has been accomplished since that 1988 publication. Nursing informatics is now recognized as a discipline by the American Nurses Association. Nurse informaticians have held two international conferences and formed computer/nursing support groups. Increasingly, nurses are integrating informatics into their daily practice. To reflect these changes, we have rethought and revised this volume, building on and adding to its strengths. Chapters carried over from the first edition have been updated; new chapters have been added in areas which have emerged or evolved since 1988.

For all its changes, the book continues to focus on how technology supports *C*linical practice, *A*dministration, *R*esearch, and *E*ducation, whose initial letters form the acronym *CARE*. Like the first edition, its aim is to emphasize how nursing *CARE* centers upon the patient.

As in the first edition, we provide author photographs at the close of the book, and to these we add electronic mail addresses. Personal networking has always been a prime force in the development of nursing informatics. That force is now strengthened by the expanding capabilities provided by high performance computing and communications.

We four editors are joined by forty colleagues to offer a view of nursing informatics today and in the near future. Each of the authors offers an expertise in the field of nursing informatics. We are privileged and pleased to share their thoughts with you.

Acknowledgments

The editors acknowledge the love and support of their families during the production of this book. Thanks go to John Ball, Rick Hannah, Cree Newbold, and Paul Douglas.

MARION J. BALL
KATHRYN J. HANNAH
SUSAN K. NEWBOLD
JUDITH V. DOUGLAS

Contents

UNIT 4   ADMINISTRATION AND NURSING INFORMATICS

UNIT 5   RESEARCH AND NURSING INFORMATICS

UNIT 6   EDUCATION AND NURSING INFORMATICS

APPENDICES

Nursing Informatics

Unit 1

INTEGRATION

Chapter 1

Integrating Nursing and Informatics

Chapter 2

Informatics and Organizational Change

Chapter 3

Informatics and Integration

Chapter 4

Health-Oriented Telecommunications

Chapter 5

Electronic Resources for Nursing

Unit 2

ROLES FOR INFORMATICS NURSE SPECIALISTS

Chapter 6

What is Nursing Informatics?

Chapter 7

Careers for Nurses

Chapter 8

The Role of the Nurse Analyst

Chapter 9

Selecting a Nursing Informatics Consultant

Unit 3

CLINICAL APPLICATIONS AND NURSING INFORMATICS

Chapter 10

Introducing NISs in the Clinical Setting

Chapter 11

Nursing's Unified Language System

Chapter 12

Nursing Data Elements and Nursing Information

Chapter 13

Point of Care Information Systems

Chapter 14

Information Management in Home Care

Chapter 15

The Automation of Critical Paths/CareMaps

Chapter 16

Clinical Imaging

Chapter 17

Usability Concepts and the Clinical Workstation

Where Caring and Technology Meet

This contents array presents the architecture of the book in reader-friendly terms. Use it to get a feel for the thrust of the units and chapters and to quickly select what you want to study in more depth.

Unit 1
Integration

Unit Introduction

Unit Introduction

The first unit of this book provides an overview of subjects that transcend the areas of nursing clinical practice, administration, research, and education. The integration of computers into the nursing discipline began almost 20 years ago. Nurses are still needed to recognize the potential of automation and to turn that potential into a reality that will ultimately improve patient care.

The first chapter by Ball, Douglas, and Newbold discusses the challenge of integrating computers into the practice of nursing. Lorenzi and Riley propose a change model to integrate automation in the organization. They discuss several roles that can be undertaken by a nurse during this integration. The reader is challenged by Gabler to rethink and redefine how healthcare problems can be addressed with the advances in technology. Skiba focuses on the emerging use of voice, data, and video communications in health care. She cites examples of this use. Newbold and Jaffe expand on the ideas of Skiba and relate reasons why the clinical, administrative, research, or education-oriented nurse should find the on-ramp for the information highway. In Appendix E, Newbold and Jaffe detail how to access nursing and health-related reference materials and provide contact information for nursing informatics support groups.

1
Integrating Nursing and Informatics

MARION J. BALL, JUDITH V. DOUGLAS, AND SUSAN K. NEWBOLD

Introduction

Integrating computers into the practice of nursing is a challenge. As we embark on this new challenge, we need to realize that nothing in life is easy. Change always elicits some fear, because it holds the unknown and unfamiliar. We prefer to look at the partially filled glass of water as half full rather than half empty. We are in for great excitement and opportunities in the nursing profession as we move toward the twenty-first century. Consider briefly the forces that are impacting nursing, both external and internal. We can then look at the new tools information technology is putting within our reach and see how those tools will help us to address those forces.

Forces Impacting Nursing

Today, evolving standards of practice increase nursing accountability. The malpractice crisis has resulted in added emphasis on complete nursing documentation. Changes in reimbursement methods are affecting nursing care delivery. Cost containment and consumerism place additional pressures on not only the individual nurse but also the entire nursing profession. The profession and its practitioners need to address, acknowledge, and prepare for the expansion and extension in nursing roles created by advances in biomedical technology. These external forces are exacerbated by internal pressures affecting the nursing environment. Hospital operations remain task oriented; systems do not promote practitioner accountability; and paperwork requirements have proliferated. These factors we cannot escape; we have to confront them and master them. How do we do so? What are the new alternatives, the new tools available to us in the late 1990s that allow us to address these forces? How can we grow in our profession and meet these challenges? The change masters, the leaders, who have networked together to produce this book will address these questions, repeatedly spiraling back to the host of issues and opportunities surrounding the use of computers in nursing care. These authors include nurses involved in every aspect of the profession, from clinical practice to education, from research to administration. They also include other professionals who have learned invaluable lessons in health care from the nursing profession and have lent their own special areas of expertise to nursing.

Stages in Integration

Whatever the use to which we put new technology in health care—clinical, nursing, hospital information systems, or elsewhere—we all pass through three defined stages before we become more or less comfortable with using the new technology. These three stages are classic in the adoption of computing and information technology.

Replacement

The first of those three stages is called replacement. Simply put, it means that when we get a new tool into our hands, the only thing that we are capable of doing with it at that stage is to try and do what we have been doing in a manual fashion. Maybe we can do it a little bit faster, a little bit more efficiently, but in effect we are replacing a function that we have done manually by this new tool, the computer.

Over the last 25 years, we have been in this first stage as we have brought computers into health care. New computer systems have been nothing more than replacements of manual systems. For example, in admissions offices, we no longer use the typewriter to enter the admissions information on a seven-part form. We brought computers into the admissions office, and we typed information into a computer terminal. We gained some advantages in that we could more easily disseminate the information or we could make changes more easily without having to use correction fluid to correct the form. We could use a little bit of the technology that made the task a little bit easier. But we were really only in the replacement stage—slowly moving into using a new tool.

Innovation

Once we became comfortable with it, we said to ourselves, "Look, we have a new tool now that's very powerful. We might be able to do something that we could not do when we didn't have this tool at our disposal." So we move from replacement into what is called the innovation stage. We have gone beyond what we could originally do manually to doing things with the computer that we could not do before. The new technology begins to be diffused throughout our profession. Computer systems become commonplace in large-scale hospital information systems, as they have in radiology and clinical laboratories.

Transformation

It is true that other industries—airlines, travel, banking—are somewhat ahead of health care and are approaching the final stage. This stage, called transformation, lies beyond replacement and innovation and involves completely revolutionizing the way business is done.

In the healthcare profession, the one area that has entered into this third stage is radiology. Radiology practices today are a transformation of those common as little as 10 years ago. Computerized axial tomography has given us the now-standard CAT scan. Even the way in which radiographs (or x-rays) are read and reported is not at all similar to what was done before new computerized capabilities were available. And, of course, every one of these instruments is based on a built-in computer. When we look at the nursing profession and its practices, it is very exciting to realize that we are going through these phases and are involved in this process. Most of us are still in the replacement stage, moving into innovation. Over the next 5 or 6 years, there will be a revolution—not even an evolution—a revolution into a transformed profession.

Information Technology Tools

Surveys by the American Hospital Association as well as by software vendors have shown that the hospital information systems (HISs) now installed in many institutions do improve communications. These systems also have the potential, when used properly, to increase access to and accuracy of data. Both are increasing in importance as we must respond to demands for more information-based reports and analysis. Hospital information systems also give us the ability to forecast by providing data gathering and storage capacities. With them, we can determine with some precision where we have been and where we are now. Software packages allow us to go beyond the present and to forecast where we will be in the future. This is particularly important in this new era of nurse involvement with overall healthcare delivery. With that as a background, let us focus on the health-care environment with which we are all familiar and on the kinds of tools that are coming into nursing.

No healthcare profession has more contact with the many aspects of patient care than does nursing. No other profession has more involvement with hospital information systems that touch all these aspects than does nursing. Unfortunately, until recently nursing as a profession was not sufficiently involved in the selection, implementation, and decision making regarding what systems are best for institutions. As a result, many of the earlier systems in the marketplace and in hospitals have not met nursing needs. Many of them have failed because of that deficiency. But there is little yield in dwelling on past failures—or even on the capabilities available at this moment in time. As Homer Warner, one of the United States' leading medical informaticians, has often remarked to the senior author, "Let's not spend all our time and resources measuring how long it takes or how much it costs to get there with today's buggy. But let us get on with the job of building tomorrow's automobile and planning where to go with it." He means, of course, that we do not need to replicate. We do not need to see how we traveled with the old horse and buggy. Our challenge is to see how we can use this new tool to innovate and to transform. Technologic advances are now available that will allow this transformation to take place. Several years ago, the senior author used to introduce to her seminar audiences a small laptop computer weighing less than 4 pounds that was carried by engineers, airline people, and academicians on the move. Now it is finding its way, not in the same form, into the working world of health professionals. Nurses no longer need to stay tied to a very large computer at a nursing station. This microchip technology is allowing us to augment as we innovate and transform by enabling us to take handheld terminals to the patient's bedside. This makes it possible to have information at hand when and where it is needed—at the patient's bedside. Truly portable, these handheld terminals are now marketed by a number of manufacturers. Models include 64K portable pocket terminals that the nurses can take to the patient's bedside for entering vital signs and some routine charting information. This frees nurses from having to jot down or remember the information until they can return to the nursing station to enter it. The tools go with the nurses who provide the care.

We also have nursing station/bedside functional systems, including among others TDS, Emtek, Sunquest, and some of the IBM PC-based systems. These represent what is now the more prevalent way of interfacing with hospital information systems development. The keyboard and the terminal remain at the nursing station, where data are entered and the charting completed. Order entries are performed at the terminal by those who are providing care for the patient, primarily by nurses and, in increasing instances, by physicians. To augment these systems, look at yet another innovation: The larger terminal may be taken away from the nursing station and placed at the bedside of the patient (Health Data Systems). This and other new ideas are being tested now. Many companies and many vendors are obviously in the business of trying to market all kinds of tools to health-care professionals.

Nursing Informatics

The nurse and all other healthcare professionals will clearly have to learn how to use these new tools. The learning process and the use that follows are covered by the term "informatics." The term "medical informatics" has been used for nearly 25 years, and it covers all the healthcare fields. Coined from the French word "informatique," the term is moving to greater use and a higher level of definition in the other healthcare professions. Informatics includes all aspects of the computer milieu, from the theoretical to the applied. It covers learning how to use the new tools and building upon the capabilities provided by computers and other information technologies.

The part of informatics designed for and relevant to nurses has been labeled "nursing informatics." This term and what it represents will clearly be part of all our professional vocabularies and practices. The term combines all aspects of nursing—clinical practice, administration, research, and education—just as computing holds the power to integrate all four aspects. Graves and Corcoran (1989) define nursing informatics as "a combination of computer science, information science and nursing science designed to assist in the management and processing of nursing data, information and knowledge to support the practice of nursing and the delivery of nursing care" (p. 227).

We could go so far as to say that nursing informatics has arrived and that the baby is starting to walk. It is exciting to see a whole new profession coming into its own. By becoming involved in the innovative phases of using the tools at our disposal, we can further nursing care and practice. Nursing informatics has introduced new challenges and opportunities along with new computer applications. For nurses, it has created a new cadre of roles and a new vision of the nursing profession. Vendors of hospital information systems now employ nurses as consultants and as nursing liaison advisors to the data processing division. Nurses are becoming programmers, systems engineers, and systems analysts, among other roles. In this volume, Hersher discusses careers for nurses in health information systems.

We may ask ourselves, "Well, isn't this just individuals changing their profession and leaving nursing?" Not quite, for it involves more. Systems analysts and engineers who come from nursing backgrounds practice their profession differently from those who come from an engineering or mathematics background. This has tremendous advantages for nurses remaining in the more traditional nursing fields. Software development is critical for nursing in that it provides the logic for applications. That logic must take into account what the profession is practicing on a daily basis, and who understands the nursing process better than a nurse? Industry has realized this and is freely hiring people with nursing degrees to be involved in software development. The technical aspects are important, because the software does in fact drive the hardware. From our point of view, though, the needs of the users are of equal or greater importance. Developers who understand the nursing profession and its needs, from abstract concepts to small details, are invaluable. Thus the evolution of professions—the hybridization of nurse and computer expert—is critical to effecting the transformation we are anticipating.

New roles evolving for nursing include consulting. Hospitals are now beginning to hire nurse consultants to assist in the design and implementation phases as well as in the process of selecting computers. They are concerned not only with input into what the software should be but also with how healthcare professionals communicate with one another and with computing professionals.

Accepting Change

One key question remains: How do we get this new technology accepted by our colleagues? No hospital information system or stand-alone surgical software system will be installed successfully, no tool used effectively, unless there is an enormous amount of preparation and training. A diffusion pathway must be laid to bring about something that will completely revolutionize the way in which all of us practice our profession. If this pathway is never built, the attempt at computerization will be a failure. We do not have to guess at this. We have seen it happen.

As a profession, we have participated in government-funded investigations on the effect of hospital information systems on healthcare delivery in nursing practice. We are progressing beyond the clinical environment and moving professionally into the establishment of a bona fide research component. We will be looking at nursing practice and nursing education and assessing the problems and issues surrounding information technology, from implementation to ergonomics. One of the biggest concerns now is that we provide strong master's and doctoral programs as well as superb bachelor's degrees in our nursing schools. Nursing informatics needs to be incorporated into the curricula offered by our schools. Only then will the nursing profession be prepared for what is in store. All areas will be freed up as we move into the era of high technology. Hands-on care, or high touch, will continue to be at the heart of the profession. Nurses in computer-aided patient care situations will become involved in administering some nontraditional therapies, such as hypnosis, therapeutic touch, acupuncture, biofeedback, or sonic vibration.

All these changes result in another professional responsibility. Nursing needs to reassess its career paths and its status and reward systems. We firmly believe that as computerization changes the profession, nursing will reappraise its value system and reward professionalism in a wide range of nursing duties not traditionally recognized. In summary, nursing will have greater diversity by virtue of employment opportunities in the health informatics field.

The Future

What will we see in the next 5 years? We will see more computer power, portable computers and handheld terminals at the bedside, voice input freeing our hands for patient care, and videodisc technology giving us vast quantities of stored data and visual information. We will benefit from expert systems, decision support systems, modeling systems, and artificial intelligence (AI) programs. The greatest benefits, however, will not come from the individual tools, as powerful and as effective as they prove to be. Nursing will reap the most from the information that these new technologies make available. Computing will be a powerful utility, fueling our healthcare information systems just as electricity fuels our operating room lights and respirators.

In electronic terms, computing is the medium, information the message. The medium is the equipment that provides the connectivity, enabling the microcomputer user to access other computers and systems. These computers link the user with colleagues, institutions, and libraries. The medium provides new tools, giving the healthcare professional new capabilities for multiple functions—education, research, clinical care, and management of all these. As we move toward integrating these functions through the computing medium, we must respond again and again to critical issues discussed by the other contributors to this book.

This new medium of computing holds our future. It is our charge to use it well, to create an information-rich environment in which patient care and all the many functions that support it are of the highest quality. As a profession, nursing can do no less.

Questions

1. What are some of the forces impacting nurses today?
2. List and define the three stages of diffusion of new technology.
3. What role is industry playing in acknowledging the new discipline of nursing informatics?
4. Take a brief look into the future and give a description of what you might be doing in your job 10 years from today. How does automation fit into this role?

References

Graves JR, Corcoran S: The study of nursing informatics. *Image: Journal of Nursing Scholarship* 1989; 21(4): 227–231.

2
Informatics and Organizational Change

NANCY M. LORENZI AND ROBERT T. RILEY

Sentimentality will always be man's first revolt against development. [However] the times have made this reaction obsolete. .... Things are happening so rapidly now that at any moment the present we're living in will be the "good old days." (Høeg, 1993, p. 381)

Change is a constant reality in both our personal and private lives. Our children grow up taking for granted such things as powerful personal computers that we could not even envision at their ages. Our societies, our professions, and our daily work lives are changing. Moreover, this pace of change appears to be accelerating, not slowing down.

The nursing profession as a whole is undergoing rapid changes, and nursing informatics—as part of health informatics in general—is a driving force in that change process. It is impossible to introduce a nursing informatics system into an organization without the people in that organization feeling the impact of change. Informatics is about change—the change of data into information with a possible evolution into knowledge. Data become information only after the data are processed (i.e., altered) in ways that make the data useful for decision making, and those enhanced decision making capabilities are inevitably going to affect the organization. Figure 2-1 shows this simple but critical circular relationship between the organization, its informatics systems, and the change process. The organization and its people influence, shape, and alter the nature and use of the informatics systems, which, in turn, influence, shape, and alter the nature, operation, and culture of the organization, and so on.

Remember the saying, "Sometimes you get the bear; sometimes the bear gets you." The analogy in change processes is that if we do not manage our change processes, they will manage us—an undesirable alternative at best. The lower our feelings of control during the change process, the lower our "resiliency" (Conner, 1994) will be—our ability to bounce back from the stresses of the change and be prepared for the inevitable next change in today's environment.

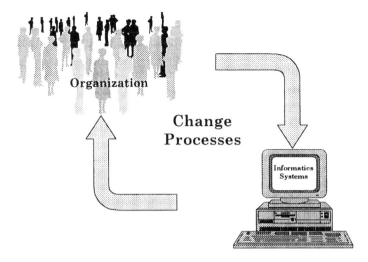

FIGURE 2-1. Circular change relationship between informatics systems and the organizations and their people.

Change and Informatics—An Example

At a 1993 conference on the topics of informatics and change, Dr. Bernard Horak, a healthcare consultant, presented an example of a professional conflict between nurses and physicians caused by the introduction of a new information technology (Draft Proceedings, IMIA, 1993). In this scenario, adapted by Lorenzi and Riley (1994), the perceived role of nurses as the integrators of patient data and information was challenged when the physicians did direct order entry.

Scenario

When using a *manual system* on an inpatient unit, the nurse usually serves as an integrator and reviewer. The physician scribbles something down on a piece of paper, which is given to a nurse, unit clerk, or paraprofessional to do something with. A nurse typically "cleans it up" and transmits the information or order to pharmacy, radiology, laboratory, dietary, etc. Occasionally the lab or pharmacy will call the physician back. However, the nurse in general serves as the conduit for the transfer of information. When nurses fill this role, they learn a lot. Moreover, they have a total view of what is happening with the patient as they filter and organize information from various sources. This is a classic work flow design. What happens when a system is implemented that calls for the physician to enter orders directly into the system?

In one hospital, the nurses did not like this type of new system. The nurses believed that the system reduced their role in the overall care process. It took them out of the reviewer, case manager, and integrator roles, which they were trained to do and which they had always done. The nurses said their two most important roles are (1) the nurse as integrator and (2) the nurse as reviewer, and this new system usurped both roles.

The nurses were very concerned. In the old system, the physicians were used to issuing vague or approximate orders. For example, the physicians would scribble "d.c." or "d/c" for discontinue. They would order "x-rays" and the nurses would figure out that a postero anterior (P.A.) and lateral chest were wanted. If the physicians tried to enter their orders as they traditionally did, they would either get nothing back or something they did not want. The physicians did not know how to order because they had not actually placed orders before. When the physician scribbled an order, the nurse knew the physician, knew exactly what was wanted, and would make it happen. With the new system, this was not possible.

There was a significant decrease of the role of the nurse as an integrator and reviewer of care. Physicians began to make mistakes that nurses had previously caught, such as ordering incorrect drugs or incorrect dosages. There was less coordination between the nursing plans and the medical care plans. In their new role, nurses tended to show less initiative in making treatment suggestions. In summary, what was lost was the second overview review and analysis by a trained professional. The "second" person had lost the overview perspective. On the other hand, some positive things did occur. Relieved of the paperwork of ordering, nurses had two to three more hours per day to spend on hands-on patient care.

Using This Scenario

The remainder of this chapter presents both theoretical concepts and practical techniques for dealing with informatics change processes. We suggest that you try to relate each of the concepts back to this scenario, especially in terms of the role of nursing and nursing informatics in the modern healthcare organization.

Types of Change

Changes within an organization can often be identified as one of four types, with the definite possibility of overlap between two or more:

- *Operational*—changes in the way that the ongoing operations of the business are conducted, such as the automation of a particular area
- *Strategic*—changes in the strategic business direction (e.g., moving from an inpatient to an outpatient focus)

- *Cultural*—changes in the basic organizational philosophies by which the business is conducted (e.g., implementing a continuous quality improvement, or CQI system)
- *Political*—changes in staffing that occur primarily for political reasons of various types, such as top patronage job levels in government agencies.

These four different types of change typically have their greatest impacts at different levels of the organization. For example, operational changes tend to have their greatest impacts at the lower levels of the organization, right on the firing line. Those at the upper levels may never notice changes that cause significant stress and turmoil to those attempting to implement the changes. On the other hand, the impact of political changes is typically felt most at the higher organizational levels. As the name implies, these changes are typically not made for results-oriented reasons but for reasons such as partisan politics or internal power struggles. When these changes occur in a relatively bureaucratic organization—as they often do—the bottom often hardly notices the changes at the top. Patients are seen and the floors are cleaned exactly the same as before. The key point is that performance was not the basis of the change; therefore, the performers are not affected that much.

Resistance to Change

It has been said that the only person who welcomes change is a wet baby. It seems to be part of the human makeup to be most comfortable with the status quo unless it is actually inflicting discomfort. Even then, people will often resist a specific change. This is probably the "devil you know is better than the devil you don't know" phenomenon. It is a shock for inexperienced managers the first time they see subordinates resist even a change that they requested.

Resistance Against What?

There can be countless reasons for resistance to change in a given situation, and the term "resistance to change" is often used broadly. One of the first aspects that must be analyzed in a given situation is the difference between

- Resistance to a particular change and
- Resistance to the perceived changer(s).

In the first case, the resistance is actually directed against the changes in the system. In the second case, the resistance occurs because of negative feelings toward specific units, specific managers, or the organization in general. In this second case, virtually any change would be resisted just because of who is perceived in favor of it. Both have to be dealt with, but it is critical that we identify the primary one.

When a new nursing informatics system is introduced, three factors are important:

• What is the general organizational climate—positive or negative, cooperative or adversarial, etc.?
• What has been the quality of the process used to implement previous informatics systems?
• What has been the technical quality of the informatics systems previously implemented?

Even if we may be new to an organization, we inevitably inherit to some degree the organizational climate and history. Negative baggage of this type can be a frustrating burden that adds significantly to the challenge of successfully implementing a new system. On the other hand, the ability to meet this type of challenge is a differentiating factor for truly skilled implementers.

Intensity of Resistance

Resistance can vary from the trivial to the ferocious. Moreover, the very perception of resistance can vary widely from one observer to another. One might perceive an end user who asks many questions as being very interested and aggressively seeking knowledge. Another might see the same person as a troublemaker who should just "shut up and listen."

We can safely assume that every significant health informatics implementation is going to encounter some resistance; however, the intensity can vary widely. In an organization with decent morale and a history of managing changes reasonably well, significant numbers of the people may be initially neutral toward a particular proposed systems change. However, there will still be a negative component to be managed. At the least, this negative component must be prevented from growing. In other situations, the proportions of positive, negative, and neutral may vary widely.

The Cast of Characters

For any given change, people can occupy a wide range of roles that will strongly influence their perceptions of the change and their reaction to it. As on the stage, some people may occasionally play more than one role. In other cases, the roles are unique. Unless we clearly identify both the players and their roles in any change situation, we risk making decisions and taking action based upon generalizations that are not true for some of the key players. The following categories provide one way of looking at the various roles involved in an overall change process.

The *initiator* or instigator perceives the problem situation or opportunity and conceptualizes the change to be made in response.

The *approver* or funder is the power figure who blesses and financially supports the proposed change.

The *champion* or cheerleader is the visible, enthusiastic advocate for the change. The champion constantly tries to rally support for the change and maintain that support during periods of adversity.

The *facilitator* attempts to assist in smoothing the organizational change process. The facilitator is sometimes involved from the beginning and sometimes is only called in for disaster relief once the change process has gone awry.

The *developer* or builder is responsible for the technical aspects of the change (e.g., developing the new informatics system). These aspects can range from the broad technical conceptualization to the narrowest of technical details.

The *installer* is responsible for implementing the change, including the necessary training and support activities.

The *doer* is the "changee"—the person who has to perform his or her work in the changed environment.

The *obstructionist* is a guardian of the status quo and typically conducts guerrilla warfare against the change. If the obstructionist is also a doer, the reason may arise from a personal fear of the change. However, the obstructionism may also arise from forces such as political infighting (e.g., who gets the credit) or institutional conflicts (e.g., union resistance to a labor-saving system).

The *customer* is the end beneficiary or victim of the change in terms of altered levels of service, cost, etc.

The *observer* does not perceive that he or she will be immediately affected by this change but observes with interest. These observations often affect strongly how the observer will react if placed in the doer role in the future.

The *ignorer* perceives that this change has no personal implications and is indifferent to it. In the broadest sense, this category also includes all those who are unaware of the change.

An overview term often applied to all these roles is "stakeholders." With the exception of the ignorers, all the categories have some stake or interest in the quality of the change and the change implementation process. The roles are subject to change, especially during a change process that extends over some time. For example, an initial ignorer might hear rumblings of discontent within the system and change to an observer, at least until the feelings of angst subside.

For those implementing change, the following steps are critical:

1. Identify what roles they themselves are occupying in the process.
2. Identify what roles the others involved in the process are playing, being careful to recognize multiple roles.
3. Identify carefully which role is speaking whenever communicating with those playing multiple roles.
4. Monitor throughout the process whether any roles are changing.

Magnitudes of Change

Change—like beauty—is in the eye of the beholder. A proposed change that virtually terrorizes one person may be a welcome alleviation of boredom to the person at the next station. In addition, the types and magnitudes of reaction are often difficult for an outsider to predict. When working with change and change management, it often helps to have a simple way of classifying the types and sizes of change.

Microchanges and Megachanges

A practical model that we frequently use divides changes into microchanges and megachanges, with no great attempt at elaborate definitions. As a first approximation, the following scheme can be used to differentiate between the two:

- *Microchanges*—differences in degree
- *Megachanges*—differences in kind.

Using an information system as an example, modifications, enhancements, improvements, and upgrades would typically be microchanges, while a new system or a major revision of an existing one would be a megachange. This scheme works surprisingly well in communicating within organizations as long as we remember that one person's microchange is another person's megachange. Later in this chapter, we will present a more rigorous analysis of the magnitude of change that can be used if necessary.

Classic Change Theories

The rate of change in virtually all organizations is escalating, and healthcare organizations—after a slow start—are no exception. The phrase "change management" has become fairly common and appears in management articles everywhere. What is change management? What is a change agent or a change management person? How does change management help people feel less threatened? How did it evolve, and why does everyone seem so fixated on it today?

Change management is the process by which an organization gets to its future state—its vision. While traditional planning processes delineate the steps on the journey, change management attempts to facilitate that journey. Therefore, creating change starts with creating a vision for change and then empowering individuals to act as change agents to attain that vision. Empowered change management agents need plans that are (1) a total systems approach, (2) realistic, and (3) future oriented. Change management encompasses the effective strategies and programs to enable the champions to achieve the new vision. Today's change management strategies and techniques derive from the theoretical work of several pioneers in the change area.

Early Group Theories

In 1974, Watzlawick, Weakland, and Fisch published their now classic book, *Change: Principles of Problem Formation and Problem Resolution*. Theories about change had long existed. However, Watzlawick et al. found that most of the theories of change were philosophical and derived from the areas of mathematics and physics. Watzlawick and his coauthors selected two theories from the field of mathematical logic upon which to base their beliefs about change. They selected the theory of groups and the theory of logical types. Their goal of reviewing the theories of change was to explain the accelerated phenomenon of change that they were witnessing. Let us briefly look at the two theories that Watzlawick et al. reviewed to develop their change theory.

The more sophisticated implications of the theory of groups can be appreciated only by mathematicians or physicists. Its basic postulates concern the relationships between parts and wholes. According to the theory, a group has several properties, including members that are all alike in one common characteristic. These members can be numbers, objects, concepts, events, or whatever else one wants to draw together in such a group, as long as they have at least one common denominator. Another property of a group is the ability to combine the members of the group in a number of varying sequences and have the same combinations. The theory of groups gives a model for the types of change that transcend a given system.

The theory of logical types begins with the concept of collections of "things" that are united by a specific characteristic common to all of them. For example, mankind is the name for all individuals, but mankind is not a specific individual. Any attempt to change one in terms of the other does not work and leads to nonsense and confusion. For example, the economic behavior of the population of a large city cannot be understood in terms of the behavior of one person multiplied by four million. A population of four million people is not just quantitatively but also qualitatively different from an individual. Similarly, while the individual members of a species are usually endowed with specific survival mechanisms, the entire species may race headlong toward extinction—and the human species is probably no exception.

The theory of groups gave Watzlawick's group the framework for thinking about the kind of change that can occur within a system that itself stays invariant. The theory of logical types is not concerned with what goes on inside a class, but it gave the authors a framework for considering the relationship between member and class and the peculiar metamorphosis that is in the nature of shifts from one logical level to the next higher. From this, they concluded that there are two different types of change: one that occurs within a given system that itself remains unchanged, and one whose occurrence changes the system itself. For example, a person having a nightmare can do many things in his dream—hide, fight, scream, jump off a cliff, etc. But no change from any one of these behaviors to another would terminate the nightmare. Watzlawick et al. concluded that this is a first-order change. The one way out of a dream involves a change from dreaming to waking. Waking is no longer a part of the dream but a change to a different state. This is their second-order change, as mentioned earlier.

- *First-order change* is a variation in the way processes and procedures have been done within a given system, leaving the system itself relatively unchanged. Some examples are creating new reports, creating new ways to collect the same data, and refining existing processes and procedures.
- *Second-order change* occurs when the system itself is changed. This type of change usually occurs as the result of a strategic change or a major crisis, such as a threat against system survival. Second-order change involves a redefinition or reconceptualization of the business of the organization and the way it is to be conducted. In the medical area, changing from a full paper medical record to a full electronic medical record would represent a second-order change, just as automated teller machines redefined the way that many banking functions are conducted worldwide.

These two orders of change represent extremes. First order involves doing better what we now do, while second order radically changes the core ways we conduct business or even the basic business itself.

There is a middle level that seems to be missing from these two extremes. Golembiewski, Billingsley, and Yeager (1976) added another level of change. They defined middle-order change as lying somewhere between the extremes of first- and second-order change. Middle-order change "represents a compromise; the magnitude of change is greater than first order change, yet it neither affects the critical success factors nor is strategic in nature" (Golembiewski et al., 1976, p. 134). An example of a middle-order change might be the introduction of an electronic mail system into an organization. There is an organization-wide impact, but there is no reconceptualization of the basic business. E-mail is more of a tool for operational and communications efficiency.

Some personality types will welcome changes that they perceive will make their jobs easier, while other personality types use their day-to-day work rituals to build their comfort zones. In the late 1960s, one unit in a medical center started to code all of its continuing medical education courses with codes in the International Classification of Disease—9th Revision (ICD 9). Even though these codes were never used and took a great deal of time to complete, the organization did not want to change the process as time passed because "we have always done it this way." The old process lasted through two directors. When a new director went to change the process, there was definite resistance to this change.

The five most important words to an individual involved in any change process are, "How will this affect me?" This is true regardless of the level or degree of change or the person's organizational position. The most traumatic changes are obviously in the second-order change category, but one person might perceive changes in the first or middle order as more traumatic than another person might perceive a second-order change. One of the challenges for the change manager is successfully managing these perceptions. How the change manager implements the process of change can have a decided effect on the resistance factors.

When the Watzlawick book was published, many people were unfamiliar with the applications of theories of change in contemporary society; thus, the book was a major contribution for alternative ways of looking at the changes that occur daily. While Watzlawick et al. comprehensively presented the theories of change and offered their model of levels of change, they did not offer practical, day to day strategies. We are interested in the effective strategies for managing change and have reviewed many social science theories to determine the psychology behind the change management concepts and strategies that are used widely today. We believe that today's successful change management strategies emanate from several theories in the areas of psychology and sociology. Small group theories and field theories provide the antecedents of today's successful change management practices.

Small Group Theories

The primary group is one of the classical concepts of sociology, and many sociological theories focus on small group analysis and interaction process analysis. These theories outline and delineate small group behavior. Small group theories help us to understand not only how to make things more successful but also how to analyze when things go wrong. For example, a practical application of small group research was presented by Bales (1954) in the *Harvard Business Review.* Bales, applying small group principles to running a meeting, makes the following suggestions:

- If possible, restrict committees to seven members.
- Place all members so they can readily communicate with every other member.
- Avoid committees as small as two or three if a perceived power problem between members is likely to be critical.
- Select committee members who are likely to participate in varying amounts. A group with all highly active participants or all low participants will be difficult to manage.

We have all seen small group behavior at work. For example, a job candidate is interviewed by a number of people. Information is then collected from the interviewers and is shared with a search committee. The search committee selects its top candidate, and that person is hired. If the person hired does not work out, a member of the search committee may very well say, "I knew that Mary would not work out, but I didn't say anything because everyone seemed to like her."

Many of the changes that new technology brings are discussed, reviewed, and debated by groups of people that usually fall within the small group framework. If negative sentiments about a product or service are stated by a member of the group who is an opinion leader, the less vocal people often will not challenge the dominant opinion. For example, a medium-sized organization was selecting a local area network (LAN) system. While the senior leader wanted one system, some of the other people not only had suggestions but documentation of the qualities of another system. During the meeting to decide which system to purchase, the senior leader stated his views first and strongly. A couple of the lower-level staff members started to confront the senior person; however, when there was no support from any of the other people present, they did not express their strong preferences for their system of choice. When the system finally arrived, the senior leader's initial enthusiasm had dwindled. He then confronted the technology people about why they had not made him aware of the shortcomings of the system selected.

These examples illustrate a key change management requirement: To manage change effectively, it is imperative for change agents to understand how people behave in groups and especially in small groups.

Field Theory

Kurt Lewin and his students are credited with combining theories from psychology and sociology into the field theory in social psychology (Deutsch and Krauss, 1965). Lewin focused his attention on motivation and the motivational concepts that underlie an individual's behavior. Lewin believed that there is tension within a person whenever a psychological need or an intention exists, and the tension is released only when the need or intention is fulfilled. The tension may be positive or negative. These positive and negative tension concepts were translated into a more refined understanding of conflict situations and, in turn, what Lewin called "force fields."

Lewin indicated that there are three fundamental types of conflict:

1. The individual stands midway between two positive goals of approximately equal strength. A classic metaphor is the donkey starving between two stacks of hay because of the inability to choose. In information technology, if there are two "good" systems to purchase or options to pursue, then we must be willing to choose.
2. The individuals find themselves between two approximately equal negative goals. This certainly has been a conflict within many organizations wishing to purchase or build a health informatics system. A combination of the economics, the available technologies, the organizational issues, and so on may well mean that the organization's informatics needs cannot be satisfied with any of the available products—whether purchased or developed in-house. Thus the decision makers must make a choice of an information system that they know will not completely meet their needs. Their choice will probably be the lesser of two evils.
3. The individual is exposed to opposing positive and negative forces. This conflict is common in healthcare organizations today, especially regarding health informatics. This conflict usually occurs between the systems users and the information technology people or the financial people.

People can easily be overwhelmed by change, especially within large organizations where they may perceive that they have little or no voice in or control over the changes they perceive are descending upon them. The typical response is fight or flight, not cooperation. Managers often interpret such human resistance to change as "stubbornness" or "not being on the team." This reaction solves nothing in terms of reducing resistance to change or gaining acceptance of it. Many managers do not accept that they are regarded as imposing "life-threatening" changes and establishing "no-win" adversarial relationships between management and those below in the organization.

Small group theory is highly applicable in nursing informatics because of the way that medical environments are organized. The care of the patient or the education of students entails many small groups. These groups converse and share information and feelings, and strong opinion leaders can sway others to their way of thinking relatively easily.

Kurt Lewin's field theory allows a diagramming of the types of conflict situations commonly found in health care. In this way, the typical approach-avoidance forces can be visualized (Lorenzi and Riley, 1994). For example, if I accept this new system, what will it mean to me and my job? Will I have a job? How will it change my role? Will this new system lessen my role? These anxieties are very clear and real to the people within the system. Remember: One person's microchanges are often another person's megachanges. So as the system designers think they are making a minor change to enhance the total system, an individual end user may see the change as a megachange and resist it vehemently. When designing the total "people" strategy for any system, it is important to involve the people from the beginning and to understand how groups function within the organization.

All of these social science theories assist the change management leader in understanding some of the underlying behavior issues as they bring health informatics technology into today's complex health systems.

Practical Change Management Strategies

Change management is the process of assisting individuals and organizations in passing from an old way of doing things to a new way of doing things. Therefore, a change process should both begin and end with a visible acknowledgment or celebration of the impending or just completed change. According to James Belasco (1990),

Our culture is filled with empowering transitions. New Year's Eve parties symbolize the ending of one year and the hope to be found in the one just beginning. Funerals are times to remember the good points of the loved one and the hope for new beginnings elsewhere. Parties given to retiring or leaving employees are celebrations of the ending of the employee's past status and the hope for the new opportunities to be found in the new status. (p. 203)

Based on our research, there is no single change management strategy that is effective in every situation. It is essential for the change management leader to take the time to know the desired state (vision-goal) and the particular organization and then to develop the appropriate strategies and plans to help facilitate the desired state.

Over the years we have evolved a core model for the major process of change management. There are many options within this model, but we believe that it is helpful for change leaders to have an overview map in mind as they begin to implement new information technology systems. The five-stage model that has proven effective for reducing barriers to technology change begins with an assessment and information-gathering phase (Lorenzi, Mantel, and Riley, 1990).

Assessment

The assessment phase of this model is the foundation for determining the organizational and user knowledge and ownership of the health informatics system that is under consideration. Ideally this phase of the model begins even before the planning for the technological implementation of the new system. The longer the delay, the harder it will be to manage the change successfully and gain ultimate user ownership.

There are two parts to the assessment phase. The first is to inform all potentially affected people, in writing, of the impending change. This written information need not be lengthy or elaborate, but it will alert everyone to the changes in process. The second part involves collecting information from those involved in the change by the use of both surveys and interviews. The survey instrument should be sent to randomly selected members of the affected group. One person in ten might be appropriate if the affected group is large. Five to ten open-ended questions should assess the individuals' current perceptions of the potential changes, their issues of greatest concern about these changes, and their suggestions to reduce those concerns. Recording and analyzing the responders' demographics will allow more in-depth analysis of the concerns raised by these potentially affected people.

In the personal, face-to-face interviews with randomly selected people at all levels throughout the affected portions of the organization, it is important to listen to the stories the people are telling and to assess their positive and negative feelings about the proposed health informatics system. These interviews should help in ascertaining the current levels of positive and negative feelings; what each person envisions the future will be, both with and without the new system; what each interviewee could contribute to making that vision a reality; and how the interviewee could contribute to the future success of the new system. These interviews provide critical insights for the actual implementation plan. Often those people interviewed become advocates—and sometimes even champions—of the new system, thus easing the change process considerably.

An alternative or supplement to the one-on-one interviews is focus group sessions. These allow anywhere from five to seven people from across the organization to share their feelings and ideas about the current system and new system.

Feedback and Options

The information obtained in the assessment step must now be analyzed, integrated, and packaged for presentation both to top management and to those directly responsible for the technical implementation. This is a key stage for understanding the strengths and weaknesses of the current plans, identifying the major organizational areas of both excitement and resistance (positive and negative forces), identifying the potential stumbling blocks, understanding the vision the staff holds for the future, and reviewing the options suggested by the staff for making the vision come true. If this stage occurs early enough in the process, data from the assessment stage can be given to the new system developers for review.

When designing your model, remember that this phase is important in order to establish that the organization learns from the inputs of its staff and begins to act strategically in the decision and implementation processes.

Strategy Development

This phase of the model allows those responsible for the change to use the information collected to develop effective change strategies from an organizational perspective. These strategies must focus on a visible, effective process to "bring on board" the affected people within the organization. This could include newsletters, focus groups, discussions, one-on-one training, and confidential "hand-holding." This latter can be especially important for professionals, such as physicians, who may not wish to admit ignorance and/ or apprehension about the new system.

Implementation

This phase of our model refers to the implementation of the change management strategies determined to be needed for the organization, not to the implementation of the new system. The implementation of the change strategies developed must begin before the actual implementation of the new system. These behaviorally focused efforts consist of a series of steps, including informing and working with the people involved in a systematic and timely manner. This step-by-step progression toward the behavioral change desired and the future goals is important to each individual's acceptance of the new system. This is an effective mechanism for tying together the new technology implementation action plan and the behavioral strategies.

Reassessment

Six months after the new system is installed, a behavioral-effects data-gathering process should be conducted. This stage resembles the initial assessment stage—written surveys and one-on-one and/or focus group interviews. Data gathered from this stage allow measurement of the acceptance of the new system, which provides the basis for fine-tuning. This process also serves as input to the evaluation of the implementation process. It assures all the participants that their inputs and concerns are still valued and sought, even though the particular implementation has already occurred.

Conclusion

It is not always easy to know exactly why a particular person or group resists change. However, experience shows that an intelligent application of the basic five-step change model—coupled with a sound technological implementation plan—leads to more rapid and more productive introductions of technology into organizations. The process can be expensive in terms of time and energy but nowhere near the cost of an expensive technical system that never gains real user acceptance.

Perhaps most important, overall success requires an emotional commitment to success on the part of all involved. The people must believe the project is being done for the right reasons—namely, to further the delivery of higher quality, more cost-effective health care. If a project is generally perceived to be aimed at just "saving a quick buck" or boosting someone's ego or status, that project is doomed to fail.

An MCI television commercial depicts a book editor—faced with adapting to major informatics changes—commenting that "Art is constant; tools change." In the same vein, the ideals of nursing are a constant; the tools change. The challenge facing nursing informatics is to implement those new tools successfully in organizations that often do not welcome them.

Questions

1. Using your own words, define change management.
2. What might be some ways to help people celebrate remembering the past and moving to the future?
3. In the cast of characters, which roles are nurses at various levels in the organizational hierarchy most likely to play? Why? What roles are nurses least likely to play? Why?
4. Why is the feedback and options phase so important in the change management model presented?
5. For the change scenario presented in this chapter, create a detailed change management plan that you think would lead to better results than those that were described in the scenario.

References

Bales RF: In conference. *Harvard Business Review* 1954; 32: 44–50.
Belasco JA: *Teaching the Elephant to Dance: Empowering Change in Your Organization.* New York: Crown Publishers, 1990.
Conner DR: Bouncing back. *Sky* 1994; September: 30–34.
Deutsch M, Krauss RM: *Theories in Social Psychology.* New York: Basic Books, 1965.
Draft Proceedings of the International Medical Informatics Association Working Conference on the Organizational Impact of Informatics. Cincinnati, OH: Riley Associates, 1993.
Golembiewski RT, Billingsley K, Yeager S: Measuring change and persistence in human affairs: Types of change generated by OD designs. *Journal of Applied Behavioral Science* 1976; 12: 133–157.
Høeg P: *Smilla's Sense of Snow*, trans. Nunnally T. New York: Dell, 1993.

Lorenzi NM, Riley RT: *Organizational Aspects of Health Informatics: Managing Technological Change.* New York: Springer-Verlag, 1994; 228–229.

Lorenzi NM, Mantel MI, Riley RT: Preparing your organizations for technological change. *Healthcare Informatics* 1990; December: 33–34.

Watzlawick P, Weakland JH, Fisch R: *Change: Principles of Problem Formulation and Problem Resolution.* New York: W.W. Norton, 1974.

3
Informatics and Integration

JAMES M. GABLER

The Challenge

With the tremendous advances in medical science, the challenge for nursing continues to be the integration of many specialized resources in the care of patients. Nursing decisions are often limited by access to necessary information available from these specialized sources; thus ease of access in a timely manner to all pertinent patient information is a necessity. Combined with business and government pressure for healthcare reform, medical informatics must economically and transparently integrate information from multiple sources in a manner that allows nurses to focus on the care being given rather than on how the information is obtained. Tremendous opportunities await those willing to rethink and redefine the problems and thus reengineer their resolutions; otherwise, "we will be limited to, at best, 20% solutions" (Simborg and Gabler, 1992, p. 200).

The Systems Problem

One limitation has been the use of a single mainframe system for all departmental functions using a single vendor's turnkey software or software developed in-house. These systems are thought to be optimal for the institution. The system is assumed to be integrated because most functions are on the same computer. Although access to many databases on the same computer simplifies sharing of collected data, it is also possible to integrate multiple systems similarly while gaining significant additional benefits.

Before exploring the multisystem approach, one must understand the weaknesses in the single-system approach. First, most existing mainframe designs have been extended multiple times to meet changing competitive requirements. Any system must have specific design goals around which compromises are made throughout the development and the maintenance and enhancement stages. Many hospital information systems have generally been designed around financial goals, such as having nurses enter orders at the nursing unit to capture charges in a more timely and complete fashion. Although these adaptations have added valuable functions, the basic design is still event focused, not value focused.

As a result, most mainframe systems' strength continues to be addressing the financial and administrative requirements. Charge events are captured, stored, and historically accessed, but the event values are viewable for limited periods. Prospective payment began—and healthcare reform has accelerated—the need for a departmental or clinical emphasis to control costs and ensure quality care. Single systems, designed for the whole institution, bias data collection processes toward their primary design focus, which has historically been finance. This requires too many compromises to capture cost and quality details accurately (e.g., submitting an all-inclusive charge and letting an accounting formula prorate cost and revenue to multiple departments based on historical, rather than actual, contributions). A multilevel design that focuses on departmental needs first and then combines subsets of the detail data from each departmental system to address institutional needs would be more appropriate in our evolving healthcare environment.

A second weakness of the single-system approach is its inability to specialize adequately. This limitation results from the three attributes that characterize hospital information processing—complexity, heterogeneity, and interdependence (Simborg et al., 1983). Individual hospital departments are more complex than their counterparts in other industries. For example, the hospital's accounts receivable department differs from that in other businesses because few of the hospital's patient customers pay their own bills. The resulting mix of insurance company payments, partial payments, and reporting requirements generates a uniquely complex environment. Another example is hospital scheduling, which must allow for unpredictable factors (e.g., when a bed will be vacated) that are not an issue with most other schedulers (e.g., airline reservations, on which seats have a fixed duration of occupancy). Heterogeneity results from the significantly different computer processing requirements of each department. For example, the primary needs in the laboratory, the radiology department, and the pharmacy are process control, text processing, and dynamic database update, respectively. Such variety results in conflicting optimization strategies for the supporting computer system. Interdependence recognizes that a given patient will involve all or many hospital departments on a given stay or visit.

A single-system approach thus forces a compromise on processing characteristics that generalizes the resulting product. In addition, these systems are basically from a single vendor that has strengths in some areas and weaknesses in others. Although the centralized approach tends to address the complexity and heterogeneity characteristics poorly, it does have the advantage, because of centralized storage, of addressing the interdependence characteristic more easily. Stand-alone systems, in contrast, address the complexity and heterogeneity characteristics extremely well because of their specialized focus and departmental heritage. The interdependence issue, on the other hand, is poorly addressed in these systems because of the technical problems involved in connecting multiple stand-alone systems (Albright and Gabler, 1986). However, multiple systems are clearly preferable in that they address more effectively the variety of processing requirements.

To summarize, a single-system simplifies institutional coordination but reduces modular departmental independence. However, modular structures can be coordinated effectively, as the following examples illustrate. First, the single-celled amoeba is not an appropriate coordination design model for the more complex human body, which includes many specialized cells grouped in modules, such as heart, hand, brain; however, the human body's skeletal, nervous, and blood systems effectively coordinate its modular specialization. Second, when the scope and span of activities exceed one person's ability, organizational structures are established to manage (coordinate) a group of people for a common purpose. Clearly, modular systems can be coordinated, but an organizational and communication structure is necessary.

The Multisystems Approach

When computer capabilities were beginning to be realized during the 1960s, computerization approaches were process oriented, characterized by the processing of data. As the value of stored data was realized, computerization designs during the 1970s and early 1980s were database oriented, characterized by the use of database management systems. In the late 1980s and into the 1990s, computerization began to connect multiple computers, creating a shift to flow-oriented systems designs characterized by the movement of data (i.e., information exchange) (Sullivan and Smart, 1987). This multisystems approach required the development of an organizational and communication structure that enabled information to be exchanged easily and multiple systems to be coordinated effectively. Although they are more common in other industries, health care is beginning to make use of these flow-oriented designs to address more effectively its multiple, uniquely specialized areas. The development of integrated delivery systems in the mid-1990s accelerates this trend, with multiple specialized departments needing to be coordinated across multiple, geographically separate entities. But coordination requires a flow design, not just the linking of computer systems to exchange information (Gabler and Lopez, 1994).

Using a hospital example, Figure 3-1 illustrates the financial information flow in hospital information systems. If this were implemented as a single centralized system, each functional ellipse in the diagram would share a

30   James M. Gabler

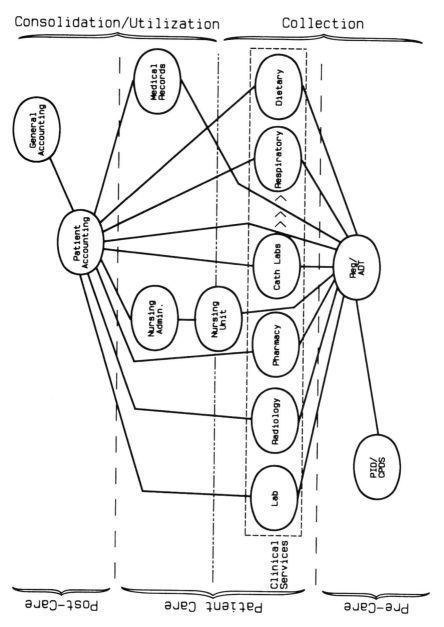

FIGURE 3-1. Financial flow.

single census file. An entry by registration/admission-discharge-transfer (Reg/ADT) is immediately available to the other functions, and charge events, once entered, are immediately available for billing (Patient Accounting); but all of the functions are locked into the single system's hardware and software environment. Conversely, if this flow were implemented as multiple departmental systems, each functional ellipse in the diagram could be a separate system module on separate hardware and software. An entry by Reg/ADT would flow to each of the other functions, and charge events would flow to patient accounting.

If the exchange protocols are standardized, an open architecture is created that allows each module to be added, replaced, or removed relatively independent of the other functions and their hardware and software environments. Although each function could be a separate quasi-stand-alone system, some functions, like patient identification (PID), Reg/ADT, and patient accounting, can be a single system in some implementations (with loss of some flexibility); however, departmental differences strongly favor separate systems for most of the other functions. Rather than consolidating all data in one database, the multisystems approach allows the relevant working data to be maintained in each functional module while focusing on the small subset of data that actually needs to flow between systems for coordination.

Since the multisystems approach requires some duplicate storage of data, special steps must be taken to address the resulting synchronization issue. First, only one system can be the official source for each information element (e.g., Reg/ADT as the official source for bed control information). Second, the duplicated data should be minimized (i.e., there should be sufficient information and identification data to facilitate patient care and to allow subsequent regrouping, or coordination, of independently generated information). For example, the medical record number, name, date of birth, sex, billing identification, and location are needed in each functional module, but insurance, guarantor, and billing information are only needed by patient accounting. Thus only a small amount of data need to be duplicated in multisystem modules for coordination and functionality.

Third, timeliness affects the synchronization strategy. If synchronization is only necessary at certain times, information updates can be transferred periodically in files or batches of data. An example of this would be nightly billing, in which charge events can be accumulated in ancillary systems (lab, radiology, etc.) and then sent to patient accounting all at once. This method is technically simple, manageable and easily recovered. However, some synchronization must take place immediately, such as patient admits, discharges, and transfers. A more sophisticated process must be established to ensure timely transfer of this time-dependent information, but a close examination of how information is actually used reveals that only the key tag information must be disseminated immediately. With tag information synchronized, batch transfers can handle the remaining flow requirements.

The synchronization process necessary for the financial flow (Fig. 3-1) allows other systems to be added that use the same collection modules (i.e., lab, radiology, pharmacy, etc.) since the tag simplifies the combination of related data subsequent to the registration process. Figure 3-2 illustrates the ability to send ancillary orders and view ancillary results. Just as bed control (Reg/ADT) was the official census source, the ancillary is the official request/result source. Figure 3-3 illustrates the ability to consolidate previously collected data for multiple purposes using the tag to combine related data. Patient accounting consolidates charge events for billing purposes, and the management reporting and archival system consolidates these performed events for costing purposes independent of billing charges. The reporting capabilities of the management reporting system allow the actual work performed to be compared to expected norms for concurrent review analysis, to various groupings for case mix analysis, to collection and charging routines for adjustments, and so on.

Figure 3-4 illustrates another data consolidation system that brings together clinical data for trend displays, clinical analysis, intervention indicators, medical decision support, and so on. This has been a major missing component of most hospital information systems but is easily added with the modular open architecture described here. Other nursing modules could be scheduling/staffing and a nursing database. The latter would be similar to the other clinical service systems (see Fig. 3-2), would maintain acuity factors, patient care data, nursing notes, care plans, and procedure manuals; and would be accessible via similar request/result (update/view) processes. The clinical database is sometimes called the computerized medical record and could be used for intervention reminders during the care of a patient. This system also requires that bedside data collection be addressed so that medication administration can be cross checked, vital signs can be captured automatically, and other nursing care information can be collected quickly and easily. Bedside terminals and/or handheld (portable) computers can then be used to facilitate the collection process. Since this flexible structure allows collected data to be reused, medical informatics can focus more productively on how data are used rather than how data are collected. Much data collection is already automated, but without a coordinated communication scheme, manual reentry inhibits full use of existing data.

The Benefits

Technical possibilities are not sufficient justification for change. There must be significant benefits to justify a multisystems approach rather than a traditional single-system, centralized database approach. These benefits can be grouped into three categories: management accountability, management flexibility, and economics (Albright and Gabler, 1986). Management accountability is limited in a single-system approach since accountability is

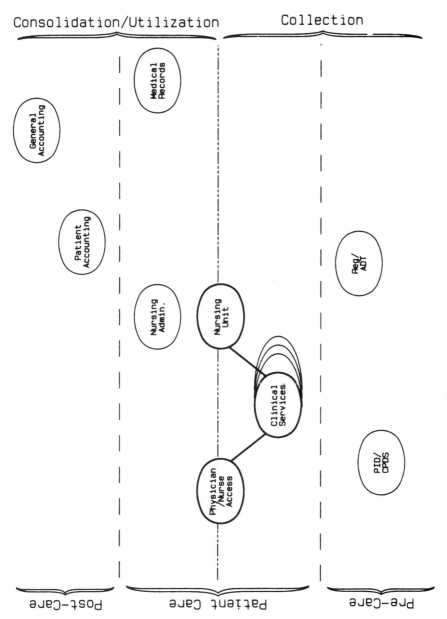

FIGURE 3-2. Communication flow.

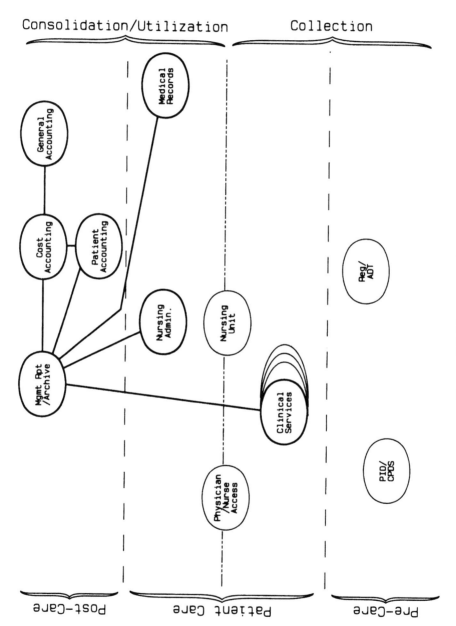

FIGURE 3-3. Management flow.

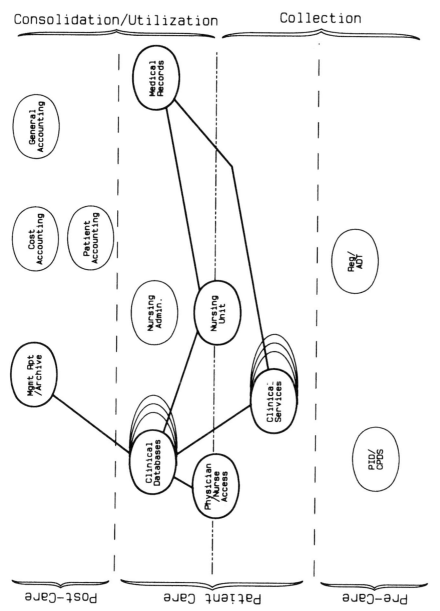

FIGURE 3-4. Medical flow.

nebulously shared by information services and the multiple user groups sharing the computer. Because the multisystems approach allows functional systems to be implemented at or below the department level, responsibility for both utilization and operation can naturally follow existing account-ability structures. These individual systems are more easily grasped and more accurately evaluated and monitored for costs and benefits without computer expertise; modular systems are simply viewed as a tool for the functional area that is relatively unaffected by other functional areas.

Because some general understanding is required to make good manage-ment decisions about technical recommendations, reducing computeriza-tion to identifiable modules allows management to make decisions without understanding all the technical details involved. One does not have to un-derstand copy machine technology to manage a copier—it is simply an issue of asking "Does it work?," "What features are needed?," "How much do they cost?," "Are they worth it?," and so forth. Management control also benefits from lower initial and incremental costs and from increased morale associated with the system's "ownership." This last point is particularly crucial because user motivation has a much greater influence on success or failure than a system's objective superiority to other systems.

Management flexibility is a second major benefit. This flexibility starts with the system selection process, since each functional area is free to choose, at any time, whatever system best fits its needs without being con-strained by previous hardware and software decisions. This flexibility con-tinues with the freedom to establish and change the implementation se-quence (priority) of each module. Initial priorities reflect the current weight of various factors when budget plans are made, but those weights will change during the budget period because of competitive pressures, govern-ment requirements, board requirements, management needs, and depart-mental readiness. These priorities are not as limited in a modular, multi-system implementation process as in traditional single-system sequential approaches. This flexibility allows management to adjust more quickly to the dynamic environment, optimizing the impact on overall enterprise ob-jectives. This becomes even more important with our rapidly evolving tech-nology. Flexibility is also realized in the natural redundancy inherent in the design. Since each system is quasi-stand-alone, it retains most of its pro-cessing capabilities even though other systems may be unavailable. For ex-ample, if the lab is down, the radiology system is unaffected; however, if Reg/ADT is down or the network is down, an ancillary system can manually enter tag information and continue processing departmental workload. Thus there is no single point of complete failure, although partial failures degrade some capabilities.

The third benefit is significant economic savings. The modular, multi-system design lowers initial and incremental costs. Total costs for multi-system approaches can be less than traditional single-system approaches due to significant advances in interface technology and true economies of scale. Interfaces have historically been discouraged, not only because they were difficult (and expensive) to develop but also because they were difficult (and expensive) to maintain over time. Their complexity increases exponentially as the number of components interfaced increases. For example, connecting two computers requires two interface programs—one in each machine to "talk" to the other. Adding a third computer requires six interface programs; four computers requires 12 interface programs, and so on. This is known as the "$N^2 - N$ problem," where N is the number of computers (Simborg, 1984). Although limiting the hardware and software involved would simplify the maintenance, it was seldom practical to interface more than two or three computers directly.

Local area networks (LANs) have simplified development and maintenance issues and costs significantly since only one program per computer is necessary for a LAN interface. The LAN simply delivers a message prepared and addressed by one computer to its destination, similar to the post office delivering mail. It is critical to note that LANs simplify only the mechanics of interfacing; the requirement for and the content of messages (data exchanged) together constitute a separate issue and must be addressed by the overall design flow. This simplification reduces costs as well. Costs are further reduced as standards evolve for the LAN interfaces. In particular, a group of hospitals and vendors have established Health Level 7 (HL7) as a de facto standard for hospital interfaces. HL7 is based on the International Standards Organization's seven-layer Open Systems Interconnection (OSI) model.

Economies of scale have also been altered by technology developments. Computer centralization is typically based on the assumption that one large computer will be less expensive than multiple smaller computers. If all computers are plotted on a single price-performance curve, the price per power measure would appear to decrease as computer power increased (Grosche's law). However, "when computers are grouped according to their size and power, Grosche's law seems to hold within each group, but not between different groups" (Ein Dor, 1985, p. 142). These groups are "microcomputers, minicomputers, small mainframes, large mainframes, and super computers" (Ein Dor, 1985, p. 145). It is important to note that a microcomputer is clearly not equivalent to a minicomputer for batch processing or intensive computations. However, if the processing can be redefined to function well on a client-server combination using computers in a lower price-performance group, the total cost will be less. Multiple units in the lower performance group can be purchased for the same or less cost as one unit in a higher performance group. Savings result when large central processor requirements decrease even though the cumulative processing power increases. Thus, it can be economical to decentralize processing into multiple modules.

Summary

The challenge for medical informatics is to rethink and redefine how problems can be addressed in view of advances in technology. Problems tend to be defined in terms of the types of tools available to solve those problems. Although one can be creative in applying tools to problems, real innovation results from redefining the problems as technology produces significantly new types of tools. For example, when arabic numbers replaced roman numerals, division was greatly simplified. Much computerization today is still based on a database approach that consolidates all data elements on a single centralized processor. This is a natural result of a legacy of interface difficulties and of a single economy of scale (Grosche's law), both of which favor increasingly larger mainframes locked into a single-system design.

Now that LANs simplify interfacing and micro- and minicomputers have reversed the economies of multiple computers, a new approach can be taken that connects multiple computer systems. Rather than consolidating all data in one database, the multisystems approach allows relevant working data to be maintained in each functional module while focusing on the small subset of coordination data that actually needs to flow between systems. In essence, each functional system becomes a replaceable component of a larger composite enterprise system that is more easily understood and managed. This becomes a flexible architectural structure that allows medical informatics to address the real patient care environment, which has been poorly addressed with single-system approaches.

Questions

1. What are the strengths and weaknesses of a single system for all hospital departments?
2. What are the strengths and weaknesses of a modular, multisystems approach for all hospital departments?
3. What characterizes information flows?
4. What are the benefits of a modular, multisystems approach?
5. How have advances in technology redefined problems and reengineered their solutions?

References

Albright J, Gabler J: Distributed processing in a large hospital. *Software in Health-care* 1986; 3: 34–37.
Ein Dor P: Grosche's law re-visited: CPU power and the cost of computation. *Communications of the ACM* 1985; 28: 142–151.

Gabler J, Lopez M: Open systems architecture: How to make it work. *Healthcare Informatics* 1994; 5: 64–70.

Simborg D: The $N^2 - N$ problem. In: Lindberg DAB, Collen MF, eds. *Proceedings of the AAMSI Congress 1984.* Bethesda, MD: AAMSI; 131–135.

Simborg D, Gabler J: Reengineering the traditional medical record: The view from industry. *M.D. Computing* 1992; 4: 198–200.

Simborg D, Chadwick M, Whiting-O'Keefe Q, Tolchin S, Kahn S, Bergan E: Local area networks. *Computers and Biomedical Research* 1983; 16: 247–259.

Sullivan C, Smart J: Planning for information networks. *Sloan Management Review* 1987; 28: 39–44.

4
Health-Oriented Telecommunications

DIANE J. SKIBA

Introduction

This chapter focuses on the use of telecommunications for healthcare applications. Telecommunications is one of the fastest growing industries in the American economy and will directly impact the delivery of health care and education. The development and expansion of the National Information Infrastructure will undoubtedly change the nature of our communications and our access to information and knowledge resources. Several authors (Center for Civic Networking, 1993; Naisbitt and Aburdene, 1990; Rheingold, 1993) believe that telecommunications will serve as a driving force for societal change. There is hardly a day that society is not bombarded with information about the Information Superhighway by both print and broadcast media. In health care, many project that telecommunications will have a profound impact on the delivery of health care and consumer and healthcare professional education (McDonald and Blum, 1992; Melmed and Fisher, 1991; Olson, Jones, and Bezold, 1992).

The definition of telecommunications is the use of wire, radio, optical, or other electromagnetic channels to transmit or receive signals for voice, data, and video communications (Witherspoon, Johnstone, and Wasem, 1994). Another definition is communications at a distance, using electric or optical means of transmission, of audio, video, and/or data between humans or computers (Strammiello, 1993). The typical telecommunications providers include telephone, cable television, broadcast and satellite companies, and, more recently, the computer industry. According to Witherspoon et al. (1994), the media of telecommunications include telephone, video, and computers whereas the means of transmission include phone lines, fiber optics, satellites, and microwave systems. Thus telecommunications applications can include voice, data, and video communications.

Another term commonly associated with the area of telecommunications is "computer mediated communication." Hiltz and Turnoff (1985) define computer mediated communication as the use of computers and telecommunications networks to compose, store, deliver, and process communication. These systems support a person's ability to exchange, edit, store, broadcast, and copy any written document, to send data and messages instantaneously, and to consult electronically (Kiesler, Siegel, and McGuire, 1984). Applications under this rubric include electronic mail (E-mail), computer conferencing, long-distance blackboards, and bulletin board systems. Computer mediated communication applications are considered a type of data communications.

For this chapter, the telecommunications classification of voice, data, and video will serve as a framework for the discussion of health-oriented applications. Given the rapidly changing technology in this area, applications in health care and education are limited to the past 10 years and serve as examples rather than an inclusive list of all available applications.

Voice Communications

Voice communications originated in basic telephone service, referred to by the industry as POTS (Plain Old Telephone Service). This telecommunications medium historically provided adequate service for voice communications. The telephone has several major advantages: ubiquity (universal telephone service was a public policy goal set over 60 years ago), relatively low cost for installation, minimal training for proper use, and a relatively low cost per use (Witherspoon et al., 1994). Telephone service can be provided via a voice/low-speed data network or a cellular network. Enhancements to the telephone service in the past decade have allowed the following services as part of voice communications: telephone conferencing, voice mail, facsimile (fax) machines, computer communication, and picture phones.

Nurses in Columbus, Ohio, use a voice communications system called Telmed to facilitate the delivery of health care to patients in their homes. The voice communications system allows nurses to consult with the system while caring for their home-bound clients. It also allows them to complete the following tasks: confirm the nurse's visit with the agency; confirm and update a preset care plan; allow voice input of patient data such as blood pressure and confirmation of injections; notify the nursing supervisor when patient data are out of limits; conduct two-way consults between nurse and doctor; chart progress notes; and initiate the billing process. According to Tanzillo (1989), "It's as close to a house call as most patients have been in decades" (p. 47).

Another voice communications system in health care is the House Calls Project instituted by Cleveland State University. House Calls is a telecommunications system for integrating patients' self-care with clinic care. The telephone messaging system empowers patients to do self-care while having the guidance of their healthcare providers (Alemi, 1993). This system allows healthcare professionals to communicate with their patients and patients to communicate with each other. The system provides patients with the following services: health education, access to healthcare providers, health reminders, social support, automated monitoring, and triage of patients (Alemi, 1993). Health education is achieved via the Voice Information System, in which patients can listen to prerecorded health education messages or can record their own health question, which is answered by a healthcare professional and recorded for later retrieval. The system's Care Mail component facilitates access to healthcare professionals and automated health reminders. Care Mail allows for the following capabilities: send health messages to lists of patients, store confidential online directory of patients, send messages to patients without knowing names or telephone numbers, integrate healthcare paging systems, and allow communication between providers and patients on the same system (Alemi, 1993). The TalkNet component allows patients to participate in telephone support groups. Patients can join support groups or receive publicly posted messages from these support groups. This component is similar to an electronic bulletin board system but makes use of the telephone rather than a computer system. Monitoring of patients is accomplished through the automated outcome evaluation component, which makes periodic calls to patients and solicits outcome information. The Triage and Risk Assessment system uses a voice-response mechanism to collect data from patients and alert healthcare providers of high-risk patients. The House Calls Project has implemented these various systems with several patient populations: pregnant mothers, mothers of newborns, and drug-abusing patients.

The GroupLink Project in California is another example of the use of voice communications as a means for support and wellness groups to function without face-to-face meetings. This teleconference system allows group facilitators and members to meet via the telephone conferencing feature of Pacific Bell's Centrex service and an 800 number access. According to Axsom (1993), "The GroupLink Project is a creative response to the human need for social support in the maintenance of mental health and physical wellness" (p. 1). The GroupLink Project is managed by Community Strategies 2000 with grants from Pacific Bell and Northern Telecom. Groups are formed with a facilitator, and a block of conference time is scheduled at a recurring time. Group members dial in at the scheduled time, and up to 30 members can participate in the conference. Support groups were formed in the following areas: teenage burn victims, Codependency Anonymous, parents of disabled children, gay and lesbian elders, women dealing with depression, men with HIV/AIDS, peer counselors for home-bound elderly, AIDS caregivers, women substance abusers, disabled women, and home-bound students. The evaluation demonstrated the efficacy of teleconferencing as a medium for support groups. The primary benefits were easy technology, reduced travel time and related expenses, no need for respite care or child care during sessions, and intact or enhanced group process due to the teleconference (Axsom, 1993).

The use of fax machines to facilitate healthcare delivery and education is also an example of a voice communications system. Staggers and Jacox (1990) reported that fax systems in the 1980s facilitated communication within an institution and outside the institution. They cited several examples of Army hospitals using fax machines to link their nursing stations with ancillary departments and hospitals connecting with rural hospitals and doctors' offices via facsimile technology as a means of communication and dissemination of information. A federally funded project in Hawaii improved medical communication through the use of a hospital fax network in the 1980s. Facsimile technology was used to connect emergency departments in hospitals across the Hawaiian Islands. It was used for telephone patient consultations, instant medical records transfer, instant electrocardiogram (ECG) interpretation, patient transfers, instant retrieval of literature, and multicenter research links (Witherspoon et al., 1994).

The federal government—in particular, the Office of Rural Health Policy—has funded several voice communications projects to support the delivery of health care in rural areas. One such voice communications project was the development of the Maine Rural Health Center Clinician Support Network. This network was created in 1991 by the Maine Ambulatory Care Coalition and their member centers, the Maine-Dartmouth Family Practice Residency and the Eastern Maine Medical Center Family Practice Residency. The network makes extensive use of teleconferencing (speakerphones) and fax transmissions and limited use of computer connections for the retrieval of literature resources via the National Library of Medicine's software, Grateful Med. The teleconferencing allows consultations among the more than 70 physicians on the network. Clinical consultations are crucial to provide support for primary care physicians practicing in rural, isolated areas. The teleconferences are also used to provide both continuing medical education and informal symposiums among the clinicians. According to Witherspoon et al. (1994), clinicians preferred teleconferencing to video conferencing because of the convenience and accessibility of telephones.

Several schools of nursing have also used audio conferencing as a technique for providing distance education to nursing students at remote sites. Audio conferences or audio teleconferences deliver two-way voice instruction over phone to distant sites, where students interact and communicate via a speakerphone. This audio-based delivery technique was used successfully by several programs (Kuramoto, 1984; Weust, 1991). According to a review by Billings and Bachmeier (1994), audio conferences are cost effective, reduce isolation, and allow for immediate feedback to students.

Data Communications

Data communications is one of the fastest growing types of telecommunications applications. Consumers, businesses, and professionals are all connecting to each other via data communications. Data communications are provided through a variety of methods: telephone service for access to dial-up lines and specialized private networks for a selected group of individuals and/or institutions. Most connections are through the use of a computer, telecommunications software, and a modem. Data communications allow computers to "talk" or access other computers located at a remote location. The three most popular uses of data communications are E-mail, computer conferences, and information access. The push to jump on the Information Superhighway has motivated many individuals to purchase the necessary equipment and services to access either the Internet (a global network of networks) or commercial networks such as CompuServe™, Prodigy™, Delphi™, and America Online™. Numerous examples of data communications applications can be found in the healthcare literature. Here are but a few applications to provide the reader with a sense of how telecommunications can be used to support healthcare professionals and healthcare delivery systems.

Electronic Bulletin Boards and Computer Conferences

In health care, the beginning of data communications occurred with the development of electronic bulletin board systems (BBSs) on the hobbyist network called FidoNet. Thousands of electronic BBSs were established across the globe, and the focus of these BBSs was on every imaginable subject. In nursing, numerous BBSs were developed as a means for healthcare professionals or students to talk with each other and to exchange information (Skiba and Warren, 1991). Most electronic BBSs consisted of E-mail facilities, discussion groups (both local and international UseNet groups), read-only text file access, and downloadable text/program files. The majority of these BBSs were targeted toward healthcare professionals and did not encourage consumer access.

Another major component of BBSs was the development of electronic support groups (Sparks, 1992). The electronic support groups provided 24-hour service in which consumers could selectively participate in discussions about their health problems. This non-face-to-face communication provided a nonthreatening environment in which to ask questions, share feelings, and communicate with others who experienced similar consequences of their specific health problems. Electronic support groups were available for a variety of healthcare problems (such as AIDS, cancer, neurotrauma, and parents of hyperactive children). One such network was the Nurse Corner, in which several electronic support groups have been flourishing for years. The philosophy of the Nurse Corner, according to Sparks (1992), "is to help participants manage situations as independently as possible, yet know when and how to get help when needed" (p. 62). The Nurse Corner participants also have access to a knowledge-based decision-support system that provides information and management options for several different healthcare problems.

As an outgrowth of these hobbyist networks, numerous electronic BBS-like systems were designed by healthcare professionals to encourage free exchange of information and to simulate the area of computer conferencing. Many systems were considered computer mediated communications projects. One such network that was publicly accessible to healthcare professionals (although it is no longer available) was designed by Sparks at the National Library of Medicine. The Educational Technology Network, or ET-NET™ as it was called, allowed professionals to dial local access numbers or the Internet to connect to a computer conferencing system and facilitate discussions of topics in the area of educational technology. Sparks (1994) stated that the purpose of ET-NET™ was to link electronically developers and users of interactive technology in health science education. ET-NET™ consisted of numerous asynchronous message areas or conferences. Users could read and post messages to a particular area, such as NUCare (Nursing Care Research). Each conference area was moderated by an organizer, who facilitated discussion and handled the logistics of the area. This successful system was available 24 hours per day, 365 days per year and had over 2000 registered users from the United States and numerous other countries.

Numerous computer communications projects were developed that combined access to a variety of information resources and computer conferencing for healthcare professionals. In Nebraska, the Synapse Health Resources Online was developed to provide timely access to information and communications research for healthcare professionals, primarily physicians. The system provided such services as access to numerous medical, nursing, and allied health journal abstract databases; E-mail; multispecialty bulletin boards; continuing education simulations; drug interaction databases; Internet resources; and various office management software. The Virtual Medical Center in Montana provides electronic information and education resources for rural healthcare practitioners across the state, including electronic mail, bulletin board systems, consultation networks, and continuing education courses. Nurses are a major user of this system, which is sponsored by two Area Health Education Centers and the State Offices of Rural Health.

In nursing, a new national computer network was created by the American Journal of Nursing. Rizzolo (1994) and colleagues developed AJN-Net to provide a variety of formal and informal continuing nursing education to nurses practicing in medically underserved areas. The electronic bulletin board system provides the following services: a nurse consultant feature, wherein users can post questions and experts will respond; text-based and computer-assisted instructional packages on-line; patient information; national and international news; conference databases; and forums for nursing discussions. The initial study offers these services to pilot sites in North Carolina, Nevada, and Wisconsin.

Community Computing

As an outgrowth of the electronic BBS movement for healthcare professionals, community computing networks were spawned. Community computing networks were different from professional BBSs in that the network was a reflection of the community and allowed public access to information and communication resources. Community computing networks, a term coined by Grundner (1991), establish a community resource that is freely accessible to the citizens through a computerized network. The community, by using a personal computer, telecommunications software, and a modem, can access the system on a 24-hour basis. The community itself defines the information resources and provides the necessary support to maintain the information resources as well as to sustain the concept of an electronic community. The first community computing system established was the Cleveland Free-Net, which started a movement that encouraged the implementation of over 20 operational free-nets to facilitate indexing across the globe and over 50 community systems in development.

The Cleveland Free-Net served as the core computer network in the seminal work conducted by Brennan and colleagues at Case Western Reserve University. Two extensive studies examined the use of an electronic network in the provision of care for both Persons Living with Aids (PLWAs; Brennan, Ripich, and Moore, 1991) and caretakers of Alzheimer's disease patients (Brennan, Moore, and Smyth, 1991). In both studies, Brennan and her colleagues investigated the use of an electronic network, ComputerLink, to bring support services into the homes of patients or caretakers. The first study was a pilot study to investigate the use of a computerized network to provide services for PLWAs. The ComputerLink system provided three basic services: an electronic encyclopedia, a decision-support system, and a communication pathway. The electronic encyclopedia was designed to meet the patient's informational needs and served as a clearinghouse for factual information about AIDS, clinical care, and local community services (Brennan, Ripich, and Moore, 1991). The decision-support tool was tailored to meet the problem-solving needs of patients and used a decision-modeling tool based on multiattribute utility theory. The communication pathway functioned as a social and professional contact to decrease the patients' social isolation needs. This pathway allowed patients to talk with their healthcare provider, each other, and other members of the electronic community served by the Cleveland Free-Net system. Within the communication pathway, patients could access the question and answer (Q&A) sections to read and post anonymous questions that would be answered by the project nurse.

In the case of caretakers of Alzheimer's disease (AD) patients, ComputerLink provided three services for the caretaker. The first service facilitated communication between the caretaker and the nurse as well as discussions among the caretakers themselves. The communication pathway was conceived as a "support group without walls" (Brennan, 1992, p. 157). The second service was an information resource that included an AD electronic encyclopedia and numerous patient educational materials. The third service was a decision-support tool similar to the one provided for the PLWAs in the previous study.

Another health-oriented telecommunications project using a community system is the Denver Free-Net. Operated by the School of Nursing at the University of Colorado Health Science Center, the Denver Free-Net is investigating ways in which an electronic healthcare community can facilitate the delivery of health care, particularly in the rural frontier areas of the state of Colorado (Skiba and Mirque, 1994). A specific goal is to provide citizens with free and open access to community information resources, particularly in health and human services. The Denver Free-Net is best conceptualized as an electronic city, in which a user enters buildings such as the post office, the schoolhouse, and the healthcare community center. It is a menu-driven system that provides information in several formats: read-only text information, databases, question and answer forums, and an online conversation mode. The Health Care Building has been developed with the Healthy People 2000 goals as a framework. The Denver Free-Net is working with the statewide library network in Colorado, Access Colorado Library Information Network, to provide consumer access to healthcare information and communication resources across the state. The statewide network will eventually allow every individual in the state to dial a local or toll-free number to access a variety of databases, including the Health Care Building of the Denver Free-Net.

Schultz, Bauman, Hayward, and Holzman (1992) have successfully used telecommunications as a means of home monitoring for patients with diabetes. In this study, patients agreed to collect their own blood glucose readings and transfer the information to their healthcare professional via a personal diary method or through an intelligent modem once a week for a specified time. A double crossover design was used to compare the two information transfer techniques. The use of telecommunications as an information transfer method demonstrated a significant improvement in serum glucose control.

Another system designed by the University of Wisconsin is the Comprehensive Health Enhancement Support System (CHESS). The four goals of the system allow consumers to communicate anonymously with each other and healthcare providers, access information in a variety of formats, assess their health risks, and decide how to regain control over their lives (Gustafson, Bosworth, Hawkins, Boberg, and Bricker, 1992). CHESS currently contains five specific health areas: Breast Cancer, AIDS/HIV Infection, Sexual Assault, Substance Abuse, and Academic Crisis.

The CHESS system offers nine distinct services: Q&A (compilation of common questions in each topic area); Instant Library (database of articles, brochures, and pamphlets); Getting Help/Support (information about how to get help and support); Personal Stories (stories written by people who are living and coping with their health crises); Expert Mail (area to ask experts anonymous questions); Discussion Group (area to discuss topics anonymously with others); Decision Aid (tools to facilitate decision making using multiattribute utility models for both specific healthcare and generic decisions); Action Plan (tools to help users analyze their plans to implement their healthcare decisions based on a change theory framework); and Assessment (a risk factors assessment tool). The authors anticipated that CHESS would have three major outcomes: improved health status (by making informed decisions, a better physical and emotional health status should be achieved), improved health behavior (tools like the decision and action analyses plus social support should facilitate the maintenance of healthy behaviors), and cost-effective service utilization (providing support for consumers to be effective users of healthcare services).

Several commercial systems are now providing similar services to consumers. These systems, modeled after many of the previously described applications, charge the user a fee to access services and an hourly rate for time connected to the system. For example, America Online™ maintains a service called Health ResponseAbility Systems' Better Health and Medical Forum. This service is an easy-to-use searchable health information database and a real-time communication and information exchange supporting thousands of individuals. This Forum allows individual subscribers to America Online the following services: full text documents and downloadable files across a vast continuum of healthcare topics, such as Lifestyles and Wellness, Senior Health, and Human Sexuality; numerous message boards for self-help and support groups; regularly scheduled real-time self-help support groups; public bulletin boards; and electronic mail. Another example is HealthOnline, an online service to improve health and quality of life. This commercial service allows users to browse through healthcare information in a virtual community and participate in informal, private, or facilitated discussions of healthcare topics.

Computer-based communications systems have also been used to provide a variety of distance education opportunities for healthcare professionals. In nursing, computer mediated conference techniques have been used for thesis advising (Thiele, 1994), graduate education (Lyness, Raimond, and Albrecht, 1994), and post-RN courses from a university in southwestern

Ontario (Cragg, 1994). In computer mediated communications systems, students access from their home or work computer a remote computer at their university. Students log in and participate in group discussions, in both real-time and delayed formats. In a real-time discussion, students could "chat" with each other or with the instructor. Delayed discussions work similarly to the computer conferences previously described. Students also have access to a wealth of course materials online and, in some cases, gateways to online library resources and the Internet.

Video Communications

Video communications is the third class of telecommunications applications. The most common video communications form is full-motion broadcast video, which is what one sees on television. Full-motion broadcast video is a form of one-way communication. The transmission signal is broadcast from the station to numerous households, but there are no capabilities for households to broadcast back to the stations. In the United States, it takes 525 lines of video scanned 30 times a second to produce the colors, brightness, and motion of the original broadcast (Witherspoon et al., 1994). Cable television operates in a similar manner. A second type is compressed video, which uses digital technology to send only those portions of the picture that change from frame to frame (Witherspoon et al., 1994). Compressed video does not require 30 frames per second for quality video. The compression of video is more efficient in terms of speed of transmission and necessary bandwidth.

A third type is slow-scan video, which allows the transmission of still pictures over traditional telephone lines. Slow scan trades capacity or bandwidth for time. Instead of 30 frames per second, it might take over a minute for a single frame of video. Slow scan has been used successfully with the transmission of x-ray images and other diagnostic images using traditional telephone lines (Witherspoon et al., 1994).

The two-way transmission of video images between distant locations is the fourth type of video communications. This type is commonly referred to as interactive video, or video conferencing systems. The real-time interactive component can be either one-way video/two-way audio or two-way video/two-way audio. Two-way video/audio systems are further divided into group systems (larger groups) and desktop systems (one-on-one systems usually connected to desktop computers). Most video conferencing systems employ the video compression techniques.

Telehealth or telemedicine applications and video conferencing are the most common applications in this arena. In recent years, numerous projects were funded to test the use of telemedicine applications. HealthNet in

Texas has integrated three demonstration projects in telemedicine to provide a variety of educational and consultation services to rural hospital sites in western Texas. This interactive video system provides clinical consultations between generalists and specialists via compressed interactive video between rural sites and a university-based health sciences center. Continuing education for nurses, physicians, and other healthcare professionals is also provided to a total of 46 hospitals across a one-way video connection with two-way audio.

Numerous statewide efforts for telemedicine and distance education for healthcare professionals are planned for the following states: Georgia, Kansas, Nebraska, North Dakota, Oklahoma, Pennsylvania, and South Dakota. Another interesting network is Oregon's RODEO Network, which provides support for mental health services in rural areas. This interactive video network provides such services as a 24-hour crisis response for persons suffering extreme emotional turmoil, mental health consultations between physicians and other healthcare professionals, preadmission services, pre-discharge interviews, and precommitment hearings. A training component is also included in this project to provide both continuing education and a post-master's degree program in psychiatric/mental health nursing.

Numerous schools of nursing are using interactive video as a distance education delivery system. The University of Hawaii at Manoa offers a Master of Science Outreach program to various locations throughout the Hawaiian Islands on its Hawaii Interactive Television System (HITS). The HITS is a combination of point-to-point microwave technology with the University of Hawaii's Instructional Television Fixed Service (Kooker, Itano, Efinger, Dungan, and Major, 1994). A similar system is being used by a consortium of schools of nursing in New York and Pennsylvania (Harrington and Baldwin, 1993). The University of Oregon Health Sciences University School of Nursing is using a two-way compressed live video for the delivery of its baccalaureate and RN/BS completion program. A similar system is used by the School of Nursing at the University of Colorado Health Sciences Center and the University of Wyoming School of Nursing (Nichols, Beeken, and Wilkerson, 1994).

Summary

Telecommunications is a powerful and useful tool that will greatly impact both the education of healthcare professionals and the delivery of health care in the United States. This chapter barely scratches the surface of all the telecommunications projects available in the areas of voice, data, and video communications. One thing is certain: More lanes will be needed on the Information Superhighway to handle the future health-oriented telecommunications applications.

Questions

1. How could the capabilities of voice communications be maximized in your organization? Would there be a benefit in using telephone conferencing, voice mail, facsimile machines, computer communications, and/or picture telephones?
2. Do you know someone who uses electronic mail in his or her work or personal life? Is the electronic mail internal to the organization and/or connected to the Internet? For what reasons is E-mail used?
3. Explain the difference between electronic bulletin board systems and E-mail.
4. Can you think of a patient or health professional subgroup that would benefit from the use of an electronic support group? How would you go about finding a group that meets your personal interests?
5. What would be the benefits and disadvantages of taking distance education classes via computer?
6. Discuss any of the telehealth applications presented in this chapter. Can you think of other applications for video technology in the healthcare arena?

References

Alemi F: Telecommunication in managed self care. In: Ferguson L, ed. *Proceedings of the First National Conference on Consumer Health Informatics.* Stevens Point, WI, July 17–18, 1993. Austin, TX: Self-Care Productions, 1993; 12–13.

A Vision of Change: Civic Promise of the National Information Infrastructure (July 1993). Cambridge, MA: The Center for Civic Networking.

Axsom D: *The GroupLink Project.* Unpublished report. San Francisco, CA: Community Strategies 2000, 1993.

Billings D, Bachmeier B: Teaching and learning at a distance: A review of the nursing literature. In: Allen L, ed. *Review of Research in Nursing Education, Volume VI.* New York: National League for Nursing, 1994; 1–32.

Brennan P: Computer networks promote caregiving collaboration: The ComputerLink Project. In: Frisse M, ed. *Proceedings of the Sixteenth Symposium of Computer Applications in Medical Care.* New York: McGraw-Hill, 1992; 156–160.

Brennan P, Ripich S, Moore S: The use of home-based computers to support persons living with AIDS/ARC. *Journal of Community Health Nursing* 1991: 8(1): 3–14.

Brennan P, Moore S, Smyth K: ComputerLink: Electronic support for the home caregiver. *Advances in Nursing Science* 1991; 13: 14–27.

Cragg C: Nurses' experiences of a post-RN course by computer mediated conferencing: Friendly users. *Computers in Nursing* 1994; 12: 221–226.

Grundner TM: Community computing at Case Western Reserve University. Unpublished report. Community Telecomputing Lab, 1991.

Gustafson D, Bosworth K, Hawkins R, Boberg E, Bricker E: CHESS: A computer-based system for providing information, referrals, decision support, and social support to people facing medical and other health-related crisis. In: Frisse M, ed. *Proceedings of the Sixteenth Symposium of Computer Applications in Medical Care.* New York: McGraw-Hill, 1992; 161–165.

Harrington J, Baldwin P: Worksite education for the BSN student. *Nursing and Health Care* 1993; 14(7): 374–377.

Hiltz S, Turnoff M: Structuring computer mediated communication systems to avoid information overload. *Communication of the ACM* 1985; 28(7): 680–689.

Kiesler S, Siegel J, McGuire T: Social psychological aspects of computer mediated communication. *American Psychologist* 1984; 39(10): 1123–1134.

Kooker B, Itano J, Efinger J, Dungan J, Major M: Interactive television: Delivering quality graduate nursing education to remote sites. *Journal of Nursing Education* 1994; 33(4): 188–190.

Kuramoto A: Teleconferencing for nurses: Evaluating its effectiveness. In: Parker LA, Olgren CH, eds. *Teleconferencing and Electronic Communications III.* Madison, WI: Center for Interactive Programs, University of Wisconsin Extension, 1984; 262–268.

Lyness A, Raimond J, Albrecht S: Descriptive study of computer mediated communication of graduate nursing students: Implications for nursing practice and life long learning. In: Grobe S, Pluyter-Wenting ESP, eds. *Nursing Informatics: An International Overview for Nursing in a Technological Era.* Amsterdam: Elsevier, 1994; 570–578.

McDonald MD, Blum HL: *Health in the Information Age: The Emergence of Health Oriented Telecommunication Applications.* Berkeley, CA: University of California, 1992.

Melmed A, Fisher F: *Towards a National Information Infrastructure: Implications for Selected Social Sectors and Education.* New York: New York University, 1991.

Naisbitt J, Aburdene P: *Megatrends: Ten Directions for the 1990's.* New York: William Morrow & Co., 1990.

Nichols E, Beeken J, Wilkerson N: Distance delivery through compressed video. *Journal of Nursing Education* 1994; 33: 184–186.

Olson R, Jones M, Bezold C: *21st Century Learning and Health Care in the Home: Creating a National Telecommunications Network.* Washington, DC: Institute for Alternative Futures and the Consumer Interest Research Institute, 1992.

Rheingold H: *The Virtual Community: Homesteading on the Electronic Frontier.* Reading, MA: Addison-Wesley, 1993.

Rizzolo M: *AJN-Net.* Unpublished document. New York: American Journal of Nursing, 1994.

Schultz E, Bauman A, Hayward M, Holzman R: Improved care of patients with diabetes through telecommunications. *Annals of the New York Academy of Sciences* 1992; 670: 141–145.

Skiba D, Mirque D: The electronic community: An alternative health care approach. In: Grobe S, Pluyter-Wenting ESP, eds. *Nursing Informatics: An International Overview for Nursing in a Technological Era.* Amsterdam: Elsevier, 1994; 388–392.

Skiba D, Warren C: The impact of an electronic bulletin board to disseminate educational and research information to nursing colleagues. In: Hovenga E, Hannah K, McCormick K, Ronald J, eds. *Nursing Informatics '91: Proceedings of the*

Fourth International Conference on Nursing Use of Computers and Information Science, Vol. 42. Berlin: Springer-Verlag, 1991; 704–709.

Sparks S: Exploring electronic support groups. *American Journal of Nursing* 1992; 92(12): 62–65.

Sparks S: The Educational Technology Network. *Nursing and Health Care* 1994; 15: 134–141.

Staggers N, Jacox A: Communications in the 1990's: A technology update. *Nursing Economics* 1990; 8(6): 408–412.

Strammiello E, ed.: *Colorado Rural Telcommunications Resource Guide.* Denver, CO: Colorado Advanced Technology Institute, 1993.

Tanzillo K: House call: Telmed provides bedside services. *Communication News* 1989; 26(6): 47.

Thiele J: Development of a thesis via electronic mail at a remote educational site. In: Grobe S, Pluyter-Wenting ESP, eds. *Nursing Informatics: An International Overview for Nursing in a Technological Era.* Amsterdam: Elsevier, 1994; 579–581.

Weust J: Learning contracts: A vehicle for increased student involvement in audio teleconferencing. *Nurse Education Today* 1991; 11: 185–190.

Witherspoon J, Johnstone S, Wasem C: *Rural TeleHealth: Telemedicine, Distance Education, and Informatics for Rural Health Care.* Boulder, CO: WICHE Publications, 1994.

5
Electronic Resources for Nursing

SUSAN K. NEWBOLD AND MIRIAM JAFFE

Computer networks have opened up a new world of communication and information for nurses. As you read this, nurses around the world are using their computers to access reference materials, to complete assignments for continuing education courses, to ask practice-related questions of colleagues they know only through electronic mail, to read messages posted to nursing-related bulletin boards or newsgroups, and to chat in real time with colleagues or fellow students. Whether you are a student nurse or a nurse in the areas of clinical practice, administration, research, education, or information systems, you can take advantage of the world of online resources to enhance your education and your career and to make meaningful connections with others who share your concern for excellence in nursing practice.

In this chapter, we focus not only on what resources are available online but also on how you can get to them. Of necessity, this is an overview since new resources are being developed and made accessible all the time. Things change so quickly in the fast-paced world of online communications that you might find electronic mail (E-mail) addresses or other references that have become incorrect since this volume was published. As an example of the immediacy of electronic communication, we have included our E-mail addresses and U.S. mail addresses in the list of contributors at the end of this volume. If you cannot get to a resource we have described in the text, send E-mail or write to us, and we will do our best to help you find it. We will take the risk that some material may be outdated because we believe there is benefit to be obtained from interacting with electronic resources. The authors refer the reader to Appendix E, "Electronic Resources," for additional information related to this chapter.

The Basics of Being Connected

We begin by defining the term "online." The term "online resource" is used to mean a resource that is accessible on a computer other than the one on which you are working (a "remote host"). You may connect to the remote host through a direct network connection (e.g., Ethernet to your campus connection to the Internet) or through a dial-up connection (phone line and modem) to a machine that is connected via a gateway to other machines and networks. The term "online" does not necessarily imply "on the Internet," though that is how the term is often used. For example, an information source like a local nursing bulletin board system (BBS) could be useful to you even if it were not networked with other computers. However, for the most part we are going to consider that you are not online to the outside world unless you have at least the ability to send and receive Internet E-mail. Many local (nonnursing specific) BBSs provide Internet E-mail access, and possibly even local "echoes" of Usenet newsgroups (see Appendix E), but few of them have full-scale Internet connectivity. The major commercial online networks—America Online™, CompuServe™, GEnie™, and Prodigy™—originally provided only E-mail access to the Internet, but all of them have either expanded their level of access or are planning to do so. New commercial vendors are expected to be added to this list.

There are many ways to get online, and some of them are free. If you are lucky enough to have a personal computer connected to a campus or institutional network that has a connection to the Internet, you can probably take advantage of the full range of online resources, from E-mail to the graphical wonders of the World Wide Web (WWW, about which there is more below and in Appendix E), and few campuses or workplaces charge their users for access. If you do not have a direct network connection at your institution, you can achieve a similar level of connectivity and access by obtaining a personal SLIP/PPP account from a local Internet Service Provider (ISP). SLIP (Serial Line Internet Protocol) and PPP (Point-to-Point Protocol) are services that permit your modem/telephone line connection to emulate a direct network connection. Other types of access include:

- A UNIX "shell" account on a host belonging to your institution (likely to be free), to a local "freenet" (free or minimal cost), or to a local or regional ISP (not free; prices and services vary)
- An account with one of the major commercial services, such as America Online™, CompuServe™, and Prodigy™ (not free)
- An account on a local bulletin board system (BBS) that has an Internet gateway (may not be free, but costs and services vary).

The type of access you have will determine the resources available to you, the interfaces you use to interact with the resources, and the costs (if any) you incur.

You do not need to have sophisticated or powerful hardware to use the majority of the resources currently available online. Electronic mail, real-time conferencing, bulletin boards, newsgroups, and retrieval of files and programs from Internet archives can all be managed adequately from a personal computer (PC) with a 286 processor, 640K of RAM, a mono-chrome monitor, and a 20- to 40-MB hard drive; many people get by with even less. Other resources, especially the commercial online services and the more graphically oriented Internet resources, require significantly more computing power. You will typically need a system with at least a 386 processor, at least 4 MB of RAM, a color (VGA or SVGA) monitor, and a 60- to 80-MB hard drive. You also need either a modem and a telephone line as well as appropriate communications software (e.g., ProComm, Cross-Talk, Kermit) to operate the modem, or a direct network connection (usually an Ethernet connection from a university or workplace) and the appropriate network software (usually the responsibility of your institution). There are millions of people communicating with 2400-bps modems, though you will find that 9600-bps, 14,400-bps, and 28,800-bps modems increase your efficiency dramatically. Accessing the World-Wide Web from home, using a personal SLIP/PPP account, requires the most computing power: a fast (minimum 33 MHz) 486 computer with at least 4 MB of RAM, and a fast (minimum 14,400 bps) modem. Macintosh computers of comparable size may also be utilized.

If you do not have access through your school or workplace, finding a provider can be difficult if you do not know where to look. The commercial networks are easy to find; in fact, their user interface software often comes preinstalled on new PCs. ISPs and BBSs are harder to locate, especially if you are not in a reasonably large city. There are so many of them springing up at such a rapid rate, that we would have to add a chapter just to list them all. In Appendix E you will find phone numbers for the commercial networks and tips to help you locate local service providers.

Uses and Benefits of Online Resources

Online resources for nursing fall into three broad categories: communication with other people, reference materials, and continuing education. Access to these online resources offers the following benefits:

- Collaboration with other professionals
- Efficient retrieval of clinical, administrative, research, and educational information
- Support, both personal and technical, for yourself, your patients, and your institution
- The ability to keep current in your field and
- The opportunity to improve the state of nursing science.

In the clinical setting, for example, a family nurse practitioner (FNP) practicing at a university-sponsored, nurse-managed center can use computer mediated communication to ask a clinical question of colleagues or to search an online database for information. Perhaps the FNP would like to know how best to care for a client with terminal cancer. She can look up current information with an online literature search, pose a question to a group of colleagues on an E-mail mailing list (see Appendix E), post queries to the Usenet newsgroups alt.support.cancer and sci.med.nursing, retrieve a care plan on "hopelessness" from the CAREPL-L database of patient care plans, and browse among the latest additions to the OncoLink WWW site.

Similarly, nurse executives can use electronic communication to access external databases for clinical and cost data from other institutions (see Shamian and Hannah, Chapter 18 in this volume) and share insights with colleagues on mailing lists devoted to healthcare management. The nurse manager can also benefit from support groups of other managers, wherein the nurse might pose a question on what computer systems are available for staffing and scheduling.

Nurse researchers employ online resources for literature searching. At the University of Maryland at Baltimore, for example, both students and faculty have access to the Health Science Library Current Contents, Medline, and a host of other reference material from the library from home as well as from their offices on campus. They can locate a book in any of the seven school libraries, reserve it online, and request that it be delivered to the nearest library. In addition, they can search publicly accessible catalogs in libraries around the world through the Internet Gopher system (see Appendix E). If they need additional material, researchers can pose questions on mailing lists or Usenet newsgroups related to their research topics. A recent discussion on one mailing list focused on software tools available to help the nurse researcher. Calls for abstracts for conferences, grant funding information, and other career-enhancing information regularly appear in online forums. Researchers with a variety of interests and at all levels of expertise can disseminate knowledge and encourage mentoring relationships and collaboration through online connections.

Nursing students and educators alike find the online world to be rich in resources. Recent topics on a mailing list for nursing educators included development of programs in community health education, production of computer assisted instruction materials, discussion of textbook choices, recommendations relating to class size, and numerous job postings.

The ability to access absolutely current information about who is doing what at schools around the world enhances decision making and allows nurse educators to share techniques and materials that work. There are exciting new developments in distance education and in delivery of continuing education online. As a caution, the nurse who utilizes online information sources needs to be able to ascertain the reliability and validity of the content of the information.

Whether you are a clinician, an administrator, a researcher, an educator, or a student, you can take advantage of the fact that your professional nursing organizations have access to the Internet. The American Nurses Association, Sigma Theta Tau International, and the National League for

Nursing all have electronic mail addresses whereby messages can be sent and received. A growing number of other nursing and healthcare publications and organizations, such as the American Journal of Nursing and the American Medical Informatics Association, are also accessible online (see Appendix E).

Communication Resources

Online electronic communication provides direct access to your colleagues, to your professional organizations, and to others (patients, family members, other caregivers) with whom you share common interests or concerns. You can communicate with people individually or in groups, in public or in private, asynchronously or in real time. In increasing order of complexity (and decreasing frequency of use), communication modes include E-mail, E-mail mailing lists, Usenet newsgroups (and their BBS or commercial service equivalents), real-time interaction (UNIX "talk," individual and multiuser chat mode on BBSs or commercial services, as well as Internet Relay Chat and other Internet multiuser applications), and advanced real-time interactive video applications (e.g., video conferencing with tools such as Cornell University's CU-SeeMe).

Electronic Mail and Mailing Lists

By far the simplest and the most widely used application, electronic mail is the gateway not only to one-on-one correspondence but also to discussion lists and other Internet applications. E-mail software is system dependent, and a technical description of how E-mail works is well beyond the scope of this chapter. If you are new to E-mail, the best way for you to learn how to use it (and how to use any other online resource, for that matter) is to obtain a user's guide from your provider and to seek the assistance of a friend or colleague who has some experience with it. A simple, one-to-one E-mail correspondence with another person is fairly straightforward, so we will not describe it in detail. The online world gets more challenging and more rewarding when you begin to use E-mail to connect with many people at once through mailing lists.

Mailing lists are an advantageous way for a group of people with common interests to meet and converse with each other. There are Internet mailing lists on just about every topic you can imagine. There are dozens of lists that cover specific medical and health-related topics (e.g., gerontologic health, traumatic brain injury, and endometriosis), and, as of this writing, 15 lists specifically for nurses and others interested in nursing issues.

Every mailing list operates basically the same way. First, after locating information about a list of interest, follow the instructions given to subscribe to the list. Messages other people are posting to the list will begin to appear in your E-mail inbox. If you so choose, you may send an E-mail message to the list address, and a copy of your message will be sent to each person who has subscribed to the list. A subscriber can reply directly to you, in which case you may begin a private conversation, or she may reply back to the list address, in which case everyone on the list receives a copy of her reply. Many people may reply to your message, and others may reply to those replies, creating a public discourse about the topic. The conversational tone varies from list to list; some are very formal, with focused discussion as you might find at a professional meeting, and some are casual, chatty, and rambling, as you might find at a social gathering. As the tone varies, so do the expectations and level of discourse. Standard net etiquette ("netiquette"), however, would suggest that you try to keep messages brief. This conserves network and personal resources, especially for those people who pay for their Internet access. It is also a good practice to sign each post, including your E-mail address. Some mailers strip such information from the headers of messages and so would prevent people from replying to you privately.

There are two types of mailing lists: manually maintained lists, in which a human being adds and deletes subscribers; and automated lists, in which members can subscribe and unsubscribe themselves, search list archives, and perform other useful functions by sending commands via E-mail to the software that manages the list. Most lists are automated, and the majority of nursing and health-oriented lists are managed by a software package called LISTSERV. Other common list managers you might encounter are called listproc, majordomo, and mailbase. The name LISTSERV, though, has become almost a generic name to refer to electronic mailing lists regardless of which software actually manages the list, much as the term "Xerox machine" refers to all photocopiers, regardless of brand.

All lists reside somewhere—that is, they are run on a specific machine (a host) somewhere on the Internet. Whether manual or automated, lists actually have two addresses each: the list address and the administrative address. The list address will be in the form listname@host, and administrative addresses will be in the form LISTSERV@host, if they are LISTSERV lists, or majordomo@host, if the list uses the majordomo list manager. As mentioned earlier, messages you intend to send to every member of the list should be addressed to the list address. Requests to subscribe to or unsubscribe from the list must be sent to the administrative address. Each list has at least one human manager, or moderator, who may or may not take an active role in online conversations but who is responsible for the smooth technical operation of the list.

As just one example, the following information describes one of the nursing-related lists you might consider joining. (See Appendix E for a description of others.) NURSERES is a list devoted to issues related to nursing research and nursing practice. Recent topics have included logistic regression, research on spirituality in nursing, protocols for Med/Surg tube feeding, and over-the-counter (OTC) drug use among the elderly. It is moderated by Linda Q. Thede, RN and has over 1000 subscribers from 19 countries.

The list is managed by LISTSERV software on a machine called kentvm.kent.edu. Thus the list address is nurseres@kentvm.kent.edu, and the administrative address is listserv@kentvm.kent.edu. If your name were Florence Nightingale and you wanted to subscribe to this list, you would send an E-mail message to listserv@kentvm.kent.edu, with the single line

```
sub NURSERES Florence Nightingale
```

Shortly thereafter, you would receive two messages from LISTSERV. The first will tell you that your request has been processed, and the second will be the welcome message that contains important information about how the list operates, including instructions on how to unsubscribe. Keep this message for future reference. Once your name is added to the subscription list, you will begin receiving messages in your E-mail inbox. Some lists (NURSENET, for example) are very prolific, separating many messages each day, so our advice is to be judicious in the number of mailing lists to which you subscribe so the mail does not become overwhelming.

Usenet Newsgroups and the Commercial Equivalents

Usenet (sometimes called Netnews) is a huge, Internet-wide system of (conceptual) bulletin boards, called newsgroups, containing "posts" from readers all over the world. In other online contexts, like local BBSs or the commercial online services, the newsgroups might be called message bases, conferences, special interest groups (SIGs), or forums. Each newsgroup covers a particular topic, some of which are very broad (rec.music, for discussions about music) and some of which are very focused (alt.support.crohns-colitis, for support and information about Crohn's disease and ulcerative colitis). Unlike mailing lists, in which a message is distributed via E-mail to a relatively small audience (usually less than a few thousand subscribers), a post to a Usenet newsgroup is distributed to every site that carries Usenet news (an estimated 260,000) and thus has a potential audience of over 10 million people. Also unlike mailing lists, in which you must subscribe and unsubscribe if you simply want to get a feel for the list, Usenet newsgroups can be browsed quickly and easily using the newsreading software available on your host system. There are a number of other important distinctions between lists and newsgroups, but conceptually they are similar. If you post a message about job prospects for new nursing school graduates, its readers can respond to you personally via E-mail or reply back to the newsgroup, thereby creating a public conversation. As with E-mail, how you actually read and post to Usenet newsgroups is entirely dependent on your type of connection and the newsreading software available to you on your system. Contact your service provider's support staff or read a user's guide to learn more about newsreaders.

There are over 10,000 newsgroups on every conceivable topic within the Usenet system, and new groups are created nearly every day. Together, the newsgroups generate over 85,000 messages a day. To make it easier for readers to navigate through that enormous volume of data, newsgroups are organized into a hierarchical structure. Each group is designated as part of a top-level category, followed by optional subcategories that, strung together, form the name of the group. The major Usenet hierarchies are

comp. (computers, hardware, software, programming, etc.)
misc. (subjects that do not fit under any other hierarchy)
news. (discussion and information about Usenet)
rec. (recreation, sports, hobbies, games)
sci. (science-related topics)
soc. ("social" topics, relating to ethnic, religious, or cultural groups)
talk. (discussions about political and social topics).

In addition, many sites carry the "alt." hierarchy, which, in addition to containing Usenet's most controversial subjects, also happens to include some of the newsgroups that may be of great interest to nurses. Other hierarchies exist as well, such as the bit.listserv groups, which are Usenet equivalents to certain LISTSERVs.

As an example of the hierarchical naming conventions of Usenet, the newsgroup for general discussions of nursing is called sci.med.nursing. Within the sci(ence) hierarchy, it is in the (med)ical topics subhierarchy and its specific topic is nursing. Other newsgroups geared specifically to nurses are bit.listserv.snurse-l (the Usenet equivalent of the SNURSE-L mailing list), for student nurses, and alt.npractitioners, for nurse practitioners. There are numerous other groups that may be of interest to nurses in specific practice areas, and some of them are included in Appendix E.

In addition to the Usenet newsgroups, some BBSs and the large network services like America Online™ and CompuServe™ have local conferences or special interest groups (SIGs) on topics of relevance to nurses. Those conferences are available only to users who subscribe to those commercial systems.

Gopher and the World Wide Web

Thus far, the term "Internet" has not been defined, possibly because the definition varies depending on how technical one chooses to be about it. For our purposes, it will be enough to describe it as an enormous, worldwide collection of computers internetworked together through the use of some common protocols, which define the way that computers exchange data. The computers, of course, are of many types, most of them normally considered incompatible (like IBM mainframes and desktop Macintoshes), but they can speak to each other because the Internet protocols serve as a translator to a common language. Running on top of these low-level protocols are applications that take full advantage of the fact that millions of machines can now "speak the same language."

Gopher is an application that lets you explore information stored on machines all over the world using a simple, menu-driven interface that looks the same whether you are seeing information on a machine in Canada or one in Australia. It was developed at the University of Minnesota in the 1990s. Thousands of schools, institutions, businesses, and organizations have each gathered together information that they feel is useful to their students, employees, members, potential customers, or to the world in general. The information is of many types, including text documents, images, software programs, library catalogs, sounds, searchable databases, and, commonly, "pointers" or "links" to interesting items stored on other machines around the world. At each site, someone organizes the information into a hierarchical structure, represented in gopher by a series of menus that you can browse using a few simple keystrokes. Since some of the menu items you choose may be (and often are) pointers to information stored on another machine, you could easily begin with your home gopher menu (information about your site) and end up reading a document that is stored on a machine in Chile, having passed through menus from two different universities in the United States and one in the United Kingdom. The fact that the machines are of different types and in distant places would be transparent to you; all you did was select interesting-sounding items from menus on your screen. The sum total of all the information in all the menus on all the thousands of machines offering information via gopher is called "gopherspace."

How you start the gopher program on your system varies from provider to provider, so once again the specifics are beyond the scope of this chapter. For the moment, let us assume that you have dialed in to your account on a UNIX system somewhere and that you have learned how to start your gopher and ask it to begin at a particular site in gopherspace, namely the NIGHTINGALE Nursing Gopher at the University of Tennessee, Knoxville. You would see the following menu:

```
        Internet Gopher Information Client v1.01

        Root gopher server: nightingale.con.utk.edu

-->  1.  Greetings!.
     2.  About NIGHTINGALE (Univ. of Tenn. nursing gopher)/
     3.  Research/
     4.  Practice/
     5.  Education/
     6.  Professional nursing communications/
     7.  Publications/
```

```
8.  Yellow Pages/
9.  Other nursing resources/
10. Other gophers and information servers/
11. Search all menus on NIGHTINGALE<?>
```

```
Press ? for help, q to Quit, u to go up a menu    Page: 1/1
```

Every choice that ends in a "/" is the name of another menu. Position the arrow at any of those choices and press enter, and a submenu will appear. At the lowest level of these menu trees are the documents themselves. For example, if you follow this menu path

```
Education/
  Online continuing education courses/
    CEU courses/
```

you will get a listing of accredited independent study continuing education courses offered through the University of Maryland at Baltimore. Select a course title, press the enter key, and the text of the document will appear on your screen. You may print the document out and take the course at your convenience. If you were to browse through the other menus on NIGHTINGALE, you would eventually come upon an item called "NURSE/"—a pointer to the other comprehensive nursing gopher on the Internet, located at the University of Warwick in the United Kingdom. (You will find the addresses of these gophers and others in Appendix E.) You may have noticed that one of the menu choices on NIGHTINGALE is called "Other gophers and information servers." Most gophers have a similar menu item on them somewhere, so once you have connected to any gopher, you can usually "tunnel" from there to any other gopher in the world.

As you might imagine, with thousands of gophers running on machines all over the world, gopherspace is very large indeed. Luckily, there is a tool that allows you to search gopherspace as if it were a giant database. It is called Very Easy Rodent Oriented Net-wide Index to Computerized Archives (VERONICA), and most gophers include a VERONICA menu item. VERONICA prompts you to enter the search terms (e.g., "nurse" or "nursing"). The search process will then return to you all the menu items in gopherspace that contain "nurse" or "nursing" in the title. This will include everything from the NIGHTINGALE and NURSE sites, which are entire gophers devoted to nursing, to listings for courses in nursing departments at universities all over the world.

The World Wide Web (WWW) is gaining rapid acceptance in the on-line world today. The Web consists of collections of hypertext and hypermedia documents stored on machines all over the world. "Hypertext" is a term used to describe documents in which words or phrases within the document can be tagged as links to other parts of the document or to other documents entirely. "Hypermedia" describes documents that can include items other than just text, such as graphics, sound, movies, interactive search interfaces, and so on. Just as gopher allowed you to browse text documents in gopherspace, so "Web browsers" allow you to view these hypermedia documents and navigate among them. And just as gopher allows a menu item on one computer to point to a collection of information on a computer in another country, so Web browsers allow the links within documents to connect to documents in any WWW collection anywhere in the world. Since the Web is a multimedia environment, most Web browsers use point-and-click graphical interfaces to display text and images. However, if all you have available to you is a basic dial-up account and a slow modem (which would preclude you from using the graphical browsers), you can still take advantage of WWW using a text-only browser. As of this writing, the two most popular graphical browsers are Mosaic and Netscape, and the most popular text-based browser is called Lynx.

When you start up a Web browser on your computer, you tell it to begin at a certain location on the Web. What appears on your screen is a document called a "Web page," and the top-level document for a site or an individual is referred to as a "home page." The document often contains images, like university logos, or photographs. Within the text of the document, some of the words or phrases will be underlined or displayed in a different color. These items are links to other pages on the Web; clicking your mouse on a link will cause the next page (which might really be on a different computer) to be displayed on your screen. Some of the links do things other than display Web pages; they play audio files or short movies (if your computer has the appropriate hardware and software installed), retrieve software and files from public file archives, display gopher menus, allow you to send E-mail to the creator of the page you are on, and so on. Simplistically, what is going on behind the scenes is that each link is associated with something called a URL, or Uniform Resource Locator, which identifies the type of resource (Web page, gopher menu, archived file, etc.), the host name (the name of the computer on the Internet where the file is stored), and the path to the resource on that host. For the most part, you do not have to think about URL, since the browser takes care of all the connections for you. However, once you know how to use your browser, if someone tells you about a new nursing resource on the Web and gives you a URL for it, you can direct your browser to point right to the URL. You will find URLs for a number of nursing resources in Appendix E. The Web is huge and growing at an extraordinary rate. Without a list of URLs, you may not know how to find information that is relevant to you. Fortunately, there are very good searching tools available that are to the Web what VERONICA is to gopherspace.

Real-Time Interaction

In addition to the many benefits to be gained from asynchronous modes of communication, like mail and news, getting online allows you to interact with your colleagues or fellow students in real time. Real-time communication allows users to "speak" to each other directly and without the delay or time lapse incurred in E-mail communication. If E-mail is analogous to an exchange of letters, real-time communication may be seen as analogous to communication via telephone, with the caveat that you can only speak as fast as you can type.

Depending on your access to the Internet and your system, various forms of real-time communication may be available for your use. The UNIX "talk" command, for instance, allows real-time interaction between two people logged in to machines running the UNIX operating system, even if those machines are on opposite sides of the world. (Nearly all ISPs run UNIX.) A talk feature is available on networks such as America Online™ and CompuServe™ and is supported on most multiuser BBSs, but you can only speak to other members of the same service.

There are also ways to interact with groups of people. Some BBSs and all the large commercial providers offer multiuser chat programs, which permit users of that system to talk with one another in groups. An example is the chat area provided by the Nursing Network Forum (see Appendix E) on Delphi™ (though Delphi™ has full Internet access, it operates more like a cross between an ISP and a commercial network). Every Wednesday there are real-time conferences with guest "speakers," and at other times members gather in the chat area for more social interaction. The most popular chat area on the Internet is the Internet Relay Chat (IRC). On IRC, people form "channels" in which they may talk about common interests, create links, or exchange ideas. There are weekly meetings of mental health professionals on the channel #interpsyc, sponsored by InterPsych (see Appendix E).

Advanced Applications

Real-time interactions that involve sound and video (the Internet equivalent of a videophone) require high-speed network connections that are presently available only at campuses and large institutions and businesses. You may be able to experiment with these types of applications, which allow you to see and/or hear someone who is sitting at a computer anywhere in the world. The rapid developments in the telecommunications industry may make these types of applications accessible to the average user within the next few years.

Reference Resources

Databases

The Sigma Theta Tau International (STTI) Virginia Henderson International Nursing Library is designed to be a comprehensive collection of databases of nursing knowledge resources. There are eight databases as of this writing:

- Demographic Information. This is a database of nurse researchers that can be initiated and updated by the researcher.
- Nurse Researcher's Projects.
- Research Dissertations.
- Research Conference Proceedings. This database contains abstracts of papers and posters presented at nursing meetings and conferences. One of the authors submitted a paper to the Sigma Theta Tau International Conference held in July 1994 in Sydney, Australia, and the abstract is available for you to access electronically.
- Research Grants Awarded by Sigma Theta Tau International. This database includes demographic and research information and abstracts about projects funded by Sigma Theta Tau International.
- Information Resources.
- Table of Contents Databases. The table of contents from *IMAGE: Journal of Nursing Scholarship* and Sigma Theta Tau monographs comprise these databases.

Another STTI initiative is the Sigma Theta Tau International *OnLine Journal of Knowledge Synthesis for Nursing.* This is the second online journal in existence. The Editor is Jane H. Barnsteiner, RN, PhD, FAAN. An individual or library can buy a subscription to either the library or the journal, which means access from home or the subscriber library. Demonstrations are available on diskette or by Internet access. Refer to Appendix E for contact information.

Archives and Databases from Mailing Lists

The archives of past postings to many nursing-related mailing lists can be searched for relevant information and thus can be thought of as online databanks. The list CAREPL-L is intended to be a searchable archive; the only messages distributed on the list are care plans. The creators/owners of the mailing list NURSERES have created a member database that serves as an excellent tool for linking nurses with similar interests. To be added to the database, members of the NURSERES mailing list complete a questionnaire from Sharon Hall (nurse039@abdpo.dpo.uab.edu). The information collected includes contact information, interests, and availability to assist with and/or collaborate on projects. Nurses seeking mentors or collaborators may retrieve the database by sending the command GET NURSERES DATABASE within the body of a message to list-serv@kentvm.kent.edu.

Software

Thousands of sites around the world maintain archives of software that is available for no charge or as "shareware," a try-before-you-buy honor system. Although there are currently few software applications geared specifically to nursing, there are some, and the wealth of applications available for personal use makes exploring these archives a rewarding endeavor. You will find all types of programs available, including educational software, planning, budgeting and recordkeeping software, and utilities to make your computer experience easier and more efficient. As new applications for nursing are developed, some will undoubtedly be made available in these file archives.

Continuing Education

There are many educational applications for electronic communication. The University of Maryland at Baltimore School of Nursing is offering continuing education credits for courses downloaded via the Internet. A student downloads the course (written instructions, reading material, a quiz, and course evaluation forms), studies the material, and takes the quiz. The student then mails in the completed quiz, along with a fee and forms, and receives credit upon successful completion of the quiz. The course materials are available through the Nursing Network Forum on Delphi™ and via WWW or gopher at NIGHTINGALE, NURSE, and the University of Maryland at Baltimore.

Distance education is being explored by several other universities for nursing-related course work. Efforts are under way at the University of Maine to develop entire courses, for full university credit, that will be delivered via computer, with the first offering during the Spring 1995 semester (L. Nicoll, personal communication, 1995).

The *American Journal of Nursing* is piloting a distance education project for rural nurses and has continuing education course materials on the AJN Network (see Appendix E) (DuBois and Rizzolo, 1994; Rizzolo and DuBois, 1994). The AJN Network was developed with the support of a grant from the U.S. Department of Health and Human Services. It is geared toward providing formal and informal continuing education opportunities to nurses in medically underserved areas. The service includes continuing education courses for credit, resource databases, message bases, a nurse consultant feature, and a chat area.

Conclusion

A wealth of material for, by, and about nurses is available online. One of the most exciting aspects of online connections is the support they offer for nurses working, teaching, and learning in isolated areas. Wherever you are in your nursing career, you can take advantage of the world of online resources to enhance your education and your career and to make meaningful connections with others who share your concern for excellence in nursing practice.

Questions

1. What are some online applications that may be of interest to you in your practice area?
2. List four benefits of using online resources.
3. Describe a scenario in which nurses in remote areas can use technology for education.

References

DuBois K, Rizzolo MA: Cruising the information superhighway. *American Journal of Nursing* 1994; 12: 58–60.
Rizzolo MA, DuBois K: Developing AJN network: Transforming information to meet the needs of the future. *Proceedings of the Eighteenth Annual Symposium on Computer Applications in Medical Care.* Philadelphia: Hanley and Belfus, 1994; 27–31.

Unit 2
Roles for Informatics Nurse Specialists

Unit Introduction

The potential exists for every nurse to integrate the use of computers in his or her practice, whether in clinical practice, administration, research, or education. Every nurse should exploit the tools of computer technology and use it to work toward the goal of improved patient care. The student nurse can utilize word processing to create scholarly papers. The nursing professor can use presentation software to make creative presentations. The staff nurse in a hospital can use a computer to view the results of a laboratory test. The nurse administrator can use a spreadsheet to manage a budget. The nurse researcher can use a database to collect data for a study and then analyze the data using a statistical package. The home health nurse or family nurse practitioner in a nurse-managed clinic can enter a patient assessment into the computer for later retrieval.

A nurse might take on a specific role dealing with computers along with current duties. That nurse might have a temporary assignment to select a documentation system for the workplace. Some nurses may decide to take on a primary role working with nursing informatics. Various roles are described in detail in several chapters in this volume.

Ball, Hannah, and Newbold delineate the historical basis for the term "informatics" and support a borrowed definition of "nursing informatics." That chapter is followed by Hersher's detailed description of career paths for informatics nurse specialists, in which she addresses the dynamic and challenging healthcare environment. Marina Douglas uses the images of butterflies, bonsai gardening, and Michelangelo Buonarroti to assist in describing the role of the nurse analyst and the balance between "high tech" and "high touch." In Chapter 9, Concordia and Hammon focus the reader's attention on the use of outside consultants to assist nursing professionals in operationalizing nursing informatics in their own work environments.

6
What Is Informatics and What Does It Mean for Nursing?

Marion J. Ball, Kathryn J. Hannah, and Susan K. Newbold

Introduction

Today, nurses around the world are rapidly increasing the extent to which they use computers and information sciences to assist them in the performance of their increasingly sophisticated and complex duties. Consequently, the field of nursing informatics is developing quickly. Because of the evolution of nursing informatics, new roles for nursing are developing in industry, research, systems development, nursing education, nursing administration, and indeed at the bedside. One need not sacrifice an avocation for direct patient care to participate in the information revolution in nursing. In fact, the reason that many nurses have ventured into the field of nursing informatics is a common vision of information systems being used to enhance the practice of nursing and to benefit the patient by extending and improving the health care received.

Developments in nursing informatics are beginning to have and will continue to have an impact on how nursing is practiced; further, this impact will be reflected in nursing education. In fact, the impact of nursing informatics ultimately will be so profound that it will be a driving force for extensive change in the nature of nursing research and administration as well. The term "nursing informatics" can be defined operationally as referring to the use of information technologies in relation to any of the functions that are within the purview of nursing and are carried out by nurses in the performance of their duties (Hannah, 1985, p. 181). Therefore, any use of information technologies by nurses in relation to the care of patients, the administration of healthcare facilities, or the educational preparation of individuals to practice the discipline is considered nursing informatics.

Graves and Corcoran (1989) offer a definition of nursing informatics as "the study of the management and processing of nursing data, information and knowledge" (p. 227). For example, nursing informatics would include but not be limited to:

- The use of artificial intelligence or decision-making systems to support the use of the nursing process
- The use of a computer-based scheduling package to allocate staff in a hospital or healthcare organization
- The use of computers for patient education
- The use of computer assisted learning in nursing education
- Nursing use of a hospital information system
- Research related to information nurses use in making patient care decisions and how those decisions are made.

In other words, advances in computing and communications are transforming health care in ways we could not predict 10 years ago. As the front line for delivering that care, nurses stand to benefit enormously from those changes and the new capabilities and opportunities they bring.

Professional meetings—and the literature to which they have contributed—have made increasing use of the term "informatics," from the French "informatique." The term first appeared in medicine, where computerization was most developed. Over the past several years, what was initially referred to as "medical informatics" has become more precisely defined. Today the literature applies the term to the full spectrum of the allied health sciences yet at the same time singles out specific areas, such as nursing informatics and dental informatics.

As all sciences, the field of informatics is continually undergoing self-analysis and redefinition to find its niche in our fast-changing world. A recent attempt at definition argues that

Medical informatics is a developing discipline, a multidisciplinary field, which has grown out of the recognition that effective utilization of computers in health care will occur only when there emerges a critical mass of individuals who understand both the fundamentals of medicine and those of engineering and information science. By medical, we do not mean M.D., but all parts of the health-care arena: allied health; biological sciences; health-care facilities; health-services research; medical specialties; and nursing. (Stead, 1987, pp. 14–15)

Stead further explains that "in the medical setting, informatics is used in a broader context than information science to include all aspects of the computer milieu," which he then itemizes as the following:

- Algorithms
- Artificial intelligence
- Biometry
- Communications
- Database methods
- Imaging and signal analysis
- Hardware design simulation
- Modeling and systems organization (Stead, 1987, p. 14).

Stead addresses the problem in interpreting the term "medical" narrowly. Many others share his concern and see a much broader orientation, with the term "health informatics" encompassing subsets such as in medicine, dentistry, nursing, and pharmacy. A move to this more global definition would clarify the place of informatics as we work to take advantage of information technology.

The growing acceptance of this concept is evidenced in the December 1986 issue of *The Western Journal of Medicine,* devoted wholly to medical informatics. In his introduction to the issue, the editor explains that

Like many of my colleagues, I had spent a fair amount of time over the past few years trying to explain the meaning of "medical informatics." When it was decided to feature this subject in the December issue of the journal, this offered an unusual opportunity to *illustrate* what medical informatics is, and to put some of its best examples on display. It also seemed useful to draw attention to the important distinction between *information* (the commodity with which informatics deals) and the *computer* as a tool for use in processing this commodity. The computer continues to be an exciting object, it is increasingly present and it rarely fails to attract attention. Unfortunately, the commodity which is processed by the computer tends to be overlooked. (Blois, 1986, p. 776)

Blois concludes his discussion of medical informatics by arguing that

what have now become necessary are better means of managing this information and locating it when needed. It is here that we have turned to computers and to information science for help. This is a major undertaking and a new adventure for medicine. Developments ... continue to break new ground so that we can look forward to an increase not only in knowledge itself but in the means of analyzing, organizing and disseminating it. (Blois, 1986, p. 777)

The Association of American Medical Colleges (AAMC) addressed these concerns for medical education. At the Association's Symposium on Medical Informatics, Lindberg (1986) proposed the "seven levels of understanding medical informatics" as a more detailed definition. This approach begins to address specifically the educational and curricular definition of "informatics." Moving from the fundamental to more complex, those seven levels are

- Computer literacy
- Independent learning
- Minimal personal skills
- Knowledgeable consumer
- See new applications
- Build a system for one's application
- Tool building (Lindberg, 1986, p. 93).

The AAMC reports agreement that today's healthcare professional must be skilled in problem solving, concept formation, data processing, and the ability to analyze, summarize, make judgments, and form valid conclusions.

The study of informatics, the AAMC argues, enables students and professionals alike to sharpen and enhance these skills. Among the contributions of informatics are the capabilities for

- Managing the information base available to treat patients
- Treating patients more efficiently and cost effectively by reference to a broad range of experiences documented in national databases
- Providing more time for physicians to spend on the important personal aspects of patient care through delegation of some information handling and processing tasks to computers
- Improving the educational process through the incorporation of information technology and decision-making science and through the utilization of computer mediated instruction
- Broadening and rationalizing the clinical experience in medical education (Steering Committee, 1986, p. 3).

The Nursing Working Group of the International Medical Informatics Association established an education task force. This task force convened in Sweden in June 1987 for the purpose of competency statements regarding nursing informatics knowledge required by nurse administrators, nurse educators, nurse clinicians, nurse researchers, and informatics nurses (Peterson and Gerdin Jelger, 1987). These competency statements are expected to be used in the formulation of educational curricula and job descriptions.

In the field of informatics—notably in the areas of dental, medical, pharmacy, and nursing informatics—we are seeing a substantial growth in the use of computers as a basic tool and integrated into the disciplines that make up these professional fields. We will see a succession of a new generation of informatics specialists develop.

The National Library of Medicine has for years funded training programs in medical informatics, and it is our prediction that the same will occur in dental, nursing, and pharmacy informatics. Two universities in the United States offer a master's degree in nursing informatics, and one of those schools offers a doctor of philosophy degree with an emphasis on nursing informatics. Academic preparation for informatics nurses specialists is discussed elsewhere in this volume.

There is no doubt that informatics as a new discipline has a bright future as the professional schools utilizing informatics in the specialty areas of nursing informatics, dental informatics, medical informatics, and pharmacy informatics become further involved. As we move into even more sophisticated uses of computers in health care, the field of informatics will thrive.

New Roles for Nurses

A side effect of the changes in health care and the evolution of nursing informatics has been the growth of new roles for nursing, as discussed elsewhere in this volume. Such roles are developing in industry, research, systems development, nursing education, and nursing administration. Nurses, most notably those with bachelor's and master's degrees, are participating in the selection and implementation of systems for use at the bedside. Nurses also articulate the information needs of healthcare professionals and of clients in clinical practice settings to the system designers and engineers. A more recent practice is the hiring of nurse consultants by hospitals to assist in the design and implementation of computer systems. The input of nurses into system selection and design is growing exponentially as healthcare facilities use computers to interpret electrocardiograms, monitor patients, and prevent drug interactions by cross-referencing drug incompatibilities and warning appropriate staff.

The Clinical Nurse

Informatics will free nurses to assume the responsibility for systematic planning of holistic and humanistic nursing care for patients and their families, for continual review and examination of nursing practice (quality assurance), for applying basic research to innovative solutions to patient care problems, and for devising creative new models for the delivery of nursing care.

The advances in the use of information technology will necessitate a more scientific and complex approach to the nursing care process. Consequently, nurses will require better educational preparation and a more inquiring and investigative approach to patient care. Nurses will also need to be more discriminating users of information. No longer will nursing practice focus on the assessment and care planning phase. Rather, it will emphasize the implementation phase. Thus, nurses will require an expanded repertoire of intervention skills. These nursing intervention skills reflect the autonomous aspects of nursing practice. Based on the body of nursing knowledge and the nurse's professional judgment, autonomous nursing interventions are complementary to, not competitive with, physician-prescribed treatments. In this context, clinical nurse specialist training at the master's degree level offers nurses the opportunity to use increased knowledge and clinical practice skills at the bedside. This intensification of the role of bedside nurse provides an alternate career path for nurses who prefer patient care to administration, research, or education.

In the delivery of health care, nurses have traditionally provided the interface between the client and the healthcare system. They are now fulfilling this function in new ways as they move into a technologically advanced environment. With nursing informatics as a guide, nurses will become increasingly more involved in the design, use, management, and evaluation of computer systems in healthcare agencies and institutions. Today, nurses are identifying and developing new ways of using computers and information science as a tool to support the practice of nursing in the performance of their duties. At the same time, computers and information science are facilitating a more sophisticated and expanded level of nursing practice. There is an interactive and synergistic effect between nursing informatics and nursing practice. The boundaries of nursing informatics are thus contiguous with those of nursing and, like them, dynamic and constantly changing.

Questions

1. Define in your own words what you understand nursing informatics to be.
2. Give the name of four or five organizations and/or monographs in which the area of informatics is being addressed as an evolving discipline.
3. What impact will informatics have on nursing as a field?
4. Where in the practice of nursing will we see caring and technology meet?

References

Blois MS, ed: What is medical informatics? *Western Journal of Medicine* 1986; 145: 776–777.

Graves JR, Corcoran S: The study of nursing informatics. *Image: Journal of Nursing Scholarship* 1989; 21(4): 227–231.

Hannah KJ: Current trends in nursing informatics: Implications for curriculum planning. In: Hannah KJ, Guillemin EJ, Conklin DN, eds. *Nursing Use of Computers and Information Science.* Amsterdam: North-Holland, 1985; 181–187.

Lindberg DAB: Evolution of medical informatics. In: *Medical Education in the Information Age. Proceedings of the Symposium on Medical Informatics.* Washington, DC: American Association of Medical Colleges, 1986; 86–95.

Peterson H, Gerdin-Jelger U: *Nursing Competencies.* New York: National League for Nursing, 1987.

Stead WW: What is medical informatics? *M.D. Computing* 1987; 4: 14–15.

Steering Committee: The evaluation of medical information science in medical education. In: *Medical Education in the Information Age. Proceedings of the Symposium on Medical Informatics.* Washington, DC: American Association of Medical Colleges, 1986; 2–61.

7
Careers for Nurses in Healthcare Information Systems

Betsy S. Hersher

Introduction

Nurses entering the healthcare information systems field will have an excellent opportunity for growth and advancement in a dynamic and challenging environment. Systems are being developed to support patient-focused care, clinical outcomes, clinical repositories, care mapping, and managed care. These systems are only the tip of the iceberg. As healthcare integrated networks evolve, information and clinical data become the key element for success. Nurses make managers and leaders. They are needed to define, design, install, develop, consult on, and market these systems.

Technology has brought about the automation of nursing information and data, and thus the advent of the nursing information systems can best be integrated into all phases of the delivery of patient care—for example, how best to deliver cost-effective care for a specified illness, how to automate all areas of documentation (care plans and assessments), how to calculate acuity, and how to use bedside point-of-care devices to facilitate collection of data.

As technology continues to evolve, nursing practice methods will also adapt to take advantage of automation. Nursing professionals will more frequently have key roles in integrating technology into patient care delivery. Not only will nurses be involved in the initial evaluation phases of information systems, but they will also play increasing roles in developing and sustaining the long-term strategy for accessing patient information.

It is desirable to complete a bachelor's degree and desirable to continue on for a master's degree in business administration or nursing for advancement into management in many of these areas. A master's degree in nursing informatics may be of great benefit in finding a position in the arena.

To move into information systems, nurses may find it helpful to act as user liaisons on any information systems steering committees and market these new systems within the hospital, where their work can serve as the transition into a new career in information systems. The experience gained combined with their nursing expertise can carry them into this new field.

77

Nurses make excellent information systems people because they are data gatherers and documenters, have global systems views, set priorities, manage all care, and understand the need to access patient information.

Where are the jobs? They are in nursing divisions; in traditional areas, like staffing, scheduling, and formulating care plans; in nursing informatics research-oriented roles; in liaison (information systems department and nursing); in clinics; in insurance companies; in utilization review organizations; in integrated health networks; and in healthcare associations and alliances. New roles in clinical information systems include the fields of epidemiology/outcomes, chief information office (CIO) clinical information liaison, network liaison, industry-outcomes review, clinical resource management, education, data repository specialization, and development and implementation of patient-focused systems (assessment-oriented systems).

User Liaison for the Hospital

When a clinical information system is installed in a hospital setting, it is necessary to coordinate the needs and staff of the institution with the capabilities of the system. Usually, a systems steering committee is formed. Participation on the steering committee is an excellent way to gain systems knowledge.

Nurses are often naturals as systems people because of their training and background. There is order and organization in nursing. Efficient and effective methods of patient care delivery are developed using a step-by-step, problem-solving approach. Automation of patient care systems effectively helps nurses analyze and handle problems. The role of the nurse includes teaching, documenting, and motivating within the patient care process.

A place on the steering committee would allow for interaction with hospital-wide users, vendors (the companies who develop and sell hospital information systems), consultants, and administrators. The role of the steering committee includes needs analysis, participation in the selection of the systems, definition of the systems, and coordination of system installation. This is an excellent place to discover if you are interested in a career in systems. As a steering committee member, a nurse has an opportunity to conduct site visits, see a variety of systems, and attend training classes given by a chosen vendor. Active participation on the steering committee makes a nurse highly visible and the obvious first choice when his or her institution is looking for a coordinator.

An ability to learn, excellent communication skills, patience, and an ability to work with ease and confidence away from the bedside are necessary. Leaving the bedside to move into the development of patient care systems is a viable transition and a move into an exciting new career. The key factor in a move such as this is to become a facilitator, using resources but not necessarily controlling or having authority over them.

Coordinator for Healthcare Institutions

In many hospitals, the patient care systems are managed by nurses. The skills required for this job are a working knowledge of systems and excellent communication and management skills. The ability to hire and supervise technical people is a plus. This position involves installing the systems and interfacing with the vendors, users, and management. This position is an excellent stepping-stone to a position with vendors, as a consultant or as vice president of information management.

Installer of Clinical Information Systems for a Vendor

The need for qualified candidates to install various components of medical information, order entry, communication, productivity, acuity, and staffing systems is growing. An installation person is often on the marketing team during and after the sale of a software package. ("Software" is the term used for the programs and operating managements that make the system run.) The installer helps the user define his or her needs and explains documentation. The main task of the installer is to train the users and help them over the rough spots during and after conversion to the new system. Many of the skills discussed earlier are operative in this job. Additionally, the installer must be a negotiator and liaison, acting as the bridge between the user and the software vendor.

Working for the software vendor adds a new dimension. Although this person is an advocate of the user's position and needs, his or her job is to have the system installed according to the design parameters. The vendor is paid as the various modules are installed. This position can sometimes be that of a juggler.

These positions often require 50% or more traveling time, a solid understanding of how hospitals work, excellent communication and presentation skills, and an understanding of systems. A move into an installation role with a vendor can lead to a number of career possibilities.

Product Manager

One of the most exciting professional moves has become available in the last few years. The responsibilities of product management/production definition are loosely defined and can change from vendor to vendor. The duties often overlap into marketing. This is a position that is beginning to be developed on the hospital side.

A person in product management is responsible for constantly updating the current product and keeping abreast of all new developments in the field. Product managers must be cognizant of the current and future needs of the clients and determine whether these needs can be or should be incorporated into the product. The people determining the product direction are the watchdogs of the product and the industry.

The characteristic role of product manager is the same in any industry. Product managers must interface with marketing staff, client, technical staff, and management to produce a usable and marketable product in a timely manner at the best price. They must satisfy the needs of one client without compromising the needs of others or the capabilities of the technical staff. This position generally begins as a staff role requiring excellent communication and negotiation skills. Product managers need to possess or acquire internal and external marketing expertise. Both vendors and healthcare organizations are under pressure to define their current and future needs accurately, and this is a key role. Success in this position can lead to high-level strategic planning positions with expanding responsibilities and compensation. Nurses will be in high demand in the development of some new applications, including decision-support systems, clinical ancillary systems, managed care, nurse staffing, productivity measures, acuity systems, and bedside and handheld terminals.

Market Support Person

Market support is defined differently in various organizations. The classic definition involves technical sales support to the salespeople and additional explanations to the client. With so many patient care and ancillary systems in development, nurses are needed to assist in closing the sale.

To be a good marketer, it is important to listen well to the needs of clients. Finding the reasons why a vendor's software products answer the needs of the clients is a key element. Market support personnel must possess excellent written and oral communication skills and understand the marketing cycle. They must be able to identify the decision makers. On some occasions, it is necessary to act as a negotiator between the clients and the salesperson.

The salesperson's role is to sell the product and close the sale. The market support person adds the technical information, often demonstrates the product, and attempts to ensure that the client is not oversold or undersold. He or she plays a key role before, during, and after the sale.

During the sale cycle, market support staff will interface with the product management team, the technical staff of the hospital, the vendor, and salespeople. In many vendor situations, market support departments will answer requests for proposals and be involved in contract negotiations.

In a software vendor situation, the move from market support to sales rarely occurs because of the additional skills required. The notable exceptions are the patient care, ancillary, and alternative delivery systems. Additionally, medical personnel often move into sales for highly technical products, such as biomedical equipment.

The move into sales from marketing should not be taken lightly. It is a rare individual who makes the transition successfully. Among the skills required are negotiation, patience, and the ability to close a sale. A successful transition can be rewarding.

Consultant

Nurses are in great demand today in most of the large consulting firms. The ideal candidate for a consulting firm has a master's degree, possesses excellent written and oral communication skills, and has a good knowledge of systems. Consultants should be analytical problem solvers, independent, creative, and assertive. Additionally, an outgoing marketing personality is a plus and would ensure growth.

Nurses make excellent consultants if they have the right personality. It is often necessary to make instant decisions based on analysis of fact. Generally speaking, nurses tend to have strong personalities, to know how to take charge and how to establish their professional credibility. These are all traits that a consultant needs.

Consulting is a high-pressure field. Assignments are not usually carried out in project teams of more than two people. Projects can range from needs analysis and selection of vendors to strategic planning, cost-benefit studies, and systems audits.

Consulting offers excellent personal growth potential. Consultants must operate independently and successfully, learn to lead projects, and be able to handle a variety of products. Consulting forces nursing professionals to stretch their ability and take on the role of liaison and expert. Some of the negatives include a heavy travel schedule and opportunity for project management but little opportunity to manage large numbers of people. In many instances, consultants make recommendations but do not remain to implement them. If a person is accustomed to follow-through, it can be difficult to walk away before the entire task is completed. A career in consulting requires a drive and ambition to seek high levels of achievement. Consulting firms hire carefully and look for candidates who will be partner material.

Sales Representative

Nurses make excellent salespeople because of their keen ability to motivate, negotiate, and be seen as credible. An additional factor in their credibility is the need to understand thoroughly a process, such as illness, and observe many signs at once. If this skill is translated into sales, nurses should be able to present the product from a sound base of understanding rather than a "smoke-and-mirrors" approach.

Because of training and experience, nurses feel the need to bring something to closure. A key requirement in sales is the skill of closure. A career in sales can be rewarding financially and lead to sales management or operational management in a vendor environment. The downside is that sales is a high-risk, high-frustration environment that requires a strong tolerance for rejection. Being tenacious is a plus.

Reengineering

A move into a reengineering or work redesign role is an excellent platform to support systems development. Nurses are excellent potential candidates for reengineering and designing systems to support patient care.

Systems Analyst/Programmer

Nurses may opt to work in a hospital's information services department as a systems analyst or programmer. A bachelor's degree is usually required as well as a working knowledge of that hospital's computer system. This person may or may not work exclusively with nursing applications.

Chief Information Officer

As nurses advance in the information systems world, they have an excellent opportunity to move into the Chief Information Officer role. This role has been expanded recently to include integrated health networks. The successful Chief Information Officer will be viewed as a leader and resource for technology. He or she must be extremely flexible and comfortable dealing with ambiguity and dramatic change; these traits allow the Chief Information Officer to respond quickly to initiatives and challenges.

Summary

It is important for nurses to upgrade their skills and goals continually, examine career options, and be flexible. This is an important point for nurses to consider before becoming actively involved in the growth of healthcare information systems. The future of the healthcare systems industry will be total systems expanding far beyond hospitals. There is and will be a greater need to provide information for decision making in the vast areas of alternative delivery, preventive medicine, industrial and occupational medicine, and adult long-term care. Large, non-healthcare corporations and business coalitions will have a strong influence on the healthcare industry. Terminals will be set up in the workplace for early detection of disease and for providing wellness programs.

Because of severe financial pressures, the healthcare industry will finally be forced to use its technology for medical research and to provide access to national databases to provide better health care and allow for prevention, early detection, and a faster cure for some diseases. The nurse consultant will play a major role in this area. This evolution will happen only over time.

As many mergers take place among the major healthcare vendors and institutions, we can only wonder what this will mean for the healthcare industry. As large consolidated corporations sort their priorities, entrepreneurs will have an ideal opportunity to use their creative ability to provide products and services to the industry. The survivors will be those firms and institutions that provide the highest quality and most flexible service at a competitive price.

In this market, the people are important. They must be global thinkers with an understanding of the present and future of the healthcare market. They must be managers who are flexible and able to use resources and technology creatively. In both a profit and nonprofit environment, these leaders will be required to be risk takers and decision makers and to operate in a proactive manner. They will need to be entrepreneurial and be open to joint venturing. The healthcare systems industry is more open to clinical specialists than ever before. This is an ideal time to consider a career as a systems specialist.

Questions

1. Given the material in this chapter on careers for nurses in information systems plus your background and skills, design a position description that describes a career move for you.
2. What have been the changes in the hospital industry that would lead to nurses playing a more predominant role in healthcare systems?
3. What are the new application areas and technical advances that nurses should be aware of? Name at least 10.
4. Why would nurses do well in sales and marketing?
5. Given the information provided in this chapter, describe at least three additional roles for nurses in information systems.

8
Butterflies, Bonsai, and Buonarroti: Images for the Nurse Analyst

MARINA DOUGLAS

What's in a Name?

The title describing the roles and responsibilities of the nurse analyst in the early 1980s was "nursing liaison" (Zielstorff, 1980). The nursing liaison specifically focused on the nursing components of a hospital information system (HIS). Whereas once systems were described as nursing information systems, the term "clinical information systems" describes more fully the systems used by nurses and clinicians in today's healthcare environment. Information required for delivery of patient care is collected from many sources. These may include laboratory, radiology, dietary, medical records, and financial systems internal to an organization. The external sources of community healthcare providers, federal agencies, and research and education databases may also be involved in the development and implementation of a patient's treatment plan. The recognition that healthcare information needs are multidimensional has expanded the role of the nurse liaison to include active involvement in nontraditional nursing systems design, development, implementation, and research (radiology, laboratory, quality assurance, etc.) in addition to increasing the nurse liaison's involvement in all aspects of the more traditional nursing applications (plan of care, acuity, assessments).

In 1993, the American Nurses Association (ANA) recognized nursing informatics as a specialty area of nursing practice. The ANA has defined the scope of practice for nursing informatics and is in the process of developing the practice standards for informatics nurses.

As a scientific discipline, nursing informatics serves the profession of nursing by supporting the information handling work of other nursing specialties. Nursing informatics is the specialty that integrates nursing science, computer science, and information science in identifying, collecting, processing, and managing data and information to support nursing practice, administration, education, research, and the expansion of nursing knowledge. It supports the practice of all nursing specialties, in all sites and settings of care, whether at the basic or advanced practice level. The practice of nursing informatics includes the development and evaluation of applications, tools, processes, and structures which assist nurses with the management of data in taking care of patients or in supporting the practice of nursing. It includes adapting, or customizing existing information technology to the requirements of nurses. It involves collaboration with other healthcare and informatics professionals in the development of informatics products and standards for nursing and healthcare informatics.

Nurses who practice in the field of nursing informatics are designated "informatics nurses." It recognizes that the person is both a nurse and an informaticist. (American Nurses Association, 1994, p. 3)

The multidimensional healthcare information needs of patients and clinicians and the specialized requirements of professional nursing pose challenges for the continued design, development, and implementation of systems. The term "nurse analyst" will be used to denote the nurse working in the healthcare information arena as an analyst supporting all healthcare information needs. The work setting may be the hospital, consulting services, or private industry.

Through education, research, and experiences, nurses have applied scientific principles, developed a body of knowledge, and made a significant contribution to the design and development of today's clinical information systems. The science of nursing and the nurse analyst must blend the technology of healthcare delivery and information systems with the patient's need for competent, compassionate care. The images of butterflies, bonsai gardening, and Michelangelo Buonarotti assist in describing the roles of the nurse analyst and the balance between the "high-tech" and "high-touch" phenomena.

Butterflies

The metamorphosis to butterfly occurs only after the caterpillar stage has been completed. For the nurse analyst, experience in the direct delivery of patient care is the essential starting point. Thoroughly schooled in the nursing process—to observe, assess, plan, implement, and evaluate—nurses utilize an analytic problem-solving approach to patient care. The nurse providing direct patient care continually assesses the status of the patient. The involvement of the patient and family in the delivery of care is fundamental. When the patient is unable to communicate or do for himself, the nurse provides care based on her best judgment, experience, and knowledge. The everyday role of the nurse providing direct patient care, therefore, requires the ability to

- Constantly observe and assess the patient and environment
- Participate in the development of the multi/interdisciplinary treatment plan based on assessed needs
- Translate the treatment plan into terms understood by patient and family

- Elicit the cooperation of the patient, family, and health care team through listening and communication skills to implement the treatment plan
- Utilize knowledge of, and experience with, both normal and abnormal physiology and the desired and adverse reactions to treatment in monitoring the progress of the patient
- Evaluate the outcomes of care relative to the treatment goal and plan.

The skills developed in the role of direct care provider form the foundation for the nurse analyst. The knowledge base of the nurse analyst expands to include the technology of information systems in conjunction with the principles and processes employed in systems analysis, development, and implementation. It is a widely held tenet that while nurses have successfully transitioned to learn and apply information systems principles and technology, those trained in computer science have been much less successful at assimilating the principles and technology of medicine, nursing, and health care to identify adequately the information needs of these professions. The metamorphosis, it appears, requires the analyst to experience the role of a nurse providing direct patient care as the prerequisite to the role of nurse analyst.

Bonsai

The practice of bonsai gardening began in Japan centuries ago. It is a living art form utilizing three horticultural practices—pruning, shaping, and containerization. The goal is to produce small three-dimensional forms of pleasing lines and aspects (Bailey and McDonald, 1972). Considerable care and commitment is required in conjunction with a long-term vision and patience. During the pruning and shapings, small cuts are taken. The future lines and the overall look of the garden are determined by these actions. The container or garden space will be a determining factor for the size of the plantings and will play an important part in the presentation of the garden. The visionary gardener plans the garden based on the desired effect of the plantings at maturity.

The nurse analyst often functions in an environment with similar constraints where nurturing and strong communication skills are essential. Managing the small prunings and the shaping of expectations during all phases of design, development, and implementation are the challenge. Fiscal limitations frequently impact the hardware and information system software selection process; it is a balance between the cost of the desired features and functions and the allocated funds. Development and implementation schedules will be dictated by the number and availability of resources to complete tasks. The nurse analyst must shape the expectations of the project team to coincide with a realistic plan while maintaining enthusiasm and a focused vision for the strategic goals of the institution and/or information system. Understanding the needs and interactions of multiple healthcare providers, balancing those needs against the fiscal and resource constraints of the institution, and delivering a functional system in a timely fashion are essential components of the role of the nurse analyst.

General Principles for Automated Systems

Just as the basic principles of health and nursing are taught and assimilated into the daily practice of nursing, the nurse analyst must learn and assimilate the general principles of automated systems. Yourdon (1989) describes four such principles. First, "the more specialized a system is, the less able it is to adapt to different circumstances" (p. 34). Helping to define system requirements requires creativity. From a system designed with flexibility and considerations of future needs comes a system in which minimal programming changes result in maximum benefits for the end users and patient care. The nurse analyst encourages users to look toward the realistic future by reviewing their current practices and future trends.

The users will likely benefit from observation skills; knowledge of industry trends in health care, information systems, and technology; relationship of the individual department to the organization; and problem-solving skills of the nurse analyst. For example, care planning software designed strictly to meet the needs of nursing may no longer meet the multidisciplinary requirements of case management. Care planning software designed with flexibility to differentiate among the care providers and their needs and to track variations between expected and actual completion dates may be adapted more easily to support the added requirements of the trend toward case management.

The second of Yourdon's (1989) automated systems principles is that "the larger the system is, the more of its resources that must be devoted to its everyday maintenance" (p. 34). The design and implementation of clinical systems must factor in system maintenance requirements. The development of policies and procedures for system operations considers the needs of patient care and the healthcare providers. Where nightly maintenance for an HIS once took 4 to 6 hours of processing, newer technologies have nearly eliminated this nightly downtime. With greater emphasis on the extraction of information (rather than simply data), development of reports and online views must consider the overall performance impact on the central processing unit. The nurse analyst ensures that the end user's response time for routine processing will not be adversely affected by new projects, report generation, or procedures.

Yourdon's (1989) third principle is that "systems are always part of larger systems, and can always be partitioned into smaller systems" (p. 35). The nurse analyst has firsthand knowledge of the smaller systems that comprise the larger healthcare organization. The challenge is to find ways to automate the smaller systems for the benefit of the larger system. Efforts to reengineer and redesign the flow of work must occur concurrently with the development and implementation of new information systems. The nurse analyst facilitates the end users' review of "the way we always do it" with an eye toward gaining efficiencies. Personnel productivity can then be focused on patient care rather than paper management.

In other instances, there may be factions of users unwilling to accept the activation of a system that is anything less than the absolute ultimate information system. While total information systems perfection has not been attained, groupings of available applications can achieve benefits for the organization in the near term. Romano (1990) points out that putting technology to practical use is innovation. The innovative nurse analyst assists in establishing development and/or implementation plans to maximize achievable benefits as soon as possible. This can be accomplished by thoughtful planning and segmenting the implementation of a total HIS into smaller activation groupings, which may include helping to evaluate the vendors' development schedule during the system selection process relative to the strategic goals of the organization and the desired implementation plan. When the organization is responsible for the development of the new system, definition of the development plan provides benefits to the end user as soon as possible. In both instances, benefits can begin accruing while the vision of attaining the ultimate ideal information system is maintained.

The fourth of Yourdon's (1989) principles is that systems grow (p. 35). The use of clinical information systems will expand greatly as healthcare networks are implemented. Traditional smaller systems (order communications, medical records, intensive care systems) will require data integration with community health information networks. The 1990 Institute of Medicine study (Dick and Steen, 1991) put forth the concept of a computerized patient record for healthcare delivery; it has become the goal for communities, hospitals, and software development. The computerized patient record initiative will provide automated longitudinal clinical information for patients. Participation in the definition and use of standard nursing nomenclature in automation will be an important first step toward the computerized patient record. Ensuring clinical data integration among the disparate systems will be the challenge and responsibility of the nurse analyst.

Buonarroti

Michelangelo Buonarroti had both curiosity and the talent for creating beauty. He began his formal art studies as an apprentice; the studies included both painting and sculpture. He studied the human form through traditional studio sessions as well as in a nontraditional manner—assisting with autopsies. By peeling back the layers, dissection of the human form provided an understanding of the form, function, and limitations of the body. In this manner, Michelangelo learned art through the combination of internal structure and external appearance. His mentor, Lorenzo the Magnificent (Mariani, 1964), provided a milieu in which curiosity and creativity were encouraged. Michelangelo's ability to blend these talents has brought enjoyment to the world for more than 400 years.

The nurse analyst approaches the design and implementation of a system in much the same manner—understanding the form and function as well as the underlying anatomy. Having actively provided direct patient care forms the foundation of knowing the healthcare delivery system and the general needs of healthcare professionals. This involves dedicated preparation and study and many long hours of direct patient care responsibilities to meet the qualifications of a registered nurse. Understanding the operational aspects of healthcare delivery assists in the design and evaluation of the system's end user interface. Exposure to administrative duties in the acute care environment provides the nurse analyst with a knowledge of the regulations and requirements often dictating hospital policy and procedure. These regulatory requirements have a significant bearing on the development and implementation of a system. Just as Michelangelo studied human anatomy to better his painting and sculpting, knowledge of the database structures, program logic, and processing requirements increases the ability of the nurse analyst to support both the end user as well as the programming resources of a system. Participation in systems analysis and development allows the nurse analyst a complete picture of a system. Development of a system requires the nurse analyst to dissect the requirements of the user, apply the rigors of systems analysis, and piece the system together in a cohesive manner that is both pleasing to the end user and programmatically efficient for the technical staff.

Systems Analysis and Development

Yourdon (1989) defines systems analysis as the study of the "interactions of people, and disparate groups of people, and computers and organizations" (p. 1). For the nurse analyst, the disparate groups of people include patients, a cadre of healthcare providers, administrators, accreditation organizations, researchers, educators, insurers, payors, software programmers, and federal and state governments, with each group identifying its own set of information requirements. In addition to the skills outlined for the direct care giver, the nurse analyst must possess the ability to think of systems in both abstract and physical terms, possess computer skills, and survive the political battles found in every organization (Gause and Weinberg, 1989; Yourdon, 1989).

Participation in the analysis and development of systems is the major component of the role of the nurse analyst. Nurses in both the hospital and community as well as in vendor and consulting settings participate in the design and development of clinical information systems (Hersher, 1985). Figure 8-1 depicts the similarities between the nursing process and the systems development life cycle. The comfort with which nurses utilize the nursing process for problem solving provides the foundation for assimilation of the systems analysis and development process. Active participation in systems analysis and development provides a detailed understanding of the needs of the end users, the information system's internal structure, and the system's limitations and potential.

The identification of system requirements is similar to the observation phase of the nursing process. The requirements of the system's users are gathered. The nurse analyst gains insight into the requirements by observing the environment in which the system operates or will operate. The information needs of the users may not coincide with the current data collected; more data may be collected than are utilized or, in other cases, insufficient data are collected. The requirements definition activities help to bring clarity to the data issues and information needs. The nurse analyst may utilize a number of techniques to define requirements. The use of decision trees, mock-ups, prototypes, and/or data mapping assists in identifying the flow of information and data elements needed. While the nurse

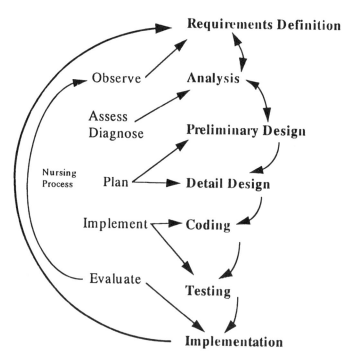

FIGURE 8-1. Comparison of nursing process to classic system development life cycle.

analyst must have the ability to conceptualize systems, the techniques provide visualization of data requirements and information flow for the end users.

During the analysis phase of systems development, the nurse analyst works closely with the technical staff to determine the feasibility of the desired requirements. Hardware and communications technologies are evaluated relative to the desired goals; financial and resource requirements are factored. The development/implementation plan is proposed. The nurse analyst communicates progress, seeks refined definition of requirements, and, where necessary, negotiates compromises.

Just as the nurse providing direct patient care continually communicates the progress of the patient's response to treatment to the patient, the health-care team, and the family, the nurse analyst is the vital communications link between the users and programmers. The abilities to assess the political environment and mediate conflict resolution are required. Coordinating meetings, tracking task completion and programming progress, and maintaining frequent and effective communication are key to successful systems development.

The requirements definition and analysis phases of systems development are most critical to the success of a development project yet frequently have the least amount of time allotted. Gause and Weinberg (1989) note that the relative cost to fix an error found when a project is in the requirements definition phase is one; in the analysis phase, the relative cost to fix an error is three to six times that of the analysis phase. The cost to fix an error increases dramatically as the project progresses, jumping to 40 to 1000 times that of the analysis phase if found after the system is operational. Collecting, collating, reviewing, refining, evaluating, and documenting the design are integral to the success of a new system. Openness to new ideas, suggestions, and surprises allows monitoring of the design and implementation of the system. The direct patient care background provides the nurse analyst a strong basis for understanding the information needs of smaller systems (nursing, radiology, dietary, laboratory, etc.), their relationship to the larger organization, and their potential impact on the new system.

The planning phase of the nursing process correlates with the development of the preliminary and detailed design phases of systems analysis and development. The nurse analyst assists by converting the desired requirements into formal specifications. The end user interface—the "look and feel" of the system—is determined. The sequencing of screens and windows, data fields, and integration points is established and refined during these phases. The understanding gained from requirements definition and analysis phases provides the nurse analyst with a strong sense of the desired sequencing and functioning of the system. The overall needs of the organization are considered as design and development of the smaller systems progress.

The coding and testing phases of systems development equate to the implementation phase of the nursing process. During these phases, the features and functions are programmed and tested. The nurse analyst seeks clarification from the end users on behalf of the programming staff. Communications during this phase are particularly important. Programmers rely on the nurse analyst for quick issue resolution; the users are consulted on issue resolution and are kept apprised of the progress of the coding. At least two levels of testing are recommended. The first level is functional testing. The individual programs are tested to assure that data are captured and processed within the individual function or application as specified. Responsibility for testing individual programs as they are completed may be shared among the programming staff, nurse analyst, and end users. During functional testing, the nurse analyst develops testing scenarios or scripts that comprehensively test each feature. The second testing phase for the newly developed programs or the implementation of the completed product is termed integrated testing. Coordinated by the nurse analyst, highly detailed testing scenarios are developed to mimic use of the functions in a production environment. Testing scripts and testing procedures are developed to facilitate utilizing the end users as testers. The focus of integrated testing is on the points of integration with other applications and the operational policies of both information systems and the end users. The testing scenarios should be executed as written, with through-put followed closely and thorough review of the output coordinated by the nurse analyst. The nurse analyst's evaluation of the success of the integrated test period has much bearing on the decision to implement the system in the production environment or to repeat testing.

The implementation of the new system equates to the evaluation phase of the nursing process. It is essentially the evaluation of the preceding analysis and development steps. The relative success of the implementation of a new system reflects the accuracy and in-depth understanding of the initial requirements and their translation into programs. As with the nursing process, the systems analysis and development life cycle will begin anew with the refining of previously defined requirements or the identification of new requirements as the system grows.

The Nurse Analyst as Project Manager

Frequently, nurse analysts are called on to serve as a design or software implementation project manager. The abilities to apply a problem-solving approach (the nursing process) to situations, to track the progress of multiple groups relative to the project's goal, to gain consensus, and to communicate issues and problems are skills the nurse analyst brings from the realm of direct patient care. The complex nature of the delivery of patient care affords the nurse analyst a solid background for assuming this role.

Summary

The role of the nurse analyst is complex and challenging. It requires observation skills with attention to detail, knowledge of healthcare delivery systems and trends, creativity in analytic problem solving, strong written and verbal communication skills, negotiation and mediation abilities, and the capability to conceptualize and communicate a vision for an information system. The nurse analyst builds from the skills and experiences of providing direct patient care. Expanding the skill set to include knowledge of information systems principles, technologies, systems analysis, and systems development begins the second level of requisite knowledge for the nurse analyst. Operating in a highly technical environment, the nurse analyst must balance the compassion of patient care needs and sometimes the perceived coldness of technology to produce an accepted and utilized clinical information system. The image of the butterfly's metamorphosis relates to the nurse analyst's prerequisite experience of providing direct patient care. Bonsai gardening teaches the need to work toward a vision fraught with constraints by using small prunings and shapings to accomplish a desired effect. Buonarroti's approach to the creation of art demonstrates the need to understand the internal structure of information systems as well as the outward appearance of the system. Systems will continue to grow and the needs of healthcare professionals will become more encompassing. The images of butterflies, bonsai, and Buonarroti provide important lessons for the role of the nurse analyst as the creation of clinical information systems progresses.

Questions

1. Discuss Yourdon's four general principles of automated systems using examples from your own setting. Are they applicable to your environment?
2. The author of this chapter contends that a nurse is in a good position to take on the role of systems analyst for the design and implementation of an automated system. Do you agree or disagree with this statement and why?

References

American Nurses Association: *The Scope of Practice for Nursing Informatics.* Washington, DC: American Nurses Publishing, 1994.
Bailey R, McDonald E: *The Good Housekeeping Illustrated Guide to Gardening* (Vol. 3). New York: Hearst Magazines, 1972; 328.

Dick R, Steen E, eds: *The Computer-Based Patient Record: An Essential Technology for Health Care*. Washington, DC: National Academy Press, 1991.

Gause D, Weinberg G: *Exploring Requirements: Quality before Design*. New York: Dorset House Publishing, 1989.

Hersher B: The job search and information systems opportunities for nurses. *Nursing Clinics of North America* 1985; 20(3):585–594.

Mariani V: *Michelangelo the Painter*. New York: Harry N. Abrams, 1964; 13–33.

Romano C: Innovation: The promise and the perils for nursing and information technology. *Computers in Nursing* 1990; 8(3):99–104.

Yourdon E: *Modern Structured Analysis*. Englewood Cliffs, NJ: Yourdon Press, 1989.

Zielstorff R: Preface. In: Zielstorff R, ed. *Computers in Nursing*. Gaithersburg, MD: Aspen Publications, 1980; x–xiv.

9
How to Select a Nursing Informatics Consultant

ELIZABETH E. CONCORDIA AND GARY L. HAMMON

When to Employ a Consultant

Hospitals, specifically nursing departments, face major decisions as they plan to meet their computing needs. It is often advisable to employ a consultant to obtain expert advice with regard to a well-defined situation or problem that is beyond the capabilities or experience of the hospital staff. At times, the hospital chief executive officer (CEO) and/or board of trustees could benefit from independent validation of a future course of action, specifically with respect to nursing informatics. Not only are sizable financial resources involved but often also the future efficiency and effectiveness of the entire hospital and nursing staff.

In considering when nursing informatics consultants should be employed, it is relevant to note what they can and cannot do. Competent nursing informatics consultants are able to review the present system and anticipate future needs. They will usually find alternative solutions for various organizational and technical problems in the nursing systems area. Consultants can hardly be expected to solve fundamental management problems in the organization, and they cannot legitimately assist in fighting private battles between or within departments in the hospital. A good consultant rarely makes definitive decisions but usually identifies a set of viable alternatives. Because professional nursing informatics consultants do not derive their income from the sale of a product, the institution must be prepared to pay for qualified consultation. To answer the question of when to employ a nursing informatics consultant, you need a well-defined goal with specific objectives. In defining the goal, consider whether the consultant is to justify the current operation of a department. The director of nursing systems may have management problems involving technical, personnel, or legal issues that require an expert opinion of a special nature. If there are major equipment decisions, reorganizations, or financial commitments in need of review, the computer department may want a different type of consultant to assist in coming to the most satisfactory solution. Another major reason for employing yet another type of consultant would be to review the current hospital or clinic situation and develop a strategic plan projecting future needs.

What to Expect from a Consultant

One of the most difficult tasks for the hospital board, CEO, or senior nurse executive is to define the mix of education and experience that constitutes the qualifications of a good nursing informatics consultant to meet particular needs. Any consultant under consideration should be evaluated using the following criteria:

• Relevant professional preparation
• Significant experience
• Recognition in the field
• Recommendations tailored to needs of the client
• Report delivered on time and within budget
• Ability to accomplish change
• Good communication skills
• Fees comparable to those of similar organizations.

Given the aforementioned characteristics, the consultant would be able to address the defined goal(s) as assigned by the board of trustees, CEO, or senior nurse executive.

How to Find a Good Nursing Informatics Consultant

Before looking for a nursing informatics consultant, the nurse manager must prepare a detailed definition of the problem(s) and the desired objective(s). The results of this definition step should be agreed on by top administration and should reaffirm the characteristics of the major problem(s), the scope of the problem(s) to be tackled, and the objective(s) to be achieved. The individual who is hiring the consultant should define precisely the parameters of the engagement. In obtaining the services of a qualified nursing informatics consultant, it is important to differentiate between the independent advice provided by a recognized consultant and the more limited opinions that vendors provide. Most representatives of both hardware and software companies are not able to provide objective advice about computerization; their job is to sell their product. Conversely, the independent advice provided by a qualified nursing informatics consultant is based on firsthand knowledge of the hospital setting gained during the consulting engagement. Of course, the consultant should also have state-of-the-art knowledge of hospital systems and their components.

One of the best ways to be assured of competent nursing informatics consulting assistance is to check with colleagues who have used a consultant who fulfilled their expectations. Subsequently, the consultant's references can be and should be checked by the prospective employer. Another approach is to work through the various national professional organizations, which are often willing to suggest several consultants who are in business for themselves or who are affiliated with a major university. A review of the literature to find authors of knowledgeable articles in the field provides another source. Organizations that may be of help include, but are not limited to, the following:

- American Association of Hospital Consultants
- American Hospital Association
- American Management Association
- American Medical Association
- American Medical Informatics Association, Work Group on Nursing Informatics
- American Nurses Association, Council on Nursing Systems and Administration
- Hospital Financial Management Association
- Institute of Management Consultants
- National League for Nursing Council on Nursing Informatics.

It is desirable to have a preliminary meeting with several nursing informatics consultants before selecting the one for the job. At this time, the prospective employer should discuss the financial arrangements and the duration of the consultation. It is important to have a written specification of the job to be undertaken that clearly describes the expected products, or deliverables, of the engagement, such as a written report, a flow diagram, or an oral presentation to the trustees. All this is essential to find the right person or firm for the job. In the overall consideration, the employer should be aware of what can and cannot be expected from a consultant.

How to Work with a Selected Consultant

Before the start of the engagement, senior nursing management should announce the planned study to avoid an uninformed adverse reaction from nursing personnel. Rumors and worries among the nursing staff can hinder and sometimes sabotage the timely completion of the task.

The competent nursing informatics consultant will be able to review the present system and anticipate future needs, both suggesting alternative solutions for various problems and offering advice on integrating the system with other systems in the organization. The nursing informatics consultant should play the role of the advisor, providing insight into alternatives and their possible consequences.

To work as a team, the hospital and the nursing informatics consultant must be sure they are working on the same problem. Since the consultant is there to assist the nursing department and the institution, it is helpful, whenever possible, to anticipate politically loaded situations and to pave the way for introductions and smooth working conditions. Timing can be the key to a constructive and successful engagement.

Conclusion

The employment of a competent nursing informatics consultant should be considered one of the wisest decisions that nursing management makes. In effect, nursing management is hiring one or more individuals who have spent a lifetime acquiring the education and experience to handle the nursing informatics problem(s) being faced by the institution. For what amounts to a minimal financial commitment, the organization will have purchased competent advice addressed specifically to its defined needs. Clearly the organization should consider the money it spends on a consultant as an investment, not an expense, and should work to quantify the return on that investment.

Although the final decision for any organizational or systems change must lie with the chief executive officer, consultants can serve as important resources, bringing valuable expertise to bear on the decision-making process.

Questions

1. What is the rationale for considering the employment of a consultant?
2. Name possible sources for locating a consultant who can be expected to address your specific requirements.
3. What are the institution's responsibilities for hiring a consultant, determining the scope of effort, and defining the deliverables?
4. What is the role of the institution's management and staff when a consultant is employed?
5. Describe the approach to the use of consultants that should maximize the investment as well as ensure a successful experience for all concerned.

Unit 3
Clinical Applications and Nursing Informatics

Unit Introduction

This unit includes eight chapters on the application of nursing informatics to clinical care. The contributors explore the many ways in which automation can be used by nurses in the clinical arena. Warnock-Matheron and Hannah begin by exploring the factors to be considered during the implementation of nursing systems within a clinical setting. McCormick provides a summary of international efforts toward developing a nursing minimum data set and a uniform nursing language. In a related chapter, Hannah and Anderson profile nursing's role in managing nursing information. They offer an international viewpoint on why it is important for nursing data elements to be collected and stored. Hughes presents major features in successful point-of-care systems and relates the benefits of this type of information system for nursing. The focus is changed from the traditional in-patient computing to home care when Hassett and Farver investigate the use of automation in this setting. Andolina furnishes a look at the use of automation in case management when she describes the automation of critical pathways. Zimmerman shares her thoughts on the application of clinical imaging and the implications for nursing. The work of Staggers concludes this unit in a call to action for the creation of usable clinical workstations.

10
Introducing Nursing Information Systems in the Clinical Setting

Ann Warnock-Matheron and Kathryn J. Hannah

The trend toward computerized systems within clinical settings changes the environment and has a major impact on nurses. Some of these changes are

1. More formalized and structured job functions, thereby reducing flexibility and autonomy
2. Newly created roles and a greater number of specialized occupations
3. Clarification of roles and departmental functions
4. Increased status differentiation (stratification) of occupations and organizational units (Farlee, 1978).

Each of these changes may be viewed by individuals and organizational units as threatening, and this can contribute to increased dissatisfaction and lower job satisfaction. Therefore, nurses need to be aware of and participate actively in the selection, implementation, and evaluation of systems. Nursing information specialists must be cognizant of the changes in procedures, functions, and roles that will result and must develop change management approaches that will promote nursing user acceptance of these systems.

Few computer systems have been installed without the staff experiencing fears and frustrations. The successful implementation of the nursing information system (NIS) can be facilitated by anticipating the potential reactions of nurses to automation. If the reasons for these reactions are identified and understood, effective strategies that will foster acceptance and support for the system from the nursing users can be developed. One strategy is to focus on the factors that make change rewarding rather than on the resistance to change. Negative perceptions may result from a failure to respond in a complete or timely fashion to concerns about computerization or, interestingly, from unrealized expectations. The balance between positive and negative reinforcement determines how the nurse will react to change. When rewards are perceived to outnumber drawbacks, acceptance will occur. Resistance occurs when the negatives appear greater than the rewards and is expressed as a desire to maintain the status quo. The manner in which such issues as security, status, and personal concerns about performance using the system are handled can tip the balance toward reward or punishment.

Based on the writings of several change theorists, three key strategies to facilitate staff adaptation, viewing change as rewarding rather than punishing, have been identified (Kirkpatrick, 1985). These are empathy, communication, and participation. Empathy is described as a means of predicting the probable perceptions of nurses of the proposed changes. A program to decrease negative perceptions and increase the positive ones will enhance the probability of a successful implementation.

Communication can be defined as the ability to create understanding. By fostering understanding, the changes may be perceived to be more positive. Communication of a change should include all of those who need to know as well as all of those who want to know.

Nursing acceptance of the new computer system can be facilitated by preparing nursing personnel for automation by soliciting their participation in the implementation process. True participation means that the users can influence the direction of the project and the change manager must be prepared to respond to the concerns of the user. Participation also requires that the change manager ensure that those concerned with and affected by the change are actively involved, thereby promoting ownership and commitment.

The introduction of a nursing information system requires that attention be paid to the hospital culture and to the human factors because organizational change and the use of technology are interdependent. To gain the organization's acceptance of the computer system, Farlee (1978) recommends that

1. Formalization be kept to a minimum
2. All occupational groups and departments be brought into the decision-making process when selecting a system and when specifying system modifications
3. Stratification be minimized
4. Good communication be maintained
5. Adherence to agreed-on plans and schedules be employed.

The aforementioned concerns may be grouped into three areas that, if addressed properly, can increase the probability for a successful implementation of a nursing information system:

1. Management of change. Successful management of change results in user acceptance of the system. Poorly managed change will generate resistance. When this occurs, attempts to circumvent changes will undermine the effectiveness of the system and the organization will fail to attain the full benefits of computerization.
2. Implementation process. A well-defined implementation process, including a project structure and formalized, detailed implementation plan, is essential.

3. Training of system users. Preparing the nursing staff for automation is crucial in establishing staff user acceptance and minimizing resistance. This can best be accomplished by designing a training program that will
   a. Provide nurses with a basic understanding of computer systems
   b. Inform staff of the benefits expected
   c. Define the roles and responsibilities of nursing personnel during and after implementation
   d. Orient staff to the use of the system.

The Project Team

The successful implementation of a nursing information system requires the participation of all affected individuals and organizational units. To integrate all these people into the project, a project team should be established. The project team will be composed of both information system professionals and user representatives. The users will play an integral role in providing functional specifications and in supporting the implementation. Unless the project is structured carefully, the diversity of views represented will result in a counterproductive environment. A project manager who possesses the required skills must be chosen to coordinate and lead the project. Posner (1987) states that "without arguing which comes first, it is clear that either (a) project managers require certain skills in order to deal effectively with the factors most likely to create problems for them in managing the project, or (b) because certain problems are most likely to confront project managers, they require particular skills in order to handle them" (pp. 109–110). Desirable project management skills include those necessary for communication, organization, team building, leadership, and coping as well as technological knowledge (Posner, 1987). Ideally, this individual should be recruited from the user community. "To handle the variety of project demands effectively, the Project Manager must understand the basic goals of the project, have the support of top management, build and maintain a solid information network, and remain flexible about as many project aspects as possible" (Meredith and Mantel, 1989, p. 101).

The Implementation Plan

Implementation of the nursing information system must compete for resources with other ongoing projects and normal work activities. Implementation processes tend to be complicated, and a plan serves as a map of the process to be followed. Kezsbom, Schilling, and Edward (1989) stress that two components that must be addressed when constructing a plan are identifying what is to be accomplished and identifying the interdependencies of the tasks to be completed. The plan must identify time frames, personnel to be involved, specification of how problems are to be documented, and strategies for assisting users when problems are encountered. An implementation timetable listing all tasks, their expected start and end dates, staffing requirements, and interdependencies provides a useful tool both for planning user involvement and for tracking progress. Successful implementation requires notifying affected personnel about the implementation plan and providing clarification if necessary.

A clear division of roles and responsibilities for all individuals involved in the process is critical to

1. Promote an effective and productive work environment
2. Prevent costly duplication of effort
3. Facilitate communication among team members
4. Ensure accountability for project tasks to be completed.

When everyone knows what has to be done (implementation plan), who is responsible (definition of roles and responsibilities), and when to do it (implementation timetable), the chances for a successful implementation are enhanced greatly.

Management of the Implementation

For the implementation to progress, a means for allocating resources, making decisions, and reviewing progress must be established. Normally, these functions are the prerogative of a steering committee composed of the upper management of all the affected organizational units. The steering committee is ideally chaired by a user with decision-making authority. User participation in the decision-making process enables the committee to direct development according to the organization's needs and priorities. Additional functions of the steering committee include setting priorities, approving any significant change to system functionality or project scope, and approving any major change in the project plan timetable.

Training

In the development of the training program, the needs of the organization, the clients to be served, and the needs and interests of the learner must be considered. The resolution of issues such as comprehensiveness of the training program and efficient performance of the graduate of the program is inherent in the developmental process.

Nurses are a traditional group and tend to view any change with a certain amount of skepticism (Ball and Hannah, 1984). It is necessary to identify common apprehensions of these nurse learners. Nurses would resist change if they believed that a patient's welfare might be endangered if they did not understand the technology adequately. Nurses would also be fairly resistant if they viewed the computer as a source of change or a threat to long-established nursing practices and procedures (Ball and Hannah, 1984). If the "machine" is viewed as a barrier in the relationship between nurse and patient, resistance will develop. The expression and/or repression of nurses' anxieties will impact training.

Nursing learners need to become competent in the use of the equipment and the performance of functions on the system. Nursing staff must be provided with information regarding the use of the nursing information system and its benefits to nursing practice so that the learners become cognizant of issues related to the computerization of patient data. Myths and misconceptions about the system can be dispelled through the presentation of facts in the orientation sessions (Zielstorff, 1976). At this time, computer terminology is defined and issues related to computerization, such as ergonomics, confidentiality, and security of patient data, are discussed.

Questions arise about whether a training program should attempt to influence nursing staff attitudes about the computer system in addition to presenting the information required to use the system effectively (Zielstorff, 1976). Zielstorff indicates that if the affective components of an introduction to automated systems are ignored, an important adjunct to orientation is bypassed. Scarpa, Smeltzer, and Jasion (1992) conclude that strategies to promote attitude change during the introduction of computerized systems are recommended. The attitude of nursing personnel toward the system and, ultimately, their morale are often a function of the quality of the training provided. Many systems professionals attribute the success or failure of a system to the degree of user acceptance achieved.

It is reasonable to assume that the target population will be adult learners who may have predetermined opinions and/or anxieties about computer training. They are mature individuals with a variety of life experiences and responsibilities. It is critical that the approaches within a training program be based on the principles of adult education. Adult learners have been described as

- Goal oriented
- Persistent
- Highly motivated
- Geared to success
- Committed to family, work, and/or other responsibilities
- Limited in time allocated to educational activity
- Best able to meet educational goals using their individualized learning style
- Best able to learn when there is direct application of theoretical concepts and skills to the work situation (Cobin and Lewis, 1983, p. 271).

More recently, Hepner (1993) outlined an approach for educating healthcare providers during implementation of a hospital information system utilizing guidelines for adult learners presented by Darkenwald and Merriam

(1982). These included active versus passive participation and presentation of information in a logical sequence to enhance the learning process (Darkenwald and Merriam, 1982).

Several factors contribute to the complexity of the task of orienting staff. The nursing staff who need to be trained in the use of the new system may consist of administrative coordinators, nursing unit supervisors, head nurses, staff nurses, and unit clerks. Presenting information simultaneously to people of widely varied backgrounds and educational levels can be considered a major challenge (Zielstorff, 1976). It is fair to anticipate that some of this group will oppose the incorporation of computers into the healthcare environment.

Defining objectives is essential not only for specifying the material to be presented but also for evaluating the effectiveness of the course. "Each objective should be clearly stated, limited in scope, and measurable, so that the learner can gauge the degree to which he or she has assimilated the material, and so that the planners of the program can evaluate its effectiveness" (Zielstorff, 1976, p. 15). Training objectives should include

1. Familiarizing the nursing learner with the use of the hardware
2. Familiarizing the nursing staff with the functions of the nursing information system
3. Providing nurse learners with basic information about computer systems, how they operate, what the benefits are to nursing, and the progress of the project to date
4. Promoting a positive attitude among the nurse learners toward computerization within the hospital environment
5. Generating feedback from the nursing staff in defining the system functions.

The training program should acknowledge the differences in knowledge and skills of the learner. By addressing these differences, providing factual information, and allowing the learner to express and interact in a stimulating environment, a training program does much more than teach nurses "how to compute." A training program provides the basis from which the learner may begin to grapple with the revolution in technology in the hospital setting and thus promotes a more sophisticated level of nursing practice.

Instructional Approaches

"Training for any system end user should be as 'hands-on' and practical as possible to aid retention and comprehension" (Hepner, 1993, p. 235). A variety of methods can be utilized in presenting the hands-on training component of the program. These include live or videotaped demonstrations followed by return practice by the learner that is guided by the facilitator. Presentation of material in a modular fashion allows the learner to control the rate of learning. Each module provides the learner with the information needed to complete the function successfully. This method of training allows for higher facilitator-to-learner ratios. To ease initial anxieties, all hands-on training exercises should be performed on fictitious patients. This allows the nurse learner to be more relaxed and provides the freedom to err without concern for patient safety. There is also no fear that the learner will corrupt real patient data during training.

Another method is computer-based training (CBT). CBT may be available from the vendor when a system is purchased. Perez and Willis (1989) cited that their organization had concerns about the traditional trainer dependent approach due to the volume of information that had to be presented. As well, the facilitators found that teaching the same class content repetitively was tedious. CBT provided several advantages in this setting from both a cost and a quality perspective. Cost savings were realized by decreasing total training time and by reducing or eliminating the one-on-one training traditionally provided in departments such as emergency.

From a quality perspective, there was increased flexibility to schedule classes for participants, and statistical data could be captured by the CBT program. Although Perez and Willis (1989) indicated that a facilitator was present at all training classes, it is feasible that participants could utilize the tool independently and work at their own pace at a time convenient to them. In addition, CBT software programs can be an advantage to the facilitator in the managing of student evaluations and in tailoring the course content to the participant's specific needs.

The training program should be designed to integrate the elements of the instructional methods discussed. This represents an attempt to meet the learner's needs while taking into consideration the resources within the hospital setting.

Preparation of Training Resources

As mentioned, to meet one of the primary objectives (i.e., the nursing learner becoming competent in performance of the various functions of the system), hands-on experience is required. This can best be provided in a training room that is located away from the patient care areas so that nurse learners are not interrupted by the demands of patient care. Training rooms should be equipped with the same hardware that learners will be required to use in patient care areas. Each learner should have an individual workstation and sufficient space for printed material and accessories. Arrangement of the workstations in a semicircle allows the facilitator to monitor several learners simultaneously.

Once the training facilities are complete, preparation of the trainers can proceed. Each facilitator should complete a basic training course and be provided with additional supervised time on the computer system. The facilitators should be knowledgeable in the content of information presented to the users so the information and examples are relevant to participants or users. Group sessions permit discussions on how to structure a session, the application of adult learning principles, and methods of dealing with a variety of situations that may arise. Each facilitator should be evaluated by the training coordinator.

The material provided to learners should include a training manual detailing the steps required to perform necessary tasks and functions on the system. It is important that the learners become familiar with this manual during orientation so that they will be able to use it efficiently in the nursing unit. Self-evaluation and facilitator evaluation tools are valuable in generating input for the refinement of the training program. Additional training tools, such as audio- and videocassettes or computer-assisted instruction modules, can be used to instruct learners on keyboard operation and troubleshooting sequences.

Scheduling of Training

The timing of the training sessions requires careful consideration. The number of staff to be trained, the physical facilities available for training, the number of trainers, and the overall staffing situation within the hospital are factors that affect the number of personnel that can be trained at any given time. Whatever the training rate, time should be blocked out immediately before implementation to allow review by the nurse learners who require or request it.

Access to the system is given when the learner has successfully completed the training program. For each training objective, minimal competency levels must be determined. Each learner must be able to achieve these levels before receiving system access. Each institution should determine what additional remedial activities will be provided should a nurse not meet the minimum standard.

In addition to the overall consideration of the development of institution-specific confidentiality and security policies and procedures, attention must be focused on reinstating access for those individual nurses absent during implementation of new functions and systems.

System Conversion

There are four basic approaches to system conversion:

1. Direct or crash conversion. This occurs when the old system is stopped and is replaced immediately by the new system. This method of conversion places the greatest stress on individuals and the organization because the change is abrupt.

2. Parallel conversion. This occurs when the new and old systems operate simultaneously for a period of time. The primary disadvantage of this approach is that the user workload is doubled. Provision should be made to have additional staff available during the conversion period in this approach.
3. Phased conversion. In phased conversion, parts of the new system are made available to users at discrete intervals. A major disadvantage is that the new system can be used for specific functions only, and other functions must be performed using the existing procedures.
4. Pilot conversion. In this method, the system is initially made available to only a small part of the organization. At intervals, other units of the organization will receive access to the system. The disadvantages of this approach are the inability to move staff freely between organization units and potential communication problems when the functions that the pilot group performs must interact with those of groups not on the new system.

The four basic conversion approaches can be combined in various ways: for example, a crash conversion for a pilot group, phased parallel conversion, or a phased conversion for a pilot group. Each of the conversion approaches has inherent problems. These problems can be minimized by giving careful consideration to the effect of the conversion method on the organization and producing a plan to address potential problems.

Postimplementation Audit

Following implementation of an automated care planning system, Allen (1991) recommends that follow-up in-services be provided to address and resolve any additional problems that may be encountered. Meredith and Mantel (1989) state that the word "audit" is usually associated "with a detailed examination of financial matters, but a project audit is highly flexible and may focus on whatever senior management desires" (p. 481). An internal postimplementation audit should evaluate, at a minimum, the following:

1. Training. The objective is to determine the effectiveness of the training program and whether users have encountered problems because of inadequate training.
2. System functionality. The overall functionality of the system is rated based on whether user requirements have been met. This will also determine what enhancements or upgrades to the system are required.
3. Implementation process. The audit process views the success or failure of the implementation primarily as a learning exercise for future implementations. The lessons learned may be applied to the implementation

of enhancements or extensions of the system. Questions that should be answered include
- Were the budget and timetable estimates realistic?
- What were the causes of missed deadlines and budget overruns?
- What obstacles were encountered?
- Does the system perform up to expectations?

4. User satisfaction. If the users are dissatisfied, they will not use the system. Factors affecting satisfaction levels include the following:
- What problems are users encountering?
- How are or will these problems be resolved?
- What suggestions for improvements have users made?
- Do the users find the system easy to use and, if not, what can be done to make it easier to use?

Problems in these areas, appropriately identified and documented, can be addressed after the review. The evaluation of these four areas is an ongoing process, and seemingly minor items of frustration can have a long-term impact on users' attitudes toward the system.

Conclusion

The implementation of nursing information systems holds great promise for nursing practice. The nursing profession will benefit from the recent advances in information technology as nurses gain the ability to access information in a timely manner, thereby enhancing the decision-making process during the provision of patient care. To realize these benefits, nursing information specialists should

1. Encourage involvement of nurses in system testing and implementation
2. Solicit feedback from nurses and respond to concerns
3. Communicate with nursing staff during implementation
4. Provide support during the implementation period.

This will enable nurses to cope with the changes in their work environment, to adapt to procedural changes, and to utilize the new tool, the computer system. By understanding the nature of user reactions to change, by communicating, by educating, and by training, nursing information specialists are able to minimize the period required to reach a high level of nurse-user acceptance.

Questions

1. Identify and describe the three elements essential to successful implementation of a nursing information system.
2. Discuss the impact of the implementation of a nursing information system on the organization.

3. Relate the principles of adult learning to the instructional approaches for training nurses to use the system.
4. Compare and contrast the four basic approaches to system conversion.
5. What is a postimplementation audit and what are its major foci?

References

Allen S: Selection and implementation of an automated care planning system for a health care institution. *Computers in Nursing* 1991; 9(2): 61–68.

Ball M, Hannah K: *Using Computers in Nursing.* Reston, VA: Reston Publishing, 1984.

Cobin J, Lewis J: Solution to a dilemma: Computer technology facilitates non-traditional post-basic nursing education. In: Scholes M, Bryant Y, Barber B, eds. *The Impact of Computers on Nursing: An International Review.* Amsterdam: North-Holland, 1983; 269–276.

Darkenwald GG, Merriam SB: *Adult Education: Foundations of Practice.* New York: Harper & Row, 1982.

Farlee C: The computer as a focus of organizational change in the hospital. *Journal of Nursing Administration* 1978; 8: 20–26.

Hepner F: Teaching/learning strategies for a successful H.I.S. implementation. *Proceedings of the 1993 Annual HIMMS Conference.* Chicago: Healthcare Information and Management Systems Society, 1993; 231–241.

Kezsbom DS, Schilling DL, Edward KA: *Dynamic Project Management: A Practical Guide for Managers and Engineers.* New York: John Wiley & Sons, 1989.

Kirkpatrick DL: *How to Manage Change Effectively.* San Francisco: Jossey-Bass, 1985.

Meredith JR, Mantel SJ: *Project Management: A Managerial Approach* (2nd ed). New York: John Wiley & Sons, 1989.

Perez LD, Willis PH: CBT product improves training quality at reduced cost. *Computers in Healthcare* 1989; 10(7): 28–30.

Posner BZ: What it takes to be a good project manager. *Project Management Journal* 1987; 18(1): 51–56.

Scarpa R, Smeltzer S, Jasion B: Attitudes of nurses toward computerization: A replication. *Computers in Nursing* 1992; 10(2): 72–80.

Zielstorff RD: Orienting personnel to automated systems. *Journal of Nursing Administration* 1976; 6: 12–16.

11
An Update on Nursing's Unified Language System

KATHLEEN A. MCCORMICK

Since 1988, there has been much progress toward a unified nursing language system (UNLS) for the nursing profession. Even more importantly, there has been significant progress within health reform and the computer-based patient record to mandate more information access, which necessitates the nursing language system and terminology for nursing with a defined structure and syntax. Progress in funded nursing research has also brought new tools in diagnosis, nursing interventions, and some outcomes of care. Further, the professional associations at a national and international level have initiated steps toward the development of a UNLS. In previous studies, the concept and advantages of building a UNLS have been described (McCormick, 1988, 1991; McCormick et al., 1994; McCormick and Zielstorff, 1993).

At an Austin, Texas, postconference following the Fifth IMIA International Conference on Nursing Use of Computers and Information Science, Clark furthered the advantages of pursuing a unified language. She stated that communicating among ourselves (in nursing) has always been important, but communicating with other people about nursing has acquired a "new urgency" since we are forced to recognize that the value of nursing is no longer apparent to those who have the power to influence our practice, make policy determinations, and allocate scarce resources (Clark, in press). Other important driving forces for this unified nursing language, according to Clark, are cost containment, resource management, and the rapidly developing science and technology of informatics, which is providing the systems necessary to support the establishment of a nursing vocabulary. Clark notes that from a survey of member countries in the International Council of Nurses, many countries collect nursing data for epidemiological and management uses. However, most of the data are not structured for use by nurses.

Mortensen and Nielsen (in press) state that surveillance of health needs in epidemiology requires nursing care data to demonstrate the people's need for nursing care and measurement of the outcome of nursing interventions. They add that since nurses contribute to between 40 and 60% of healthcare costs (in Europe), it is imperative to ensure that information on the care of this sector of health providers is acquired.

Casey (1994), from the United Kingdom, notes that the development of standardized terminology in that country is driven by a quest for information systems that support patient care and improve quality. Integral to the provision of quality care are three provisions: (1) that the practitioners are able to measure their effectiveness with accurate information about patient care and outcomes, (2) that the practitioner has ownership and control over the process of care and information about quality of care, and (3) that the improvements in quality do not occur in isolation but through a process of assessing and improving care alongside measurement and improvement in all aspects of care, treatment, and supporting services. Casey further notes that standardized language will facilitate care plans, protocols, decision support, research, audits, central planning, management, and epidemiology.

Holzemer, Henry, Reilly, and Miller (1994) state that the advantage of uniformity is the undergirding of the profession's ability to delineate the relationships between the cost and quality of nursing care. They further attest that cost and quality judgments rest on the state of nursing's data.

This update chapter will extend beyond the previous discussions of the need, necessity, and advantages of a UNLS and will update

- Advances in the nursing profession
- Classification schemes recommended for the UNLS
- An integration of UNLS into the unified medical language system (UMLS)
- Other U.S. research initiatives toward language development
- Other international research initiatives toward language development
- International workgroup progress
- Future directions needed.

Advances in the Nursing Profession

The American Nurses Association (ANA) Cabinet on Nursing Practice mandated the formation of a Steering Committee on Databases to Support Clinical Nursing Practice. The steering committee, chaired by Dr. Norma Lang, has manuscripts in press describing the output of the committee work (Lang et al., in press; McCormick and Zielstorff, in press; McCormick et al., 1994). The monograph developed by the ANA contains the concepts endorsed by the committee and the four classification schemes recognized by the committee as nursing language with sufficient scientific validity and reliability to be entered into the unified medical language system (UMLS) to become a unified nursing language system (UNLS). The committee first endorsed the 1991 ANA practice standards, which expanded the concept of nursing process from four levels to six: assessment, diagnosis, outcome identification, planning, implementation, and evaluation. Then the committee and ANA resolutions endorsed the Nursing Minimum Data Set (NMDS) and the 16 items identified in it to guide the collection of nursing data in any healthcare delivery system. These elements include four nursing care elements, five patient or client demographic elements, and seven service elements. The four nursing care elements that are important to the UNLS are nursing diagnosis, nursing intervention, nursing outcome, and patient intensity.

Another concept that the committee endorsed was coordinating development of the UNLS with the National Library of Medicine's UMLS (Lindberg, Humphreys, and McCray 1993). The concept of the UNLS is based on the same principles as the UMLS and includes semantic typing for the concepts and identification of semantic relations with mapping of terms from different vocabularies by relating them to each other or by acknowledging them as synonyms of the same concept.

To recognize schemes of nursing classification and vocabularies that may be appropriate to recommend for a UNLS, the committee established criteria to select them. Table 11-1 lists the criteria that have been used by the committee. These criteria expand those defined by McCormick in the original 1988 publication of *Nursing Informatics: Where Caring and Technology Meet*. The purpose of the criteria was to analyze the internal consistency of the classification schemes and determine the scientific rigor that went into developing them, in addition to determining if a commitment toward updating the product was made by the developers.

Classification Schemes Recommended for the UNLS

Using the criteria, the committee has recognized four nursing classification schemes that span diagnosis, interventions, and some outcomes. The utility of the schemes has been described for the acute care environment, home health, community health, and long-term care. The four classification schemes recognized by ANA and recommended for inclusion into the UNLS are the North American Nursing Diagnosis Association (NANDA)

TABLE 11-1. The Criteria Used by the ANA Database Committee to Recognize a Nursing Classification Scheme

1. Be clinically useful for making diagnostic, intervention, and outcome decisions.
2. Be stated in clear and unambiguous terms, with terms defined precisely.
3. Demonstrate evidence of testing for reliability.
4. Have been validated as useful for clinical purposes.
5. Be accompanied by documentation of a systematic methodology for development.
6. Be accompanied by evidence of process for periodic review and provision for adding, revising, or deleting terms.
7. Provide a unique identifier or code for each term.

(NANDA, 1992); *The Omaha System: Applications for Community Health Nursing* (Martin and Scheet, 1992); The Home Health Care Classification (Saba et al., 1991); and the Nursing Interventions Classification (NIC) (McCloskey and Bulechek, 1992). The data element components of each of these are described in a new ANA monograph (ANA, in press).

An Integration of UNLS into UMLS

The UMLS is a project of the NLM that includes concepts, terms, and strings. It includes semantic relationships and mapping of terms from different vocabularies by relating them to each other. The NLM has made a commitment to the ANA to include classification schemes recognized by the committee in the UMLS. The nursing classification schemes can then be utilized by the nursing profession to pull them away from UMLS to form a UNLS. As described previously, in the 1988 McCormick article and in a recent paper by McCormick et al. (1994), the advantage of integrating nursing terms with the UMLS is a multidisciplinary language, which depicts the environment in which we practice, document care, and strive to reach quality outcomes in patient care.

To date, the NLM has added three of the classification schemes recognized by the committee to the UMLS: NIC, NANDA, and the Home Health Care Classification. As of this writing, the NLM was in the process of adding the Omaha System. The inclusion of these classification schemes in the UMLS represents the addition of nursing diagnosis, interventions, and some outcomes to the UNLS. However, by far the weakest component of the UNLS is the area of outcomes. While several concept papers have described classifications of outcomes of care that nurses are engaged in achieving, no classification scheme has been developed based on valid and reliable methods.

Other U.S. Research Initiatives Toward Language Development

Other nurses have recently been involved in determining linkages of nursing terminology with other medical data sources. Zielstorff, Cimino, Barnett, Hassan, and Blewett (1992) conducted a pilot analysis of whether nursing terminology could be found in the UMLS before the addition of the four nursing classification schemes. It was found that direct matches were possible 10% of the time with NANDA and the Omaha System lists of terms. When terms were split to separate major concepts from modifiers, there was at best a 32% match between concepts. The authors concluded that the nursing terms were not well represented in the UMLS and recommended expansion of the UMLS.

Grobe (1992) has developed important research on a natural language processing method to analyze and classify statements of nursing interventions in home health. This study was supported by the NLM and was reviewed by the steering committee, which found that the statements reflect higher level organizing concepts of the interventions that nurses prescribe in home health. The ANA database committee also reviewed the ANA mental health practice group nursing classification and recommended further definition of terms such that the terms would then represent a nursing classification scheme.

Henry, Holzemer, Reilly, and Campbell (1994) described the feasibility of using the Systematized Nomenclature of Medicine (SNOMED III) to represent nursing terms. The authors matched terms used in the care of patients with pneumocystis carinii pneumonia. Nurses used nursing diagnosis terms (NANDA) for documentation of care, and direct matches with SNOMED III were 30%. In their subset of terms, the authors found that nursing terms matched SNOMED III terms 69% of the time when different combinations of SNOMED terms were used.

Another research project that is supported by the University of Virginia, Thomas Jefferson University Hospital, and the University Hospital Consortium attempts to develop a set of terms to represent nursing diagnoses, nursing intervention, and patient outcomes (Ozbolt, Fruchtnight, and Hayden, 1994). Ozbolt and colleagues used Saba's 20 home health components to classify the following: 209 nursing diagnostic terms, 545 interventions, and 122 expected outcomes identified from seven nursing units in two hospitals. The intent of the project is to determine what the most frequently occurring clinical problems are, what activities nurses engage in to solve the problem, and what outcomes are achieved. In addition, the group attempts to determine the relationships between productivity and quality and to link these relationships to costs.

A San Francisco group has classified nursing interventions for persons with AIDS (Holzemer et al., 1994). In a three-hospital study with 201 patients, 21,492 nursing activities were coded by nurses. The major nursing activities were patient interview, nursing interview, intershift report, and chart audit.

In a U.S. hospital on the Texas-Mexico border, a group implementing a hospital information system with nursing documentation developed standard nursing care plans based on assessment, NANDA nursing diagnosis, patient outcomes, nursing interventions, evaluation of whether outcomes were met, and reassessment if necessary (Taylor, Scholten, Cassidy, and Corona, 1994). They found that the nursing process with the nursing minimum data set as a structure was missing the demographic component of culture of poverty, issues of nationality, and entitlements added to the elements of race and ethnicity. They also found that when evaluating care based on patient outcomes, it was clear that a classification or taxonomy of patient care standards or outcomes had to be developed so that the entire construct of the nursing process could be articulated. While their interventions were not following the NIC intervention classification, Taylor et al. (1994) found in retrospect that there was remarkable consistency between the interventions stated by their hospital nurses and the McCloskey and Bulechek (1992) list.

Other International Research Initiatives Toward Language Development

International projects that have been published include those in the United Kingdom, Sweden, Belgium, Denmark, and Australia. In the United Kingdom, Casey (1994) reports on the Terms Project. The primary aim of this project is to produce a thesaurus of healthcare terms, coded (in Read Codes) for use in computer systems and mapped to the International Classification of Disease—9th Revision (ICD). The project incorporates nursing terms, including terms for midwifery and visiting nurses. Currently over 20,000 terms have been identified as unique to nursing. This work is being translated into education through a Strategic Advisory Group for Nursing Informatics (SAGNIS) to get information management and information competencies and the support of the standardized vocabulary into the mainstream of nursing education. Following identification of terms, the project will define terms and classify concepts, which are steps toward an agreed-on language.

In Sweden, Ehnfors (1994) has extended research on uniform key words used to document nursing practice in a new model called VIPS. The Swedish authorities have described the utility of the patient record to support health professionals in the delivery of care, to serve as a basis for quality care, to be the reference point for judgments and choice of interventions to be implemented by health providers, to be a tool in quality assurance, to be the basis for audit and control, and to give the patient insight into the treatment and care he or she has received. (In Sweden, the patient has a right to his or her medical record.)

The VIPS model was used for documentation of nursing care on seven wards in two hospitals in Sweden (Ehnfors, 1994). The process model governing the development of terms includes nursing history, nursing status, nursing diagnoses, goals, nursing interventions, nursing outcomes, and nursing discharge note. The key nursing interventions are participation, information, education, support environment, general care, training, observation, special care, continuity, and coordination. One hundred forty patient records were reviewed before and after structured nursing documentation with uniform key words and nursing educational seminars. Criteria were developed to rate changes in documentation before and after intervention on a five-point scale ranging from (1) the problem is described in the problem list or intervention or outcome to (5) the problem is described with relevance to nursing. After the planned intervention, the number of records with notes and the number of notes per record increased with respect to all parts of the nursing process except goals. The greatest increase was a fivefold increase in the discharge note, followed by a threefold increase in the use of nursing diagnoses and almost a doubling of the use of nursing outcomes. The numbers of notes per record increased for nursing interventions.

In another project initiated by Spri in Sweden, Sahlstedt (1994) describes the results of common language in computers in 200 installations throughout Sweden. The key words of Ehnfors (1994) with definitions served as the language, and nursing process served as the structure for nursing documentation. The project was introduced into acute care, psychiatric, geriatric, and primary community care environments. Four key concepts were used: patient well-being, respect for integrity, prevention, and safety. Nursing history included admission, health situation, hypersensitivity, previous health care, social history, and life style. Nursing status was represented by the terms communication, breathing/circulation, nutrition, elimination, skin, activity, sleep, pain, sexuality, psychosocial, spiritual, and, finally, well-being. Nursing interventions were classified the same way as in the project described by Ehnfors (1994). Use, satisfaction, and quality of notes were evaluated and shown to be improved with the uniform nursing language and computerized nursing process.

The Nursing Minimum Data Set has been required by law to be collected four times per year in Belgian General Hospitals since January 1, 1988 (Sermeus and Delesie, 1994). Inherent in the collection of minimum nursing data has been the need to develop a uniform nursing language. In 1985, the Belgian Nurses Association developed a list of 111 nursing interventions. This list has been pared down to 23 nursing interventions for sampling purposes; these were found to contain 80% of the statistical information in the whole list of 111. In Belgium, the essential elements in defining patient population and variability have been attributed to identifying the diversity of the patient population (medical diagnosis, age, degree of dependency on daily activities found in the nursing notes), and variability of practice (23 nursing interventions, length of stay, number of nursing staff, level of qualifications of the nursing staff). A listing of these interventions is provided in Table 11-2 (Vandewal and Vanden Boer, 1994). In the majority of Belgian hospitals, the reliability of nursing intervention data collection is about 80%, with emotional support and patient teaching being only weakly reliable. NMDS data in Belgium have also been linked with the San Joaquin Patient Classification System (Vanden Boer and Vandewal, 1994). The four categories of intensity that have become standards in the country are no help, average, more than average, and intensive care. These four classifi-

TABLE 11-2. The 23 Minimal Nursing Activities Found in Belgium Hospitals since 1987 (Vandewal and Vanden Boer, 1994)

1. Hygiene care
2. Mobility care
3. Elimination care
4. Feeding care
5. Gavage feeding
6. Complete care of mouth, nose, eyes
7. Decubitus preventive care
8. Assisting in getting dressed
9. Attending tracheostomy or ventilation
10. Interviewing patient or relatives
11. Teaching individual patients or relatives
12. Supporting patient/highly emotionally disturbed
13. Supervision of mentally disturbed patients
14. Isolation
15. Monitoring of vital signs
16. Monitoring of clinical signs
17. Attending continuous traction or cast
18. Drawing of blood specimens
19. Medication IM, SC
20. Medication IV
21. IV therapy
22. Surgical wound care
23a. Surface of the traumatic wound
23b. Traumatic wound care

cations of patients coincide with the NMDS national map, separating patients into self-care, care oriented needing complete help, or cure oriented needing complete help.

Data have been chosen to be collected cross-sectionally rather than longitudinally. Two national presentations have been used to describe data: the fingerprint and the national map. The fingerprint gives a picture of individual ward data, and the national map depicts all nursing units in the country. An important element of the Belgian collection of data is the feedback that is given through the publication of a booklet titled "National Statistics," published by the Ministry of Public Health. In addition, a computer diskette is developed for each hospital to identify its nursing units compared to the whole country. An educational program has been developed with seven Belgian universities to educate nursing directors and head nurses on how to work with the program and read their fingerprints and the national map. At a governmental level, there is a proposal to use the NMDS information to determine the hospital's budget.

A European Union (EU) program called Advanced Informatics in Medicine (AIM) initiated a program called TELENURSING in 1991 "to promote standardization of definitions, classifications and codings of essential nursing care data in order to further the development of internationally comparable minimum data sets in nursing based upon uniform definitions of data items" (Mortensen and Nielsen, in press). The sole contractor for this project is the Danish Institute for Health and Nursing Research in Copenhagen, Denmark. The group of nurses in Europe hopes to establish a Euro-Nursing Health Data Base. The overall objectives of TELENURS-ING are listed in Table 11-3. To carry out these objectives, nursing will (1) distribute a questionnaire with three dimensions: (a) a professional dimension (including nursing process), (b) a technical dimension (including documentation, definition, coding, classification, standardization, and a Nursing Minimum Data Set), and (c) a decisional dimension (including from a national to a ward level); (2) prepare a TELENURSING proposal to develop a European Standard Data Sheet to collect essential nursing data on patient problems/nursing diagnoses, interventions, and patient outcomes; and (3) collect data for and create a minicomputerized European Nursing Health Data Base (CAN—Computerized Availability of Nursing Care Data) in accordance with the European Standard Data Sheet (Mortensen et al., 1994). The first CAN project included a European Standard Data Set to collect data on feeding problems and verbal communications. Later the group will expand to sleep, elimination, pain, and emotion. From the pilot results of the CAN data sheet, a formal proposal will be made to Telematics for Health Care in the European Union.

The European group envisions definitions in nursing to consist of nursing terms: (1) derived from the nursing process, (2) derived from clinical practice, and (3) derived from the literature of nursing theorists (Mortensen and Nielsen, in press). Overriding the nursing process are the terms assessment, problem/nursing diagnosis, goal, intervention, and outcome.

Findings as of this writing indicate that nurses in Europe are committed to the nursing process. Moreover, there is a tendency to define nursing

TABLE 11-3. The Overall Objectives of TELENURSING (Mortensen and Nielsen, 1994).

1. To create a European Platform for nurses interested in classifications of patient problems/nursing diagnoses, interventions and outcomes, and minimum data sets, taking into account modern information technology.
2. To create a European network of nurses interested in health care informatics and willing to participate in EU Health Telematics consortia.
3. To create awareness among nurses of standardization efforts in health care informatics, e.g. CEN/TC/251 with regard to items of TELENURSING: definition (terminology) coding and classification.
4. To link the technical approach of CEN/TC/251 with the professional approach of WHO and ICN with regard to development of classifications in health care, including the development of an International Classification for Nursing (ICNP).
5. To develop nursing tasks to be included in the workplan accompanying the program on Telematics within the 4th EU Framework Program based upon TELENURSING requirements for computerized accessibility of samples for a European Nursing Health Data Base.

terms for problems/nursing diagnoses, interventions, and outcomes with more definitions from theory rather than practice when defining patient problems/nursing diagnosis.

The application of such nursing standards is believed to improve availability, quality, and comparability of nursing data. In addition, it is the hope of the European group to coordinate its efforts with the AIM committee, which has been working on the European Standardization Committee (CEN); the Technical Committee (TC251), which has been working since April 1990 to develop standards in healthcare informatics; and the International Council of Nurses (described later in this chapter).

In addition, the European World Health Organization/Europe (WHO/ EURO) initiated a multinational study in 1981 called "People's Need for Nursing Care," which collected data to demonstrate nursing's contributions toward physical, mental, and social well-being in care (Ashworth et al., 1987). More recently (1993), WHO/EURO has proposed a European strategy for continuous quality improvement to identify the specific physical, mental, and social well-being health indicators related to nursing (Mortensen et al., 1994). For each of these projects, a data set of nursing has been indicated for adequate information systems.

Foster and Conrick (1994) and Gliddon and Weaver (1994) state that a Community Nursing Minimum Data Set exists in Australia and is being pilot tested. They describe a project that involves defining standard terms at a national level for a national minimum data set (including an Australian Thesaurus, an Australian Taxonomy, data definitions and classifications, and a data format) before developing an NMDS. The Australia NMDS includes 18 nursing elements, and a recent book has been published containing the data dictionary and guidelines (CNMDSA, 1994).

International Workgroup Progress

American representatives (Lang et al., in press) have been reporting the progress of the ANA Database Committee to the International Council of Nurses (ICN) related to the recognition of nursing classifications and integration into a UNLS. Activities in the international arena have focused on integrating nursing classifications with the International Classification of Diseases (ICD) and establishing an International Classification of Nursing Practice (ICNP).

The ANA submitted the NANDA classification in 1989 to the National Center for Health Statistics, Public Health Service, U.S. Department of Health and Human Services, World Health Organization, and the North American Collaborating Center for inclusion into ICD. The goal was to have NANDA represented in the ICD-10-CM, which is the U.S. version. The NANDA classification was modified to conform with ICD-10 coding, and a new classification concept was added to ICD-10 called *The Family of*

Disease and Health-Related Classifications (Fitzpatrick et al., 1989). This concept enabled nursing diagnosis to be added to ICD even though the terms do not always depict disease conditions. The classification was approved, endorsed, and forwarded to the WHO for approval by other member countries. The WHO nursing unit and ICN were charged with obtaining endorsement by the nursing organizations from around the world. WHO consisdered international agreement on nursing diagnosis classification essential before endorsing its inclusion in the ICD framework.

In 1993, a draft classification scheme was proposed at the ICN meeting. The ICN is composed of 105 member national nursing associations (NNAs) and 21 WHO Collaborating Centers for Nursing (Clark, in press). Three consultants were named to conduct a literature search, and three small surveys of member associations identified classifications systems in use or being developed around the world (Wake et al., 1993). The draft-proposed classification scheme is called the International Classification of Nursing Practice (Table 11-4) and includes not only the four classification schemes recognized by the committee but also others developed internationally. The Professional Services Committee of the ICN has been developing this proposed classification (Clark and Lang, 1992). The framework for this classification scheme includes three elements: (1) nursing problems/diagnosis, (2) nursing interventions, and (3) outcomes. Each of the elements is alpha-

TABLE 11-4. The Proposed International Classification of Nursing Practice (Reproduced with permission from JAMIA, 1(6), 425. Hanley & Belfus, Inc., Philadelphia.)

System	Author(s)	Country	Language	Type
Ambulatory Care	Verran	US	E	I
Australian	Jones et al.	Australia	E	P,I
Belgian	Sermeus et al.	Belgium	F,FL,E	I
Danish	Danish Institute	Denmark	D,E	P,I,O
Henderson*	Henderson	US	E,F,S,G	P
Iowa	McCloskey & Bulechek	US	E	I
Lang & Marek	Lang & Marek	US	E	O
NANDA	NANDA	US	E,F,P,S	P
Nursing Lexicon	Grobe	US	E	I
Nursing Minimum Data Set	Werley & Lang	US	E	I,O
Omaha	Martin & Scheet	US	E	P,I,O
Répertoire diagnostics infirmiers	Riopelle et al.	Canada	F	P
Saba	Saba	US	E	P,I
Swedish	Ehnfors et al.	Sweden	Sw,E	I

*Available in 26 different languages.
Languages:
D = Danish, E = English, F = French, Fl = Flemish, G = German, P = Portuguese, S = Spanish, SW = Swedish.
Types:
P = problem/diagnosis, I = intervention/treatment, O = outcome.

betized and compared to terms used in member countries. This process is compounded by the fact that the ICN officially recognizes three languages: English, French, and Spanish (Clark, in press). In addition, Clark suggests that the ICN will be challenged to transcend the boundaries of countries and continents with different races and cultures. These elements were also found to need expansion in the NMDS in the project described by Taylor et al. (1994) in implementing nursing standards and the NMDS in a Texas-Mexico border hospital.

The goal of the ICN project has broadened the initial attempt to add only nursing diagnoses to ICD. Through this effort, compatibility of nursing classifications will have an international representation and will be compatible with other WHO classifications. The goals of this project are to (1) develop a specified process and product, (2) achieve recognition by national and international nursing communities, (3) ensure compatibility with other WHO classifications, (4) achieve utilization for the development of national databases, and (5) establish an international minimum data set. The criteria for inclusion of terms into the ICNP are presented in Table 11-5.

These goals are not new to the ICN. Eighty-six years ago, a participant reporting on an ICN meeting in Paris said the following:

While attending a special meeting of the ICN in Paris, I was naturally at once struck by the fact ... that the methods and the ways of regarding nursing problems were, in many respects, as foreign to the various delegations as were the actual languages, and the thought occurred to me that if ... we hoped ever to actually realize the aims of the International Council, one of which is: to confer upon questions relating to the welfare of their patients, sooner or later we must put ourselves upon a common basis, and work out what may be termed a "Nursing Esperanto" which would, in the course of time, give us a universal nursing language, and methods for all our affiliated countries. (Hampton Robb, 1909)

Perhaps the most important vision that Robb had in addition to recommending that nursing needed an ICNP was that the affiliating countries

TABLE 11-5. Proposed Criteria Required by Terms in ICNP (Reprinted with permission of Clark, in Press)

1. Broad enough to serve the multiple purposes required by different countries;
2. Simple enough to be seen by the ordinary practitioner of nursing as meaningful description of practice and a useful means of structuring practice;
3. Consistent with clearly defined conceptual frameworks but not dependent upon a particular theoretical framework or model of nursing;
4. Based on a central core to which additions can be made through a continuing process of development and refinement;
5. Sensitive to cultural variability;
6. Reflective of the common value system of nursing across the world as expressed in the ICN Code for Nurses; and
7. Usable in a complementary or integrated way with the family of disease- and health-related classifications developed within WHO, the core of which is the ICD.

needed the methods. That the methods needed are methods to contribute toward developing a universal language in the affiliated countries is an assumption that this author makes.

Recent advances in the ICNP project have also included the establishment of a technical advisory group of nurses from Israel, Nepal, Chile, Kenya, Jamaica, and Japan, who are testing the feasibility and applicability of the work to date at a global level (Clark, in press). Three presentations were made at the Quadrennial Congress of the ICN in Madrid in June 1993. These were well attended, which demonstrated to the participants that there is an interest and enthusiasm for ICNP by nurses from many countries. Finally, most recently, in Mexico, an advisory meeting funded by the W. K. Kellogg Foundation proposed future directions needed for nurses to use the ICNP in primary health care (ICN, 1994). The meeting brought together selected nurses from Africa, North America, and South America. A meeting of consultants and technical advisers was scheduled for Geneva in August 1994 to prepare a first draft of an ICNP.

Thus far, based on surveys and consultative meetings, two broad starting points have been achieved for which there is consensus: (1) that the nursing process is a means of structuring practice, and (2) that the focus must be on basic needs, functional patterns, or activities of living. The latter focus is derived from the work of Henderson (1977) which has been translated into 26 languages, with several more translations into Eastern European languages in preparation (Clark, in press).

Future Directions Needed

Any commitment toward the development of nursing classification systems, nursing vocabulary, or unified nursing language systems is a commitment toward update, continual review and revision of the process, criteria, and revision of content. Every language and classification scheme developed for health care has become an investment in keeping the content updated, new terms added, new concepts added or deleted, new research initiatives added, and new classifications with new and advanced information systems integrated. Maintenance includes addressing the issue of missing terms or new terms to be added by the nursing profession or other health professionals.

At the national and international level, when a unified nursing language becomes a uniform nursing language, the terminology needs to converge. The process for this convergence in the business industry is called harmonization. In the harmonization process, the codes of one country are linked to codes in another country under a uniform standard classification system. These codes are used for country import/export classifications of commodities. For example, what is called a "sweater" in the United States is called a "jumper" in Australia. Yet both codes sit side by side in the apparel section of the international codes. A corollary for nursing informatics is that one country might call a patient symptom an "alteration in comfort" whereas another country could call it "pain." Both terms could be harmonized to a coded term. This harmonization of terms requires specialized procedures. The maintenance and update of the harmonized terms require national or international committees to oversee the harmonization of terms. The conflict between local use of terms and universal or international use of the nursing language will remain until harmonization is attempted beyond national boundaries. In medicine, this is done through the ICD coding structure, with committees nationally and internationally.

A further issue is that nursing lacks protocols or methods to set boundaries in developing classification schemes. The developers of language systems have complete latitude, with no boundaries on development, testing, and updating. National and international standard protocols or methods need to be developed to guide the developers so that their end products will be usable in national and international classification schemes. If the end products of nursing terminology and classification schemes are to be used nationally and harmonized into an international classification, then protocols and methodologies for development are critical.

Research will be required into the twenty-first century on the development, validation, and reliability testing of nursing language systems. Model criteria need to be developed and quantitated. Model development paradigms need to be developed and evaluated. The application of terminology to improved monitoring of costs, efficiencies, effectiveness, and outcomes is important. Studies done on the reliability of terms in nursing diagnoses/problem lists and interventions will need to intensify.

Summary

The concept of the unified nursing language system is steadily making progress in the United States and is being discussed on the international level. The United States has made great strides in identifying criteria for selection of nursing classification schemes and recommending those schemes for inclusion in the unified medical language system, to become a part of a unified nursing language system. Now the challenge is in research to develop protocols for further nursing classification systems, evaluate the utility of the nursing language system developed in the UNLS, evaluate and quantitate the use of criteria to select classification schemes, and develop update procedures.

The next advances at an international level will not only facilitate the description of nursing's contributions toward health care but also begin to link us intellectually. Without a unified nursing language integrated into other healthcare standard initiatives, the nursing profession will not be able to use the standard language developed in corollary health reform initiatives.

Questions

1. What four nursing classification schemes have been recognized by the U.S. ANA?
2. Name at least five criteria used to select classification schemes for recognition and inclusion in the UMLS.
3. How does a UNLS differ from a UMLS?
4. How will international use of classification schemes benefit the nursing profession?
5. What research and developments are needed to move further toward a UNLS?
6. What international progress is being made toward proposing a unified nursing language system?
7. Why is there a need for continuous maintenance and update of the content in a UNLS?
8. Describe the concept of convergence or harmonization.
9. Discuss at least one other initiative in nursing research that evaluates classification schemes.
10. How are nursing language systems related to other healthcare standards initiatives?

References Cited

American Nurses Association: *Nursing Data Systems: The Emerging Framework.* Washington, DC: American Nurses Association, in press.

Ashworth P, et al: *People's Need for Nursing Care: A European Study.* Copenhagen: World Health Organization, 1987.

Casey A: Nursing, midwifery and health visiting terms project. In: Grobe SJ, Pluyter-Wenting ESP, eds. *Nursing Informatics: An International Overview for Nursing in a Technological Era.* Amsterdam: Elsevier, 1994; 639–642.

Clark J: An international classification for nursing practice (ICNP). In: *Proceedings of a Postconference on Informatics: The Infrastructure for Quality Assessment and Improvement in Nursing.* Austin, Texas, June 23, 1994, in press.

Clark J, Lang NM: Nursing's next advance: An international classification for nursing practice. *International Nursing* 1992; 39: 109–112, 128.

Community Nursing Minimum Data Set Australia: *Version 1.0: Data Dictionary and Guidelines* (CNMDSA). Canberra: Australian Council of Community Health Nursing Services, Inc., 1994.

Danish Institute for Health and Nursing Research Information and Diagnosis: Copenhagen: 1991.

Ehnfors M: Nursing information in patient records: Towards uniform key words for documentation of nursing practice. In: Grobe SJ, Pluyter-Wenting ESP, eds. *Nursing Informatics: An International Overview for Nursing in a Technological Era.* Amsterdam: Elsevier, 1994; 643–647.

Fitzpatrick JJ, Kerr ME, Saba VK, Hoskins LM, Mills WC, Rott Kamp BC, Warren JJ, Carpenito LJ: Translating nursing diagnosis into ICD code. *American Journal of Nursing* 1989; 89: 493–495.

Foster J, Conrick M: Nursing minimum data sets: Historical perspective and Australian development. In: Grobe SJ, Pluyter-Wenting ESP, eds. *Nursing Informatics: An International Overview for Nursing in a Technological Era.* Amsterdam: Elsevier, 1994: 150–154.

Gliddon T, Weaver C: The community nursing minimum data set Australia: From definition to the real world. In: Grobe SJ, Pluyter-Wenting ESP, eds. *Nursing Informatics: An International Overview for Nursing in a Technological Era.* Amsterdam: Elsevier, 1994; 162–168.

Grobe SJ: Nursing intervention lexicon and taxonomy. In: Lunn KC, DeGoulet P, Piemme TE, Rienhoff, O, eds. *MedInfo '92.* Amsterdam: Elsevier, 1992; 981–986.

Hampton Robb I: *Reports of the Third Regular Meeting of the International Council of Nurses.* Geneva: International Council of Nurses, 1909.

Henderson V: *Basic Principles of Nursing Care.* Geneva: International Council of Nurses, 1977.

Henry SB, Holzemer WE, Reilly CA, Campbell KE: Terms used by nurses to describe patient problems: Can SNOMED represent nursing concepts in the patient record? *Journal of the American Medical Informatics Association* 1994; 1: 61–74.

Holzemer WE, Henry SB, Reilly CA, Miller T: The classification of nursing interventions for persons living with AIDS. In: Grobe SJ, Pluyter-Wenting ESP, eds. *Nursing Informatics: An International Overview for Nursing in a Technological Era.* Amsterdam: Elsevier, 1994; 687–691.

International Council of Nurses: *Nursing's Next Advance: An International Classification for Nursing Practice (ICNP).* Working paper, October 1993.

International Council of Nurses: *Report of Advisory Meeting on the Development of Information Tools to Support Community Based and Primary Health Care Nursing Systems.* February 1994.

Lang NM, Hudgins C, Jacox A, Lancour J, McClure ML, McCormick KA, Saba VK, Stenvig TE, Zielstorff R, Prescott P, Milholland K, O'Connor KS: Toward a national database for nursing practice. In: *Nursing Data Systems: The Emerging Framework.* Washington, DC: American Nurses Association, in press.

Lindberg DA, Humphreys BL, McCray AT: The unified medical language system. *Methods of Information in Medicine* 1993; 32: 281–291.

Martin KS, Scheet NJ: *The Omaha System: Applications for Community Health Nursing.* Philadelphia: W.B. Saunders, 1992.

McCloskey JC, Bulechek GM, eds: *Nursing Interventions Classification (NIC).* St. Louis, MO: Mosby-Year Book, 1992.

McCormick KA: A unified nursing language system. In: Ball MJ, Hannah KJ, Gerdin-Jelger U, Peterson H, eds. *Nursing Informatics: Where Caring and Technology Meet.* New York: Springer-Verlag, 1988; 168–178.

McCormick KA: The urgency of establishing international uniformity of data. In: Hovenga EJS, Hannah KJ, McCormick KA, Ronald JS, eds. *Nursing Informatics '91: Proceedings of the Fourth International Conference on Nursing Use of Computers and Information Science.* Berlin: Springer-Verlag, 1991; 77–81.

McCormick KA, Zielstorff R: Building a unified nursing language system. *Nursing Data Systems: The Emerging Framework.* Washington, DC: American Nurses Association, in press.

McCormick KA, Zielstorff R: Building a unified nursing language system. In: *Papers from the Nursing Minimum Data Set Conference.* Edmonton, Alberta: The Canadian Nurses Association, 1993; 127–133.

McCormick KA, Lang N, Zielstorff R, Milholland LC, Saba V, Jacox A: Toward standard classification schemes for nursing language—Recommendations of the American Nurses Association Steering Committee on Databases to Support Nursing Practice. *Journal of the American Medical Informatics Association,* 1994; 1(6): 421–427.

Mortensen R, Nielsen GH: TELENURSING and CAN: Clinical Nursing Vocabulary as part of two European studies. In: *Proceedings of a Postconference on Informatics: The Infrastructure for Quality Assessment and Improvement in Nursing.* Austin, Texas, June 23, 1994, in press.

Mortensen R, Mantas J, Manuela M, Sermeus W, Nielsen GH, McAvinue E: Telematics for health care in the European Union. In: Grobe SJ, Pluyter-Wenting ESP, eds. *Nursing Informatics: An International Overview for Nursing in a Technological Era.* Amsterdam: Elsevier, 1994; 750–752.

North American Nursing Diagnosis Association: *NANDA Nursing Diagnosis: Definitions and Classifications.* Philadelphia, PA: North American Nursing Diagnosis Association, 1992.

Ozbolt J, Fruchtnight JN, Hayden JR: Toward data standards for clinical nursing information. *Journal of the America Medical Informatics Association* 1994; 1: 175–185.

Riopelle L, Grondin L, Phaneuf M: *Répertoire des Diagnostics Infirmiers selon le modèle conceptuel de Virginia Henderson.* Montreal, Quebec: McGraw-Hill, 1986.

Saba VK, O'Hara PA, Zuckerman AE, Boondas J, Levine E, Oatway DM: A nursing intervention taxonomy for home health care. *Nursing and Health Care* 1991; 12: 296–299.

Sahlstedt S: Computer support for nursing process and documentation. In: Grobe SJ, Pluyter-Wenting ESP, eds. *Nursing Informatics: An International Overview for Nursing in a Technological Era.* Amsterdam: Elsevier, 1994; 648–652.

Sermeus W, Delesie L: The registration of a Nursing Minimum Data Set in Belgium: Six years of experience. In: Grobe SJ, Pluyter-Wenting ESP, eds. *Nursing Informatics: An International Overview for Nursing in a Technological Era.* Amsterdam: Elsevier, 1994; 144–149.

Taylor ME, Scholten R, Cassidy DA, Corona DF: Using nursing standards as a basis for reporting care using a computer. In: Grobe SJ, Pluyter-Wenting ESP, eds. *Nursing Informatics: An International Overview for Nursing in a Technological Era.* Amsterdam: Elsevier, 1994; 625–629.

Vanden Boer G, Vandewal D: Linkage of NMDS-information and patient classification systems. In: Grobe SJ, Pluyter-Wenting, ESP, eds. *Nursing Informatics: An International Overview for Nursing in a Technological Era.* Amsterdam: Elsevier, 1994; 158–162.

Vandewal D, Vanden Boer G: NMDS-information for the allocation of budgets to nursing units. In: Grobe SJ, Pluyter-Wenting ESP, eds. *Nursing Informatics: An International Overview for Nursing in a Technological Era.* Amsterdam: Elsevier, 1994; 129–133.

Wake M, Murphy M, Affara F, Lang N, Clark J, Mortensen R: Towards an international classification for nursing practice: A literature review and survey. *International Nursing Review* 1993; 40: 77–80.

Zielstorff R, Cimino C, Barnett G, Hassan L, Blewett D: Representation of nursing terminology in the UMLS metathesaurus: A pilot study. In: Frisse ME, ed. *Proceedings of the Sixteenth Annual Symposium on Computer Applications in Medical Care.* New York: McGraw-Hill, 1992; 393–396.

12
Determining Nursing Data Elements Essential for the Management of Nursing Information

KATHRYN J. HANNAH AND BETTY J. ANDERSON

This chapter explores nursing's role in managing nursing information. It focuses on international efforts at identification of essential nursing data elements, development of minimum health data sets, and use of nursing information. Factors related to the role of the nurse in information management and obstacles to effective nursing management of information have been detailed elsewhere in this book as well as in other publications (Hannah and Anderson, 1994). The issues for all nurses relate to information and information management, and the salient issue is identification of nursing data elements that are essential for collection and storage in national health databases.

Nurses must be able to manage and process nursing data, information, and knowledge to support patient care delivery in diverse care delivery settings (Graves and Corcoran, 1989). To accomplish this goal, nurses must attend to the content (the data) contained in local, regional, national, and international information systems. For some time, nurses have been distracted by the technological aspect of information management at the expense of the data. In fact, the initial systems for gathering minimum uniform health data can be traced back to systems devised by Florence Nightingale over a century ago (Verney, 1970). Despite Nightingale's early attempts to develop a nursing database, nurses in most countries have yet to define the minimum set of data elements essential to describing the practice of nursing.

At the time this chapter was written, nursing data elements were not being collected and stored in Canada in any jurisdiction, either regionally or nationally, for use in decision making related to health policy or resource allocation. The patient discharge abstracts prepared by medical records departments across Canada and the United States currently contain no nursing care delivery information. The abstracts therefore fail to acknowledge the contribution of nursing during the patient's stay in the hospital. This omission is important because the abstracts are used by many agencies for a variety of purposes, including funding allocation and policy making. Much information vital to determination of the costs of hospitalization and the effectiveness of nursing care in achieving appropriate patient outcomes is being lost. Given the current status, anyone looking back 500 years from now at national health databases would never know that nursing took place in North America during the twentieth century.

Fortunately, these data gaps have been recognized, and nurses have developed a heightened awareness of the importance of collection, storage, and retrieval of nursing data. Attention is now being directed at initiating the process by which the nursing profession will begin to address the essential data needs of nurses in all practice settings. This awakening is coinciding with an increasing international thrust for healthcare reform and restructuring, which has generated an increased awareness of the need to develop national health databases as a foundation for rational decision making. It is important that a minimum number of essential nursing elements be included in such databases.

The nursing profession must provide leadership in defining appropriate nursing data elements to be included in national health databases, specifically through patient discharge abstracts or summaries. In Canada, these nursing data elements are beginning to be referred to as the Nursing Components of Health Information. Such a set of data elements would be similar to the uniquely nursing elements included in the nursing minimum data set (NMDS) currently being tested in the United States. The purposes of the NMDS are "to establish comparability of nursing data across clinical populations, settings, geographic areas, and time; to describe the nursing care of patients and their families in both inpatient and outpatient settings; to show or project trends regarding nursing care needs and allocation of nursing resources according to nursing diagnoses; and to stimulate nursing research" (Werley, Devine, and Zorn, 1988, p. 1652). Such data are essential because they allow description of the health status of populations with relation to nursing care needs, establish outcome measures related to nursing care, and investigate the use and cost of nursing resources.

Thus, the salient issue in information management for nurses is identification of nursing data elements that are essential for collection and storage in national health databases. These data elements must reflect the data that nurses use to build information that is the foundation for clinical judgment and management decision making in any setting in which nursing is practiced.

Contextual Factors Influencing Development of Health Information in Canada

There are several factors influencing the development of the nursing components of health information. These include initiatives to facilitate the evolution of a national system for health information built on essential and comparable data; increasing drug costs; new technologies and treatment modalities that are driving up healthcare costs; changing demographics as a result of an aging population; rising healthcare costs resulting in alternative approaches to managing hospitals and a drive to find alternative funding mechanisms; a trend toward patient-specific costing of health services and analysis of health services in terms of patient outcomes; a shifting paradigm in terms of the value and emphasis placed on community-based practice as opposed to acute care hospital-based practice; examination of the roles of healthcare providers and organizations to eliminate duplication of services and functions; and the trend toward consumerism. There need to be ways in which nurses can be more efficient and more effective as well as maximize the quality of care that is available to patients within available resources. There is also a need to identify strategies to provide enhanced information management to facilitate use of the ever-diminishing resources.

These are some factors influencing the drive toward identification of essential nursing data. The information revolution has prompted initiatives by healthcare organizations to develop or acquire automated information systems focused on the utilization of data for the purposes of resource allocation, patient-specific costing, and outcomes of services. The information revolution has also been a driving force in the evolution of national systems for health information.

Information and information management will become increasingly important in the future. Nurses must demonstrate that nursing makes a difference to patient outcome and must provide quantitative evidence to support this claim. We need nursing information to facilitate articulation of our professional scope of practice and of our authority and responsibility within the healthcare system. We must determine the essential data elements required for inclusion in national, multidisciplinary, patient-focused health data sets.

Background on Health Minimum Data Sets

A national health data set containing a minimum number of elements with uniform definitions and classifications was first developed in the United States in 1969 (Murnaghan and White, 1970). Similar health data sets have been developed and implemented in the United Kingdom and Canada. The historical background on the development and implementation of minimum health data sets has been described elsewhere (Anderson and Hannah, 1993). These data sets include almost no nursing data. The authors are aware of only one health data set that focuses on nursing data. This is the nursing minimum data set (NMDS) developed by Werley and colleagues in the United States.

The NMDS is defined by Werley and colleagues as a "minimum set of items of information with uniform definitions and categories concerning the specific dimensions of professional nursing, which meets the information needs of multiple data users in the health care system" (Werley, 1988, p. 7). This data set consists of nursing care elements, including nursing diagnosis, nursing intervention, nursing outcome, and intensity; patient demographic elements, including personal identification, date of birth, sex, race, ethnicity, and residence; and service elements, including health record number, principal nurse provider identification, admission date, discharge date, disposition of the patient, expected principal source of payment, and facility number. In addition to development of uniform definitions for the data elements, standard classification systems are being developed and tested (Delaney, Mehmert, Prophet, and Crossley, 1994; Vanden Boer and Sermeus, 1994; Werley and Lang, 1988). Research activity continues to be directed at the development of standardized taxonomies for nursing diagnosis, interventions, and outcomes to be used in describing the nursing care elements in a data set (Bulechek and McCloskey, 1990; Grobe, 1990; Jenny, 1989; Lang and Marek, 1990; McCloskey et al., 1990; McLane, 1987; North American Nursing Diagnosis Association, 1989).

The gaps in nursing data elements in national health information sets have been recognized by nurses in many countries, as evidenced by the activities currently ongoing in countries outside the United States. European nurses also recognize that their health systems need to include nursing data elements that are significant in the nursing decision-making process. A research initiative entitled "A Concerted Action on European Classification for Nursing Practice with Special Regard to Patient Problems/Nursing Diagnosis, Nursing Intervention, and Outcomes," known as TELE-NURSING, was launched in 1991. The objectives of TELENURSING are to create a network of nurses interested in classification of patient problems/ nursing diagnosis, nursing interventions, and nursing outcomes; to establish minimum data sets and healthcare informatics; to raise awareness among nurses of standardization efforts in healthcare informatics; and to link the technical approach of national groups and the professional approach of international groups with regard to development of classifications of health care. The TELENURSING group has established evidence of an interest in developing data standards and a nursing minimum data set. The next step is to promote standardization of definition, classification, and coding of data as initial work that may contribute to the development of internationally comparable nursing minimum data sets (Mortensen et al., 1994).

Australian nurses recognize and support the need for integration and standardization of data from all disciplines involved in the provision of health care. To this end, Australian nurses are participating in the development of a national healthcare data dictionary of standard definitions and the nursing data element identification and classifications based on these standard definitions. At present, Australian nurses have developed a national minimum data set for community nurses based on the work of Werley and colleagues in the United States. As of this writing, this data set is in the pilot stage (Foster and Conrick, 1994).

Canadian Initiatives Directed at the Development of HI:NC

In Canada, many nurses recognize the need to identify the nursing components of health information to facilitate development of a national health information system at a time when provincial health information systems are being reengineered. To have nursing data incorporated into a national health information system, nurses must take a proactive stance and mobilize resources to ensure the identification of those data elements that are essential to nurses in all practice settings in Canada.

In meeting this challenge, the Canadian Nurses Association responded to a resolution calling for a national consensus conference "to develop in Canada a standardized format (Nursing Minimum Data Set) for purposes of ensuring entry, accessibility, and retrievability of nursing data" (Canadian Nurses Association [CNA], 1990). The Nursing Minimum Data Set (NMDS) Conference was held in Edmonton, Canada on October 27–29, 1992. The overall objective of this working conference was to develop an NMDS in Canada to ensure both the availability and accessibility of standardized nursing data. Due to a recognition of the paucity of dialogue that had taken place on the topic among Canadian nurses and the inappropriateness of attempting to achieve consensus on the topic at such an early stage, the invitational conference brought together those individuals best able to formulate a plan for initiating the development of an NMDS in Canada. The NMDS conference culminated in identification of the elements, displayed in column on the left in Table 12.1, for inclusion in a national health data set. These nursing data elements are proposed for addition to the Health Medical Record Institute (HMRI) database, displayed in the column on the right in Table 12.1, as a next step toward a cross-sectoral, multidisciplinary, longitudinal national health database in Canada (CNA, 1993). Group deliberations on each of the data elements are summarized elsewhere (CNA, 1993).

At the provincial level, the Alberta Association of Registered Nurses (AARN) has actively participated in supporting the development of an NMDS. A strategic plan has been endorsed and an ad hoc committee struck to guide initiatives related to development of an NMDS. In developing the strategic plan, the committee deliberated over the name "NMDS," which some individuals perceived as portraying a stand-alone nursing data set. In Canada, it is essential that the nursing data elements constitute one component of a fully integrated health information database. Therefore, the committee members recommended that the nursing data

TABLE 12-1. Elements of HI:NC and HMRI Data Sets

HI:NC[1]	HMRI[2]
Care Items	Care Items
Client status (nursing diagnosis)	Medical Diagnosis (most responsible,
Nursing interventions	primary, secondary)
Client outcomes	Procedure & dates
Nursing intensity	
Patient Demographics	Patient Demographics
Unique lifetime identifier	Health care number
	Date of birth & age
	Sex
Race, ethnicity	
	Weight (newborn & infants < 28 days)
Unique geographical location	Postal Code
Language	
Occupation	
Living arrangement	
Home environment including physical structure	
Responsible caregiver upon discharge	
Functional health status	
Burden on care provider	
Education level	
Literacy level	
Service Items	Service Items
	Prov./institution #
	Chart #
Principal nurse provider	Most responsible doctor
Unique nurse identifier	
	Most responsible consultant
	Admission date & hour
	Admission category
	Admit by ambulance
	Discharge date & hour
	Length of stay
	Institution to alive/death codes
	Responsibility for payment
	Main patient service

[1] *Papers from the Nursing Minimum Data Set conference.* (pp. 153–154), CNA, 1993, Ontario, Canada.
[2] *HMRI Abstraction Manual* (pp. 5.5–5.6), Health Medical Records Institute, 1991, Ontario, Canada.

elements be renamed Health Information: Nursing Components (HI:NC). This name change was endorsed by a resolution passed at a CNA meeting in 1993.

The strategic plan for HI:NC endorsed by the AARN Ad Hoc Committee has three major goals:

1. To facilitate the identification of the HI:NC in Alberta
2. To facilitate the utilization of the identified nursing components of health information in Alberta
3. To refine further and maintain the data elements.

Strategies implemented to date directed at achieving these goals include convening HI:NC workshops in June 1993 and November 1993 in Edmonton and Calgary, respectively; developing and distributing information pamphlets about Health Information: Nursing Components; disseminating information through armchair sessions at conferences and poster presentations at conferences; and providing talks, teleconferences, letters to key education contacts, and articles on HI:NC.

The HI:NC workshops are being held for the purpose of disseminating information about HI:NC and stimulating the dialogue necessary to expose issues related to the minimum essential nursing data elements. HI:NC workshops will continue to be held to stimulate ongoing dialogue about nursing data elements throughout the province of Alberta. It is expected that the HI:NC workshops will culminate in the achievement of consensus on those nursing data elements considered essential for inclusion in a national health data set. The two objectives of the HI:NC workshops are to examine critically the identified nursing component elements from the national NMDS conference and discuss issues related to the nursing component element. Attendees are provided with background information on HI:NC, after which considerable time is allowed for deliberation on those nursing care elements considered essential for inclusion in a Canadian national health data set. The nursing care elements include client status, nursing interventions, nursing intensity, and client outcomes. Proceedings from the HI:NC workshop, including a summary of group deliberations on nursing care elements, have been published and disseminated as a discussion document (AARN, 1993).

In summary, participants at the HI:NC workshops have voiced general agreement on the essential nature of the four nursing care elements: client status, nursing intervention, nursing intensity, and client outcomes. Group deliberation on these nursing care elements has exposed some important issues that require examination.

Client status is broadly defined as a label for the set of indicators that reflect the phenomena for which nurses provide care, relative to the health status of clients (McGee, 1993). Although client status is similar to nursing diagnosis, the term "client status" was preferred because it represents a broader spectrum of health and illness and is perceived to be less problem oriented than the term "nursing diagnosis." Several issues were deliberated in relation to client status. While many nursing diagnostic taxonomies are deemed useful to describe client status, the need for considerable research directed at enhancing these taxonomies was identified. With the focus on a multidisciplinary approach to client care, it was felt that a common label "client status" should be used because it incorporates all disciplines. Finally, with the move toward "hospitals without walls" and a continuation of services throughout the entire spectrum of care, the question arose regarding the point in the continuum of care at which the data element would be collected.

Nursing interventions refer to purposeful and deliberate health-affecting interventions (direct and indirect) based on assessment of client status, which are designed to bring about results that benefit clients (AARN, 1992). Concern was voiced that a focus on interventions could perpetuate professionally focused health information as opposed to patient-focused information. However, emphasis on the client and not the professional when the nursing interventions are identified was deemed to overcome the tendency to concentrate on professional disciplines.

Group deliberation culminated in three major issues. The first issue was the need to utilize and develop existing nursing intervention taxonomies rather than start all over again from the beginning. The second issue was the need to ensure linkages between all elements of the data set. The third issue is that with the emphasis on a multidisciplinary approach to client care, the overlapping of professional boundaries with respect to interventions must be acknowledged.

Client outcome is defined as "client's status at a defined point(s) following health care [affecting] intervention" (Marek and Lang, 1993, p. 100). While agreement was achieved regarding the essential nature of this data element, issues arose relating to how the data should be collected. The attendees identified the need to define what data to collect and at what points along the continuum of care this data element is to be collected. Once these issues are resolved, the reliability and validity of the data must be established. Then attention must be directed at the aggregation of the data element independently and interdependently with other elements in the health data set.

Nursing intensity "refers to the amount and type of nursing resource used to [provide] care" (O'Brien-Pallas and Giovannetti, 1993, p. 68). The issues related to this data element include the absence of a consistent methodology for measurement and collection of nursing intensity data and the lack of availability of computers in all healthcare settings to facilitate collection of this data element. Emphasis was also placed on the need to establish the reliability and validity of nursing intensity data.

As nurses in Canada embark on development of the nursing components of health information, several issues germane to the development of minimum data sets emerge, including data integrity (Giovannetti, 1987) and the scope of data to include in a minimum data set (Murnaghan, 1978). Other technical issues of relevance relate to aspects of data linkage (Hannah, 1991). Once the nursing components of health information are developed, three issues emerge:

1. Promoting the concept to ensure widespread use
2. Educating users to ensure the quality of the data that are collected
3. Establishing mechanisms for review and revision of the data elements (Murnaghan, 1978).

Considerable discussion has occurred surrounding the essential nursing data elements for inclusion in a health data set. A think tank in the fall of 1994 focused on exploration of the taxonomies for use in describing each of the nursing data elements. Conference participants were challenged to explore and debate the existing nursing diagnosis, nursing intervention, and nursing outcome taxonomies for inclusion in HI:NC. A comprehensive review of these taxonomies was prepared as background information to stimulate a discussion of the issues surrounding use of these taxonomies to describe nursing data elements (AARN, 1994). Substantial discussion occurred about the standardization of nursing language in Canada. On the one hand, standardization of nursing language is criticized because of the inflexibility of standardization, the belief that a standard language is not clinically useful, and the fear of eroding clinical nursing judgment through the encouragement of a "cookbook" approach to nursing documentation. On the other hand, standardization of nursing language is promoted to further the development of nursing information systems, to communicate the nature of nursing, and to expand nursing knowledge (McCloskey and Bulechek, 1994).

Initiatives Directed at Development of Standardized International Nursing Data Elements

Although considerable work has been invested in the identification of and achievement of consensus on essential nursing data elements for inclusion in national health data sets, the linkages to an international nursing data set are only beginning to be explored. The American Nurses Association Steering Committee on Databases to Support Clinical Practice has begun initiatives to develop a uniform language for nursing and is working with the International Council of Nurses to promote the inclusion of nursing data in the World Health Organization's Family of Disease and Health Related Classifications (an internationally used classification system) and to develop an international language that describes nursing care, the International Classification of Nursing Practice (McCormick et al., 1994; Zielstorff, Lang, Saba, McCormick, and Milholland, 1995). There are issues related to the development of an international nursing classification system that have been debated from a philosophical and a professional perspective. Yet if the universal reason for developing an international classification system for nursing is to promote clinical reasoning in nursing and improving nursing care decisions in an effort to improve the quality of patient care (Mortensen, 1993), this is hardly a point with which nurses are expected to take issue.

There is much work to be done on the development of an international classification system for nursing data. Nurses in all countries must raise their awareness of this important work. Linkages need to be created among national and international initiatives to facilitate identification and resolution of issues related to the development and use of these standardized languages among nurses. It is imperative that efforts not be duplicated.

Implications of Nursing Data

In the absence of a system for collection, storage, and retrieval of nursing data, it is evident that much valuable information is being lost. This information is important to demonstrate the contribution that nursing makes to the care of patients and to demonstrate the cost effectiveness of nursing care (Werley et al., 1988; Werley, Devine, Zorn, Ryan, and Westra, 1991). The trend is away from nursing-specific models of patient care delivery to patient-focused models that emphasize collaboration of disciplines, multi-skilling of healthcare providers, standardization of care, and streamlining of documentation through charting by exception. In this move, it is imperative that nurses be able to articulate what is and is not nursing's role. Furthermore, nurses will be asked to demonstrate nursing's contribution to patient care in terms of outcome measures that are objective and measurable. Nurses require nursing data to identify outcomes of nursing care, defend resource allocation to nursing, and justify new roles for nursing in the healthcare delivery system (Gallant, 1988; McPhillips, 1988; Werley et al., 1991). Similarly, nurses need to understand and value nursing data so that, in the selection and implementation of information systems for their organizations, they insist that nurses play a major role and that nursing data needs are incorporated in the selection and implementation criteria. For greater detail on the selection and implementation of information systems, see Hannah, Ball, and Edwards (1994).

Although nursing must preserve its professional identity, this must be balanced against professional compartmentalization. Collection and storage of essential nursing data elements that are not integrated as components of a national data set will serve to ghettoize nursing. This is dangerous at a time when significant emphasis is being placed on multidisciplinary collaboration, patient-focused care, and patient outcomes. In view of priorities such as these in health care, the need for integration of data elements could not be clearer.

Nurse clinicians need to know what nursing elements are essential for archival purposes so that nursing documentation includes data related to these elements. With the move toward standardization of care through the use of care maps, it is essential that outcomes of nursing care are determined and included. As healthcare organizations embrace the concept of charting by exception in an effort to decrease the valuable hours spent by healthcare workers in documentation, nurses must be sure that the tools that outline the inherent patient care delivered are not devoid of nursing's contributions. If there are no data that reflect nursing activities, there will be no archival record of what nurses do, what difference nursing care makes, or why nurses are required. In times of fiscal restraint, such objective nursing data are necessary to substantiate the role of nurses and the nurse-patient ratios required in the clinical setting.

Nurse researchers need a database composed of essential data elements (1) to facilitate the identification of trends related to the data elements for specific patient groups, institutions, or regions, and (2) to assess variables on multiple levels, including institutional, local, regional, and national (Werley et al., 1988). Collection and storage of essential nursing data elements will facilitate the advancement of nursing as a research-based discipline (Werley and Zorn, 1988). Nurse educators need these essential nursing data to develop nursing knowledge for use in educating nurses and to facilitate the definition of the scope of nursing practice (McCloskey, 1988).

Finally, definition of nursing components of health information is essential to influence health policy decision making. Historically, health policy has been created in the absence of nursing data. At a time of profound healthcare reform, it is essential that nurses demonstrate the central role of nursing services in the restructuring of the healthcare delivery system.

Clearly, a priority for nursing is the identification of the nursing components of health information—those essential nursing data elements that must be collected, stored, and retrieved from a national health information database. There is much work to be done in the brief span of time that is available to ensure that nursing data elements are included in national health databases. The challenge for all nurses is to identify their role in helping to define the nursing elements essential for inclusion in such a database. The time to respond to this challenge is now, for if we do not, the essential nursing data elements will either be defined by someone else or will remain absent from national health databases.

Questions

1. Why is it important for nursing data elements to be collected and stored?
2. Briefly discuss some of the worldwide initiatives in nursing that are working toward the development of nursing data elements. Consider work from Australia, Canada, and the United States. How do the initiatives differ? How are they similar?

References

Alberta Association of Registered Nurses (AARN): *Scope of Nursing Practice.* Alberta: AARN, 1992.

Alberta Association of Registered Nurses (AARN): *Papers from the Alberta Association of Registered Nurses Health Information: Nursing Components Working Session.* Alberta: AARN, 1993.

Alberta Association of Registered Nurses (AARN): *Client Status, Nursing Intervention and Client Outcome Taxonomies: A Background Paper.* Alberta: AARN, 1994.

Anderson BJ, Hannah KJ: A Canadian Nursing Minimum Data Set: A Major Priority. *Canadian Journal of Nursing Administration* 1993; 6: 7–13.

Bulechek GM, McCloskey JC: Nursing interventions: Taxonomy development. In: McCloskey JC, Grace HK, eds. *Current Issues in Nursing* (3rd ed.). St. Louis: Mosby, 1990; 23–28.

Canadian Nurses Association: *Papers from the Nursing Minimum Data Set Conference.* Ottawa: Author, 1993.

Canadian Nurses Association: *Report of the Resolutions Committee.* Unpublished report, June 1990.

Delaney C, Mehmert M, Prophet C, Crossley J: Establishment of the research value of nursing minimum data sets. In: Grobe SJ, Pluyter-Wenting ESP, eds. *Nursing Informatics: An International Overview for Nursing in a Technological Era.* Amsterdam: Elsevier, 1994; 169–173.

Foster J, Conrick M: Nursing minimum data sets: Historical perspective and Australian development. In: Grobe SJ, Pluyter-Wenting ESP, eds. *Nursing Informatics: An International Overview for Nursing in a Technological Era.* Amsterdam: Elsevier, 1994; 150–154.

Gallant BJ: Data requirements for the Nursing Minimum Data Set as seen by nurse administrators. In: Werley HH, Lang NM, eds. *Identification of the Nursing Minimum Data Set.* New York: Springer Publishing, 1988; 165–176.

Giovannetti P: Implications of Nursing Minimum Data Set. In: Hannah KJ, Reimer M, Mills WC, Letourneau S, eds. *Clinical Judgment and Decision Making: The Future of Nursing Diagnosis.* New York: John Wiley & Sons, 1987; 552–555.

Graves JR, Corcoran S: The study of nursing informatics. *Image: Journal of Nursing Scholarship* 1989; 21: 227–231.

Grobe SJ: Nursing intervention lexicon and taxonomy study: Language and classification methods. *Advances in Nursing Science* 1990; 13: 22–33.

Hannah KJ: The need for health data linkage hospital/institutional needs: A nursing statement. In: *Papers and Recommendations from the National Workshop on Health Care Data Linkage.* Don Mills, Ontario, Canada: Hospital Medical Records Institute, 1991; 17–18.

Hannah KJ, Anderson BJ: Management of Nursing Information. In: Kyle M, Hibberd J, eds. *Management for Nurses: A Canadian Perspective.* Toronto: W.B. Saunders, 1994; 516–533.

Hannah KJ, Ball MJ, Edwards MJ: *Introduction to Nursing Informatics.* New York: Springer-Verlag, 1994.

Jenny J: Classifying nursing diagnoses: A self care approach. *Nursing and Health Care* 1989; 10(2): 82–88.

Lang NM, Marek KD: The classification of patient outcomes. *Journal of Professional Nursing* 1990; 6: 158–163.

Marek K, Lang N: Nursing sensitive outcomes. In: Canadian Nurses Association (CNA), *Papers from the Nursing Minimum Data Set Conference.* Ontario: CNA, 1993; 100–120.

McCloskey JC: The Nursing Minimum Data Set: Benefits and implications for nurse educators. In: National League for Nursing, *Perspectives in Nursing 1987–1989.* New York: National League for Nursing, 1988; 119–126.

McCloskey JC, Bulechek GM: Standardizing the language for nursing treatments: An overview of the issues. *Nursing Outlook* 1994; 42(2): 56–63.

McCloskey JC, Bulechek GM, Cohen MZ, Craft MJ, Crossley JD, Denehy JA, Glick OJ, Kruckeberg T, Mass M, Prophet, CM, Tripp-Reimer T: Classifications of nursing interventions. *Journal of Professional Nursing* 1990; 6: 151–157.

McCormick KA, Lang N, Zielstorff R, Milholland DK, Saba V, Jacox A: Toward standard classification schemes for nursing language: Recommendations of the American Nurses Association Steering Committee on Databases to Support Clinical Nursing Practice. *Journal of the American Medical Informatics Association* 1994; 1(6): 421–427.

McGee M: Response to V. Saba's paper on Nursing Diagnostic Schemes. In: Canadian Nurses Association (CNA), *Papers from the Nursing Minimum Data Set Conference.* Ontario: CNA, 1993; 64–67.

McLane AM: Measurement and validation of diagnostic concepts: A decade of progress. *Heart & Lung* 1987; 16: 616–624.

McPhillips R: Essential elements for the Nursing Minimum Data Set as seen by federal officials. In: Werley HH, Lang NM, eds. *Identification of the Nursing Minimum Data Set.* New York: Springer Publishing, 1988; 233–238.

Mortensen R, Mantas J, Manuela M, Sermeus W, Nielson GH, McAvinue E: Telematics for health care in the European Union. In: Grobe SJ, Pluyter-Wenting ESP, eds. *Nursing Informatics: An International Overview for Nursing in a Technological Era.* Amsterdam: Elsevier, 1994; 750–752.

Mortensen RA: A common language for nursing practice: A persistent dilemma. *Varda Norde* 1993; 4: 18–24.

Murnaghan JH: Uniform basic data sets for health statistical systems. *International Journal of Epidemiology* 1978; 7: 263–269.

Murnaghan JH, White KL: Hospital discharge data: Report of the Conference on Hospital Discharge Abstracts Systems. *Medical Care* 1970; 8(Suppl.): 1–215.

North American Nursing Diagnosis Association: *North American Nursing Diagnosis Association: Taxonomy I: Revised 1989.* St. Louis: Author, 1989.

O'Brien-Pallas B, Giovannetti P: Nursing intensity. In: Canadian Nurses Association (CNA), *Papers from the Nursing Minimum Data Set Conference.* Ontario: CNA, 1993; 68–76.

Vanden Boer G, Sermeus W: Linkage of NMDS-information and patient classification systems. In: Grobe SJ, Pluyter-Wenting ESP, eds. *Nursing Informatics: An International Overview for Nursing in a Technological Era.* Amsterdam: Elsevier, 1994; 158–163.

Verney H: *Florence Nightingale at Harley Street.* London: Dent & Sons, 1970.

Werley HH: Introduction to the Nursing Minimum Data Set and its development. In: Werley HH, Lang NM, eds. *Identification of the Nursing Minimum Data Set.* New York: Springer Publishing, 1988; 1–15.

Werley HH, Lang NM: The consensually derived Nursing Minimum Data Set: Elements and definitions. In: Werley HH, Lang NM, eds. *Identification of the Nursing Minimum Data Set.* New York: Springer Publishing, 1988; 402–411.

Werley HH, Zorn CR: The Nursing Minimum Data Set: Benefits and implications. In: National League for Nursing, *Perspectives in Nursing 1987–1989.* New York: National League for Nursing, 1988; 105–114.

Werley HH, Devine EC, Zorn CR: Nursing needs its own minimum data set. *American Journal of Nursing* 1988; 88: 1651–1653.

Werley HH, Devine EC, Zorn CR, Ryan P, Westra BL: The Nursing Minimum Data Set: Abstraction tool for standardized, comparable, essential data. *American Journal of Public Health* 1991; 81: 421–426.

Zielstorff RD, Lang NM, Saba VK, McCormick KA, Milholland DK: Toward a uniform language for nursing in the U.S.: Work of the American Nurses Association Steering Committee on Databases to Support Clinical Practice. In: Greenes A, Peterson H, Protti D, eds. *Proceedings of MedInfo '95.* Edmonton: International Medical Informatics Association, 1995; in press.

13
Point-of-Care Information Systems: State of the Art

Shirley J. Hughes

Introduction

Requirements for patient care documentation and information access by healthcare professionals have changed dramatically over the past few years. The nursing professional has always needed to document care given and to review patient information to make care decisions; but in the current health-care environment, where inpatients are more acutely ill, staffing is minimized, and care is more integrated across disciplines and care settings, the documentation requirements are much more intense and the need to access meaningful information in a timely manner is much more urgent. As stated in the findings of the Institute of Medicine's study of the patient record, current patient records cannot adequately manage all the information needed for patient care. Future records must be computer based and used actively in the clinical process (Dick and Steen, 1991). In other words, to-day's healthcare environment demands that healthcare professionals have more and better automated information tools to provide quality patient care. These tools must be available and used as an integral part of the patient care setting, whether at the inpatient bedside, the physician's office, or the patient's home.

The technology, communications, and software challenges involved in providing computer-based patient records and useful automated information systems tools to healthcare professionals are not insignificant. A number of hospitals, healthcare professionals, and systems and technology vendors have invested a good deal of time and effort in developing, refining, and expanding on early product offerings. Although the technology is still evolving and the software solutions still growing in depth and breadth, there are a number of good systems that provide real benefits to clinicians today. These systems tend to be focused, at least initially, in specific care settings such as critical care, general medical surgical inpatient units, the physician's office, and home health care. Most, however, are based on technologies that support integration with other systems; some have already been net-worked with other products to provide an enterprise-wide information system solution; and others are being expanded to address the specialized needs of multiple care settings.

Productivity and Quality Improvements

Collecting and recording data about the health status of the patient and communicating that data to other healthcare professionals is one of the important roles played by the professional nurse on the healthcare team. The recording function, however, has historically been a time-consuming and paper-intensive task. Communication methods intended to convey accurate information to other healthcare professionals in a timely manner have not always been reliable. The nurse often spends significant time away from direct patient care simply trying to make sure the patient's needs are communicated and the orders carried out. Increasingly more healthcare enterprises are looking to point-of-care automation to simplify and make these functions much more effective and available across the continuum of care. Point-of-care systems are seen as a way to allow nurses to get back to direct patient care. The goals most often identified by those moving to point-of-care systems are as follows:

- To minimize the time spent in documenting patient information
- To eliminate redundancies and inaccuracies of charted information
- To improve the timeliness of data communication
- To optimize access to information
- To provide the information required by the clinician to make the best possible patient care decisions.

Capturing data at the source is the first step in minimizing time spent charting and in eliminating redundancies and inaccuracies. When a single data entry can be entered directly into the patient's electronic chart at the point of care, either by the clinician or via a medical device (i.e., hemodynamic monitors, infusion pumps, ventilators), and made immediately available (perhaps in multiple formats and automatically trended or compared with other data elements) to all others involved in that patient's care, then time is saved and data have been transformed accurately into useful information. With this type of functionality incorporated into point-of-care information systems, nursing productivity is maximized, data are more accurate, and information is more usable and accessible.

Productivity is also improved when access to patient information is made easy. With a point-of-care information system, there are, in effect, multiple copies of the patient's chart, one at every terminal. The nurse is no longer the "gatekeeper" of the chart and no longer needs to spend precious time tracking down and filing paper documents, phoning test results, and dealing with interruptions to convey information already documented. The nurse also has immediate access right at the point of care to information documented by others and needed for decision making.

Proper administration of treatments and medications requires that the care provider have complete and accurate information available at the point of care related to the physician's orders and to guidelines for carrying out complicated procedures. Additional assistance, such as dosage calculations and potential drug or allergy interactions, may be needed for medication administration. An automated point-of-care information system can provide this information to the clinician along with prompts to ensure that the proper schedule and/or sequence of events is followed. These types of features provide busy clinicians with valuable quality checks and balances— balances that not only result in higher quality patient care and improved patient satisfaction but also have the potential to lower risk and the costs of liability insurance.

Timely access to online reference databases, incorporation of standards of care and best practice protocols into the patient's care planning process, and use of standard terminologies and data storage techniques allowing for quality studies and research are all important quality enhancement capabilities that computers can offer the healthcare environment and that the paper approach of the past could never achieve. As data are gathered in real time at the point of care and stored in usable format in the computer-based patient record, not only is the patient's record more complete and accessible for those providing care but this wealth of data can be used by nursing researchers to help nurses learn how to do what they do better. Future patients will benefit, as will the nursing profession.

User friendliness and ease of data entry are especially important concepts when applied to point-of-care systems. At the point of care, the clinician's primary focus must be on the patient, not on the computer system. An automated point-of-care system requiring more documentation or time than a manual system will not enhance the time spent with the patient, only the time spent in the patient's room. The most effective point-of-care information system is intuitive to the clinician, requires minimal time to use, and presents a minimal amount of intrusion into the patient environment. Neither the patient nor the clinician should be inconvenienced. They should instead perceive the system to be beneficial to the care process.

Hardware

The hardware solutions used for point-of-care information systems have varied greatly. This variety has a good deal to do with the specific needs of the care settings (i.e., critical care, home health) but probably more to do with the uncertain and evolutionary state of technology. Most would agree that a portable, real-time communication device with multiple reliable input technologies (i.e., touch, pen, voice), the ability to display all of the patient information needed, the appropriate graphics and trending capabilities, a quick and easy documentation method, battery power to last at least 16 hours, and batteries that fit easily into the pocket would be ideal for most care settings and clinical users. Technology is moving very fast and we will no doubt be using this device one day, but it is not easy to find all of these features in one terminal suitable for all care settings today. We see, instead, mostly full-sized personal computers (PCs) and workstations, some laptop computers, and a variety of portable terminals, most in the developmental stages of use. Besides the standard keyboard data entry, most of these systems offer some sort of pointing devices and some offer touch screens.

Portable interactive terminals can give the nursing professional the best of all possible worlds, especially for the inpatient medical/surgical and home health environments. Portable devices with quick and easy data entry capabilities, such as bar code readers, pens, and touch screens, can be very user friendly and not at all intrusive in the patient environment (Fig. 13-1). Portability truly allows the nurse to remain at the point of care and still access the computer-based chart. There may be disadvantages to this approach if the portable devices prove to be too heavy, cumbersome, or restrictive in function for the nurse to use them easily.

The wireless communications technologies required for real-time interaction between the portable point-of-care terminal and the computer-based patient chart are available today and being used reliably in healthcare environments. For less intensive care (i.e., home health), downloading of

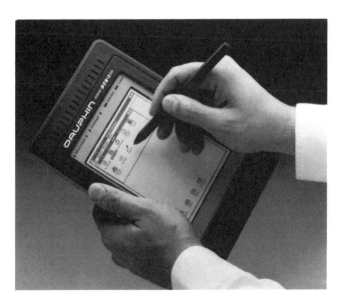

FIGURE 13-1. Portable terminal with pen technology for use with point-of-care systems. Reprinted with permission of Dauphin Technology, Inc.

patient records into a portable terminal for reference by the caregiver and then periodic updates back to the central computer database via modem is an alternative communication strategy that seems to be working well.

It is evident that there will be many new hardware and technology options available for use with point-of-care systems in the future. Most vendors offering clinical applications have announced a portable terminal option, either available now or in the future (Andrew, 1994). It is very probable (and for good reason) that a combination of terminal solutions will be used with point-of-care systems. These different approaches may be important for the differing care settings, and even for different caregivers (i.e., physicians and nurses).

Moving the HIS to the Point of Care

A common first step toward bedside information solutions in the acute care medical/surgical setting has been to move to the bedside the standard CRT or PC used at the nursing station to access the hospital's Hospital Information System (HIS). This is the most expedient approach, for it provides at the bedside the same functionality that nursing is accustomed to at the nursing station and involves minimal development effort and no additional user training. A centralized database is a key advantage with this approach. Data are available to all members of the healthcare team from any terminal location in the hospital.

There are, however, some disadvantages. The patient environment is invaded by a high-tech but not necessarily high-touch solution. The software solution developed for use at the nursing station is not necessarily the quick and easy tool needed for the point of care. Some of the features required at the point of care that may not be included in a system designed for the nursing station include security, confidentiality, quick data entry techniques, specific functions such as validation of therapies, and expeditious retrieval of critical patient information. There are also the physical problems associated with placing a full-sized terminal into an already crowded patient care area. Both space and location are significant considerations. Since the terminal is a stationary device, no matter where it is located the nurse must leave the patient to go to the terminal to look up or to chart information at least some of the time. The humming noise usually associated with CRTs and PCs may not be noticeable at a busy nursing station but can be very irritating to a sick patient. In addition, the costs of wiring each patient room should not be overlooked.

From a systems viewpoint, there is also the danger that the HIS expanded to the bedside without sufficient design enhancements may not be able to accommodate the additional workload and expanded numbers of simultaneous users. The result may be an irritatingly slow system response time to the clinician at the point of care.

In some cases, the HIS vendors have offered new terminals specially designed for use at the bedside. These special terminals and some modification of the user screens can satisfy physical space limitations and provide for quick and easy data entry. With special function keys and specially designed menu selection screens for which minimal typing is required, the task of documentation can be made more efficient. This will accomplish the goal of saving time and, if not too limiting in its functionality, maintain the completeness of the information.

The commercially available SMS System is an example of an HIS for which the functionality has been moved to the bedside with specially designed stationary terminals or standard PCs used. Nursing documentation is supported as well as data review and all HIS functionality.

The TDS System, an HIS well known for its clinical applications, uses standard PCs with light pens as pointing devices. Some hospitals have moved the TDS System terminals to the bedside or at least distributed them around the nursing units and therefore made them more accessible to clinicians from the point of care.

The Ulticare System offered by Health Data Sciences includes a full HIS software system designed specifically for use at the bedside. It uses a standard fully functional CRT in the patient room. Nurses may sit or stand at the terminal, which is mounted on a hydraulic lift in an alcove, in or near the room, or placed on a cart.

Point-of-Care Systems on Medical/Surgical Units

Systems designed specifically for use in the medical/surgical inpatient setting at the point of care generally are more focused on quickly capturing information normally jotted down by the nurse on the paper worksheet. Reminders of treatments and medications to be administered are provided to the nurse by the automated system. Validation of these therapies and/or warnings of potential error conditions are highlighted. Data access shortcuts are provided to facilitate quick access to critical information. Although these systems are designed specifically for the bedside, charting and data review may also be done at central locations, often using standard terminals or PCs. These systems are typically also tied into the HIS so that the need for data accessibility throughout the hospital is satisfied.

CliniCom's CliniCare System is an example of this type of system. It uses a portable touch screen terminal with backlighting in the patient room that includes a bar code reader (Fig. 13-2). The portable terminal rests in a recharger unit mounted on the wall in the patient's room when not in use. The portable terminal communicates in real time to a central database via radio frequency technology. A standard CRT or PC may be used at central locations. The CliniCare applications are focused primarily at this time on

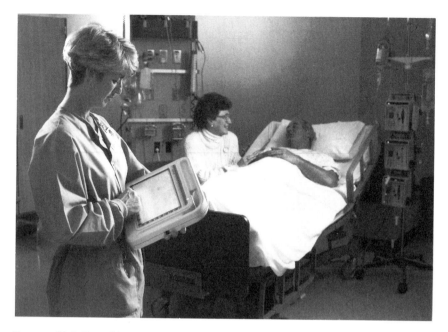

FIGURE 13-2. Portable terminal used in an inpatient room. Reprinted with permission of CliniCom Inc.

documentation of care and retrieval of patient information. This system can be interfaced to the hospital's HIS for access to results and orders.

The Medtake System by Micro Health Systems, Inc. uses a specially designed stationary terminal at the point of care. A small footprint terminal with function keys and a numeric keypad replace the complex keyboard of most CRTs. Menu-driven screens are used extensively. This system provides the nursing documentation functions at the bedside and communicates this information to a PC located at the nursing station. Additional information can be added to the charting at the nursing station, and chart documents can be printed.

Point-of-Care Systems in Critical Care

Point-of-care information systems designed specifically for use in critical care settings have, for the most part, used PCs or workstation devices at the point of care. These systems are designed to manage and display large amounts of data on critically ill patients and interface to medical devices to collect data automatically. The user interface is most often flowsheet oriented and provides numerous graphical and data trending capabilities. Many of these systems use distributed architectures with perhaps multiple servers and redundant processors to ensure maximum system availability and quick response times for the users. They are normally interfaced to the hospital's HIS and laboratory systems to gather test results and provide access to orders.

The EMTEK System 2000, an example of this type of system, has a fully distributed database and uses networked workstations to capture and present flowsheet information at the point of care. Graphics are used to display information and to aid in documenting observations and care (Fig. 13-3). The Hewlett Packard System, CareVue 9000, the CliniComp Clinical Information System, and the Quantitative Sentinel System offered by QMI are other examples of critical care systems.

The aforementioned critical care systems are beginning to be expanded to support additional inpatient areas, such as the general medical/surgical units, the operating rooms, and postanesthesia recovery areas. Some of the systems described as addressing the medical/surgical areas are also expanding to address the needs of the critical care areas. The clinical users and information systems support staffs often prefer a single vendor solution for all point-of-care needs within the same institution. These vendors will no doubt continue to expand their applications to address additional inpatient settings in an attempt to offer that single solution.

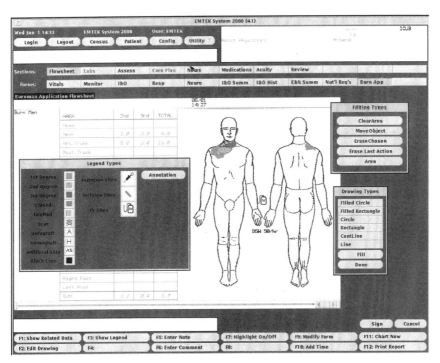

FIGURE 13-3. Use of graphics in critical care systems. Reprinted with permission of EMTEK Health Care Systems, Inc.

Point-of-Care Systems in the Physician's Office

Point-of-care systems in the physician's office are new and not widespread. There are, however, some good examples of comprehensive applications offering a completely computerized patient record. Easy-to-use applications provide nurses and doctors with templates and standard terminologies to facilitate documentation of history and physical examinations, observations, orders, and prescriptions. The availability of an online view of all of the patient's visits and phone contacts, instructions given, and reminders for follow-ups and immunizations is a major improvement in these care settings. The office triage nurse is much better prepared to make decisions and provide advice to patients with a point-of-care system that provides immediate access to the patient's complete online record.

For example, the Epic Systems Corporation's EpicCare Electronic Medical Records System is used in a number of clinics and networked physician office environments. A PC is located in each examining room and physician office and at other central areas within the clinic. All are networked to a central database, where the electronic patient record is stored. No matter which physician or nurse the patient sees, the same record is accessed and updated. The system offers a friendly graphical user interface designed specifically for clinicians and has, therefore, been readily accepted by most. Clinics have seen improved efficiency and believe the quality of care delivered has also improved.

Point-of-Care Systems in Home Health

The information challenges facing home health professionals, who often spend most, if not all, of their time working remotely (perhaps going into the office only once a week, and in rural settings maybe not even that often), include administering care without ready access to the patient record (it is usually several miles away at the central office), spending hours catching up on the growing documentation requirements (often long after the patient care is delivered), and attempting to keep the billing records up to date and accurate. Again, the nurse is spending valuable time tending to information management problems instead of providing patient care. Point-of-care systems based on a central database and portable terminals have been proven to enhance greatly the efficiency of the home healthcare provider and improve the timeliness and accuracy of the patient and billing information documented. With the patient record readily available, the appropriate care can be delivered and more informed patient care decisions made.

Patient Care Technologies, Inc. (PtCT) is an example of a point-of-care system developed for home health care. It uses a small portable terminal that weighs less than 1 pound, with applications specifically designed to support home health documentation requirements and patient chart review (Fig. 13-4). The data are stored in the portable terminal and then transferred periodically by the users to the central database via phone modem.

Summary

Point-of-care information processing is not a new requirement, but a long-established one to which new technologies are now being applied. The major features included in successful systems are fast and easy data entry, data accessibility across care settings, quality checks for accuracy of patient care, and, most importantly, nurse and patient friendliness. Computerized point-of-care information systems are still relatively new to health care. The healthcare institutions that use these systems have, however, shown that point-of-care systems can provide significant quality and productivity improvements for nursing. Systems that enhance the safety of patients and

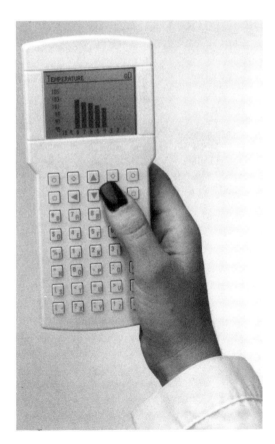

FIGURE 13-4. Portable terminal for home health care application. Reprinted with permission of Patient Care Technologies, Inc.

increase the efficiency of nurses can be cost effective in today's healthcare environment (Ball, Douglas, O'Desky, and Albright, 1991).

The databases of patient records resulting from point-of-care documentation provide a means for nurses to study processes and outcomes and learn more effective ways of caring for patients and promoting wellness. Over the next several years, as the various point-of-care approaches and technologies in use today evolve, as new technologies are introduced, and as the computer-based patient record is established, nurses will find many opportunities to participate in and benefit from these systems. The challenge will be in effectively packaging the technology, clinical applications, and information management and storage capabilities into usable and reliable tools that are readily adopted by clinicians in patient care settings.

Questions

1. List the benefits of a point-of-care information system for nursing.
2. What benefits specifically are realized by capturing data at the source?
3. List three quality features typically provided by point-of-care systems.
4. Describe the pros and cons of stationary versus portable terminals for point-of-care systems.
5. What considerations do you feel are important for the patient environment when considering a point-of-care information system?

References

Andrew WF: Point-of-care systems review. *Healthcare Informatics* 1994; 11: 33–48.
Ball MJ, Douglas JV, O'Desky RI, Albright JW: *Healthcare Information Management Systems: A Practical Guide.* New York: Springer-Verlag, 1991.
Dick RS, Steen EB, eds.: *The Computer-Based Patient Record: An Essential Technology for Health Care.* Washington, DC: National Academy Press, 1991.

14
Information Management in Home Care

MARGARET M. HASSETT AND MARJORIE H. FARVER

Introduction

Nurses are experiencing patient care situations in the home setting that, until recently, would only have occurred in an acute care setting. While new medical skills and technologies have made it possible for patients to recuperate faster and for surgery to be less traumatic, cost containment, diagnostic related groupings (DRGs) with the associated decreased length of hospital stay, consumer preference, and healthcare reform are supporting the move toward patient care at home. Information technology can provide the home healthcare professional with data at the point of care in a format that improves home care practice, creates clinical documentation, and generates data for payroll and billing.

History and Growing Pains

Home health care, while being the oldest type of healthcare delivery, has been a small segment of the healthcare delivery system in the United States throughout the nineteenth century and most of the twentieth century. The beginning of home health's exponential growth dates from 1966, with Medicare and Medicaid reimbursable home care benefits. The second significant growth period occurred after 1983, when Medicare implemented prospective payment, DRGs, leading to a significant decrease in hospital length of stay. The number of home health agencies has grown from 1700 home health agencies in 1967 to 10,000 agencies in 1992 (Harris, 1988; Klein, 1993; National Association for Home Care's Information Resources and Quality Assurance Committee, 1994). Home health care has now become an integral component of between 8 and 15% of hospitalizations (Klein, 1993) and is recognized as an essential intervention in most critical pathways of coordinated care. Acute care facilities, rehabilitation centers, and other providers have developed pathways that include home healthcare services.

HCFA Definition of Home Health Care

Home health care, as defined by the Health Care Financing Administration (HCFA), includes skilled nursing, physical therapy, occupational therapy, speech therapy, medical social work, and home health aide services. The goals of home care are restorative; to increase self-care knowledge and ability and improve function. Home health agency services are highly regulated. The *Federal Conditions of Participation* dictate that a patient must be home-bound and require skilled professional services (not custodial) under a physician's direction, services must be intermittent, and a caregiver must be available. Ancillary services, although not as heavily regulated, are also important in the total care of a patient at home. These services include respiratory and durable medical equipment, infusion and pharmacy, and hospice.

Inaccessibility of Information in Home Care

The home care provider and hospital professional require similar information to deliver the necessary patient care. Both practitioners require patient demographic data, past medical history, diagnoses, laboratory and x-ray test results, and a treatment plan. In addition, patient teaching materials, policies and procedures, drug and treatment information, technical data, available community services, and updated phone lists facilitate the delivery of patient care either at home or in the acute care setting.

The point of care in home care is the patient's home. However, the patient's medical record, policies and procedure books, teaching materials, and clinical reference books are inaccessible because they are kept at the agency office. The practitioner, who is already carrying assessment equipment, dressing supplies, infection control supplies, and other equipment, must also carry information. Condensed drug and treatment references, copies of the patient's medical record, new procedure documentation, and patient teaching materials are taken on home visits.

Another missing link in home care, traditional in the hospital setting, is collaboration with peers during the delivery of patient care. Case management conferences are necessary to ensure continuity of care between professional disciplines in home care. Scheduling these conferences is often difficult due to variations in working hours and dependence on staff who work for more than one agency.

Documentation in Home Care

Quality documentation is vital in the billing process for home care services. However, the documentation of the patient visit is traditionally accomplished in the home, car, or other convenient location, challenging the practitioner to deliver the patient documentation to the agency office in a timely fashion.

The financial burden of Medicare's documentation requirements has a significant impact on a home care agency's costs. The HCFA 485 forms impose a great burden on most home health agencies. Excess Medicare documentation wastes 25 to 33% of a home health nurse's time (Hoyer, 1990). Previsit and postvisit preparation time exceed the time spent in the home with the patient, with up to 50% of the nurse's total time spent on paperwork. Documentation required for Medicare (compared to non-Medicare) home care visits requires eight minutes more per visit, or a 36% increase in time expenditure (Storfjel, 1989).

Technology

Clinical Technology in Home Care

Clinical technology has changed home care practice, just as it has changed hospital practice. Management of intravenous (IV) therapy, chemotherapy, pain management, enteral and parenteral nutrition, and ventilator dependence are therapies delivered in the home on a regular basis. The equipment and technology are portable, simple to use, and reliable. Teaching and support are given by an intermittent visiting professional. Emergency service is always available, enabling the patient or a caregiver to participate in therapies formerly delivered in an intensive care unit of the hospital.

Telecommunications

During the early 1990s, a home care professional gained access to improved communication with supervisors in the main office through display beepers and car phones. Today, portable computers, notebooks, or handheld devices continue to improve this communication. Telecommunication to the agency database gives clinicians current information concerning new admissions or emergency visits. This eliminates a visit to the home office or jotting information on a scrap of paper during a telephone call. Complete, accurate demographic and clinical information can be telecommunicated to a portable computer.

The home health professional's day starts with a download of patient information from the agency's main office into a portable computer via a telephone line. The information provided informs the practitioner not only of daily assignments, previous assessments, actions, and plans prescribed by other professionals involved in a patient's care but also of office communication regarding meetings and in-services. In addition to patient care information, the portable computer contains the agency's policy and procedure manual, a database with medication teaching materials, and a program to analyze electronically the home care patient's medication profile for drug interactions.

Portable computer systems are enhancing both the collection and communication of data and information gathered in the practice area. Telecommunications is a form of communication and information technology that is developing rapidly and can facilitate home healthcare practice using a computer and modem. Communication is accomplished regardless of location or time of day.

Electronic mail (E-mail) enhances the communication abilities of the home care professional by providing notices, messages, announcements, changes in policies or procedures, and other information to the home health agency workers. Home health professionals are able to send messages regarding patient treatment plans, case management issues, agency expectations, and case review comments.

Electronic bulletin board systems (BBSs), which function in a similar fashion to a wall corkboard, provide a means by which both practitioners and patients can post and respond to notices. These communications are important resources for healthcare professionals. The BBS provides a means of communication with experts in the field. New developments can be compared and problems and care situations discussed as well. This reduces the isolation felt by a home health professional by promoting peer collaboration.

Patients are also beginning to use this medium by participating in electronic support groups (ESGs). These groups are an outgrowth of the BBS and are providing participants with an electronic means to obtain the information and support they may need to stay in the home (Sparks, 1992). Unlike face-to-face communications, ESGs are

1. Available for access on a 24-hour basis
2. Accessible by the visually or physically handicapped
3. Able to link participants locally and worldwide
4. Anonymous and private.

Computerlink is a project in Cleveland that has been helping Alzheimer or AIDS patients cope by linking them with caregivers in an electronic support group. It has been found that the network provides the participants with information, decision support, and communication abilities not previously available to them. It is operated by Case Western Reserve University and runs with the Cleveland Free-Net, a public access computer network in operation since 1988 (Brennan, Ripich, and Moore, 1991).

Computer Networks

Telecommunications technology makes a wide area network (WAN) a practical choice for large metropolitan area agencies. A single patient information database can service a large geographical area or provider network. Information is available to a nurse on call, regardless of the location of the nurse, branch office, or patient. Operational costs are reduced since one or two nurses can cover a large area for after-hours telephone support.

One such application of this technology is used by the Visiting Nurse Association of Washington, DC and suburban Maryland (VNA of DC). The VNA of DC runs on a LAN/WAN (local area network/wide area network) with six sites tied together by FNS circuits[1] and T1 links. Five file servers and an IBM AS/400 are used in this network to provide

1. Clinical and scheduling modules run under Novell NetWare
2. A gateway to file servers and the AS/400 for the E-mail connection to other corporation hospitals and facilities in the Washington area
3. Network printers at each site
4. Updating of data on the AS/400 and clinical databases nightly after data are sent in by modem from clinical staff
5. A bank of five computer motherboards with 28,800-bps modems to allow modem access for the clinical staff to upload visits and communicate on a daily basis.

The IBM AS/400 manages billing and payroll functions while producing statistical information necessary for the management of the home health agency. Clinical field staff dial in to the data center to upload the day's activities at the end of day. Billing and payroll information is transferred to the AS/400, and the remainder of the clinical visit information is transferred to the Novell NetWare file server. Data entry is nearly nonexistent with full computerization; payroll, billing, and clinical information are transferred electronically.

Rural home care agencies with branch offices that are widely distributed across counties or states use a LAN in each branch for the collection and aggregation of clinical, statistical, and billing information. The VNA of Butler, Pennsylvania, operates its seven offices on such LANs. The benefits they have realized are

1. Reduction in number of offices maintained
2. Reduction in operating costs
3. Better access to information for clinical staff
4. Reduction in staff meetings (biweekly or weekly).

Referral information, payroll, billing, and statistical information are entered on the IBM AS/400 during the day and updated on a nightly basis. Clinical information uploaded from the practitioners' portable computers generates verbal interim physician orders and recertifications (HCFA 485), integrated clinical care plans, medication profiles with written teaching instructions to be given to the patient on the next visit, physical assessments,

[1]FNS (FDDI network services); FDDI (fiber data distribution interface, ANSI defined standard specification 100 megabits per second token passing network).

visit records, interdisciplinary case conferences, and E-mail to the supervisor or peer, which optionally can be attached to a patient's medical record.

Scheduling Software

Home health scheduling software is used to schedule the hourly work of home health aides, nurses, and visiting staff. A Windows™ environment enables the scheduler to work on the schedule of several patients and employees at one time. Preferences, service requests, and time frames are set up in the database in conjunction with the geographical location of the care provider and the patient. Another benefit of the scheduling software is that upon verification of scheduled activities, payroll and billing information is generated, minimizing or eliminating manual data entry.

Data Storage and Structures

Databases represent electronic storage of gathered data. Data must be stored, formatted, and easily retrievable to be transformed into useful information. Information provides management and clinicians with knowledge, insight, and power in decision making, problem solving, and planning. The practitioner can better control and influence the care of the patient regardless of the patient's and practitioner's locations. The practitioner requires three kinds of data: patient-specific data such as treatment plans prescribed and the patient's progress; agency-specific data on types and locations of patients serviced and the length of service necessary for a specific diagnosis; and domain-specific data such as patient outcomes related to specific nursing interventions over time (Zielstorff, Hudgings, and Grobe, 1993).

For data to be collected in a database, structured languages must be developed to facilitate the formatting of the nursing information for entry into a database. The American Nurses Association has established a steering committee that is addressing the issue of selecting and supporting the development of such languages enabling the inclusion of nursing data in various databases. Refer to the McCormick chapter in this book (Chapter 11) for more information on the steering committee.

Finally, the continued development of computer interfaces will provide for linking different databases, such as the home health agency patient database and the hospital patient database. This will enable a seamless electronic discharge from the hospital and admission to home healthcare service.

Nursing Minimum Data Set

The nursing minimum data set (NMDS), developed by Dr. Harriet Werley and Dr. Norma Lang, represents a basic or minimum set of data elements that can meet the different information needs of nurses and illustrate the nursing practice across time, settings, and populations. Sixteen data elements comprise the NMDS. The elements are categorized as nursing care elements, patient demographic elements, and service elements (Table 14-1). These elements form the basis for aggregating data to allow for the description of a population's health status and investigation of nursing diagnosis, interventions, outcomes, and cost (Werley and Lang, 1988).

National Association for Home Care

The National Association for Home Care (NAHC) has recognized the need for home health to develop a structured language and has formed an Information Resources and Quality Assurance Committee with a similar goal of defining a home care minimum data set

1. To establish comparability of data across agencies, geographic regions, and time
2. To describe home and hospice care
3. To allow for more reliable research findings
4. To provide data to facilitate and influence health policy decisions.

The preliminary results of the committee's work on a home care and hospice minimum data set categorize data by the organizational level and the individual patient/client level (Table 14-2).

North American Nursing Diagnosis Association

The North American Nursing Diagnosis Association (NANDA) focuses on developing and testing nursing diagnoses. The nursing diagnosis is a statement describing a patient's response to an actual or potential health problem reflecting the clinical judgment gained through systematic data collection and analysis. The diagnosis is the basis for determining nursing

TABLE 14-1. Nursing Minimum Data Set Elements

Nursing Elements	Patient Demographic Elements	Service Elements
Nursing diagnosis	Personal identification	Unique facility or service agency number
Nursing intervention	Date of birth	Unique patient health record number
Nursing outcome	Sex	Unique number of principal RN
Intensity of nursing care	Race and ethnicity	Episode admission or encounter date
	Residence	Discharge or termination date
		Disposition of patient
		Expected payor for most of bill

162   Margaret M. Hassett and Marjorie H. Farver

TABLE 14-2. Draft Uniform Data Set for Home Care and Hospice

Organizational Level			
Organization/ Services	Utilization	Financial	Personnel
Type of home care programs	Unduplicated patient census	Gross revenue	Number of employees
Ownership of organization	Duplicated patient census	Net revenue	Number of independent contractors
Control of organization	Number of nonadmissions	Other revenue	Number of subcontract workers
Controlling organization		Bad debt expense	Number of volunteers
Profit status		Charity care	
Number of branches		Total payroll costs	
Services		Benefits and payroll tax expense	
Programs		Total expense	
Certification		Annual capital expenditures	
Licensure		Gross accounts receivable	
Accreditation		Net accounts receivable	
Service area		Days sales outstanding	
		Operating income	
		Cost per unit of service	
		Charge	

Individual Level: Patient/Client Data			
Demographic Items	Clinical Items	Service/Utilization Items	Defer for Further Study
Personal identification	Medical diagnoses	Provider identification	Functional status
Date of birth	Surgical diagnoses	Admission date	Nursing diagnosis/ patient problem
Race		Discharge date	Patient classification
Ethnicity		Episode of care	Intervention
Sex		Length of stay	Outcome
Location of residence		Number of hospital admissions	Discharge status
Type of residence		Discharge reason	
Living arrangements		Discharge disposition	
Caregiver availability		Expected payor	
Caregiver		Unit of service-visit	
Preadmission location		Unit of service-hour	
		Units of service per discipline	
		Number of days per level of hospice care	

treatment. Diagnoses accepted by this group are considered useful for practice and research in a variety of settings (Milholland, 1992).

Omaha

The Omaha System offers a model for classifying client data in the home care setting. It supports the database design by providing home health practitioners with an efficient, research-based, reliable, and valid method for capturing, sorting, and analyzing data collected by the home care providers. The three components of the Omaha System are

1. The problem classification scheme
2. The intervention scheme
3. The problem rating scheme.

These schemes are all computer compatible and therefore promote the transformation of data into information via databases and automation (Martin and Scheet, 1992).

Home Health Classification Method (Saba)

The Home Health Classification Method (HHCM) is designed by Saba (1994) to predict home care needs and resource use for the Medicare population. Four sets of nursing parameters categorized by 20 healthcare components are used not only to assess but also to code and classify care. Care is determined by classifying healthcare needs, nursing diagnosis, and interventions. Resource use is predicted considering providers such as speech therapists, nurses, occupational therapists, and social workers. Finally, the medical assessment parameters and sociodemographic data elements are correlated with the clinical nursing parameters. The structure of classification systems has facilitated the recording of the clinical process throughout an entire episode of home health care by incorporating critical care maps (Saba, 1994).

Nursing Interventions Classification

Nursing Interventions Classification (NIC) is the result of work begun at the University of Iowa in 1982 by Bulechek and McCloskey and continued by a large research team. The purpose of the project was to define and relate nursing interventions. The result is a list of 336 intervention labels, each with a set of nurse activities (McCloskey and Bulechek, 1992).

The VNA of DC is using the NIC in care plans and as library text available for selection by nurses documenting home visits on portable computers. In time, this will give validity to clinical data and will be a resource for retrospective research.

Implementation Planning

Analysis of the present information flow (paper or existing computer system) should focus on identifying priorities and redundancies within the work flow. A result of the analysis may be reengineering of the organization. If reengineering is indicated, it should be completed prior to implementation to reduce the amount of stress in the organization and achieve stability in paperflow systems (Hammer and Champy, 1993).

Adequate resources, especially personnel, must be assigned to the computer implementation process to assure success. Temporary workers may be required to perform the existing work in the agency while agency employees learn the new system.

Clinical Field Staff Implementation and Training

The most efficient and effective method for training is a phase-in approach utilizing super users from within the organization. Super users can be supervisors, team leaders, well-placed staff, or clinicians. The program includes training the super users initially, enabling them to train other staff later. By scheduling the training for various times during a week and over a several-week period, clinical staff (employees, nurses, therapists, and social workers) are able to complete 40 hours of training and achieve a goal of computer literacy while continuing with their patient visits.

This type of training schedule has been used successfully by the VNA of DC; VNA of Butler, Pennsylvania; VNA of Southwestern Missouri; and VNA of Boulder, Colorado.

Administrative Implementation

A clinical system that drives the financial modules is ideal, especially in home health. When data are transferred electronically from the clinician's computer to the home health agency system, timeliness and accuracy are no longer problems. Automation represents a significant capital expense. However, the clinical and financial records are relatively inexpensive to maintain as compared to the staff needed to create and maintain clinical and financial records manually. A wide range of quality assurance (QA) reports is possible. Clinical or financial reports can be designed based on QA indicators, and the clinical and financial information can be linked.

Electronic claims can be processed for half the cost of paper claims. Electronic billing is required by Medicare. This is far less expensive for the government as well as for the home health agency. Medicaid and commercial insurance companies can be billed electronically as well. Days outstanding for accounts receivable should be reduced with the speed and efficiency

TABLE 14-3. Effect of Electronic Billing on Days Outstanding

	Agency 1	Agency 2
Electronically billing	85%	70%
Hand-billing	00%	30%
Computer-printed bills	15%	00%
Number of billing staff	1	10
A/R days outstanding	45	80
Annual visit count	113,500	170,000

A/R = accounts receivable.

of electronic billing. A comparison of two agencies shows the effect of electronic billing on the days outstanding (Table 14-3).

Conclusion

Health care is becoming increasingly competitive. Automation is the marketing edge that home health agencies will need to survive. The benefits of an integrated home health system include complete timely clinical documentation and improved patient care due to having resources available at the point of care in the home. Employee satisfaction and retention are enhanced due to ease of documentation and communication. Physician satisfaction is enhanced due to improved communication and better patient outcomes. Management and quality assurance flexible reports are readily available. Financial impacts include increased reimbursement due to quality and timeliness of clinical documentation, reduced accounts receivable due to electronic billing and payment, and decreased overhead due to the need for fewer branch offices.

Questions

1. Discuss the problems of not being able to access information on a home care visit. How can information technology be used to help solve these problems?
2. How do you envision patients and their families being able to use technology in the home for patient care?
3. What are the types of software packages that may help store data in the home health environment?
4. Discuss the nursing minimum data set (NMDS) as a model for collection of data in the home care environment. What inroads have been made to categorize data in home health care?
5. Discuss some of the implementation planning suggestions that were presented in this chapter. Would they work in your environment?

References

Brennan PF, Ripich S, Moore S: The use of home based computers to support persons living with AIDS/ARC. *Journal of Community Health Nursing* 1991; 8(1): 3–14.

Hammer M, Champy J: *Reengineering the Corporation: A Manifesto for Business Revolution.* New York: HarperBusiness, 1993.

Harris MD: *Home Health Administration.* Owings Mills, MD: National Health Publishing, 1988.

Hoyer RG: Coming to grips with the paperwork burden. *CARING* 1990; 9: 36–40.

Klein E: Automating technology's impact on home healthcare providers. *Healthcare Informatics* 1993; 8: 22–28.

Martin KS, Scheet NJ: *The Omaha System: Applications for Community Health Nursing.* Philadelphia: W. B. Saunders, 1992.

McCloskey JC, Bulechek GM: *Nursing Interventions Classification.* St. Louis, MO: Mosby, 1992.

Milholland DK: Naming what we do: Nursing vocabularies and databases. *Journal of AHMIA* 1992; 63(10): 58–61.

National Association for Home Care's Information Resources and Quality Assurance Committee: Draft uniform data set for home care and hospice. *CARING* 1994; 13(6): 10, 11, 69–75.

Saba VK: A home health classification method. In: Grobe SJ, Pluyter-Wenting ESP, eds. *Nursing Informatics: An International Overview for Nursing in a Technological Era.* Amsterdam: Elsevier, 1994; 697–701.

Sparks S: Exploring electronic support groups. *American Journal of Nursing* 1992; 12: 62–65.

Storfjel JL: Home care productivity: Is the home visit an adequate measure? *CARING* 1989; 8(9): 60–65.

Werley HH, Lang NM: *Identification of the Nursing Minimum Data Set.* New York: Springer Publishing, 1988.

Zielstorff RD, Hudgings CI, Grobe SJ: *Next-Generation Nursing Information Systems.* Washington, DC: American Nurses Publishing, 1993.

15
The Automation of Critical Path/CareMap® Systems

Kathleen M. Andolina

Care delivery is moving beyond that defined by strict boundaries of geography, tradition, and discipline and into multidisciplinary, collaborative relationships with a focus on coordinated, patient-centered care. In fact, managed care coordinated by clinician providers represents the latest advance in care delivery. Provider-controlled managed care means that clinicians have accountability and authority for achieving both cost and quality outcomes for the patient populations they serve directly. This is illustrated by the leadership roles that nurses and physicians find themselves in as caregivers or as managers of projects that impact on such populations as cardiac surgical, orthopedic, and frail elderly.

The cost and quality outcomes of care, as indicated in Table 15-1, require that clinicians have access to better information systems, restructured job descriptions, and creative management tools, such as critical path and CareMap® tools (CareMap® is a trademark and concept of The Center for Case Management, South Natick, Massachusetts) that support collaborative, coordinated practices. Provider-controlled managed care is a new and exciting evolution for healthcare practices.

The effect has been synergistic, producing care outcomes that are realistic in terms of patient and family needs, more predictable, and, in many instances, better than if care had been conducted in its usual manner. When care is managed, outcomes are defined for the average population, accountability is clarified, and care is individualized according to patient needs. The new emphasis on collaborative, coordinated care systems comes at a time when technological capability is catching up with the demand for automated information systems (ISs). Automation is required for provider-controlled managed care systems for numerous reasons:

1. To foster collaboration, communication, and collaboration among care providers on a team
2. To track resource use

TABLE 15-1. Provider-Controlled Managed Care Focuses on Both Cost and Quality Outcomes

Cost Outcomes	Quality Outcomes
• LOS within norm • Resource use stable • Process inefficiencies reduced • Extended stays in expensive care areas avoided • Complications, accidents avoided or minimized • Ineffective treatments avoided • Restrictive, outdated regs eliminated • Complex psychosocial needs anticipated • Treatment at least cost to individual and society	• Prevention via early detection, intervention • Access to services, providers • Stabilization, improvement • Minimize or reduce effects of complications • Pt/Fam representation, inclusion, informed along the way, participates in care, goal planning • Treated in the appropriate time • Least Restrictive Alternative • Effective Self-Management/ Supervision • No injury, incidents

Reprinted with permission from The Center for Case Management. Copyright, The Center for Case Management

3. To measure care results in terms of effectiveness, efficiency, and appropriateness
4. To allow caregivers to monitor the present patient/family status as compared to a predicted status for an average population
5. To keep documentation fast, relevant, and focused on what is important
6. To use single-entry data in multiple ways
7. To retrieve data for retrospective quality improvement
8. To give case managers and others the overall plan.

More then ever, the possibility for an automated solution for thorny, persistent problems in managing and documenting care is nearing. With the confluence of managed care pressures, technology capability, and increased demand from clinicians, the question is not if to automate, but when to do so.

Despite the progress, however, a single, fully integrated automated product will continue to elude organizations looking for an immediate strategy. This preautomation period is experienced as both a chaotic and invigorating time for health care. It is a time when new relationships between people and technology continue to emerge, producing different methods of healthcare delivery in their wake and at the same time improving healthcare outcomes by getting focused information to the caregivers at the right time.

Examples of this are evident in the numerous critical path/CareMap® initiatives implemented throughout the world. Yet to appreciate where automated information systems will fit or what they will support, the connection between technology and outcomes-based practice must be described.

Outcomes-Based Practice

Outcomes-based practice is a multidisciplinary practice method that supports achievement of both cost and quality outcomes with the patient and family as the unifying concern. It includes collaborative practice behaviors and a continuum view, uses tools and systems, yields data, and focuses on intentional, proactive practice (see Table 15-2). The structure for achieving patient-centered outcomes does not just happen. Initiatives start with an agency's commitment to cost and quality management and a realistic model for outcomes-based practice with concrete care delivery structures. These care delivery structures include models for professional care with high degrees of authority and accountability for results. Examples of this are primary nursing, clinical case management, or other high-accountability/high-authority professional care delivery models. Figure 15-1 illustrates that outcomes-based practice structures are the foundation for the practice database, the map, and the outcomes. The critical path/CareMap® is the planning grid that integrates the practice standards with the population needs. Through its actual use in guiding patient care, it yields data on cost and quality outcomes of that care.

Outcomes-based practice will look different within actual care delivery frameworks but always rests on some combination of caregivers with superb clinical skill, care management tools such as critical path or CareMap® tools, and systems that support the process of care and position the patient squarely at the center of concern. As recent reports from multiple healthcare facilities suggest, experiences with these models have produced such striking results that they often become the genesis for healthcare redesign initiatives, changing whole systems of care delivery both structurally and operationally. Agencies with fully collaborative practices and an outcomes focus will not make change decisions based on old rehashed data acquired through retrospective means, reactivity to current market pressures, fear,

TABLE 15-2. Definition of Outcomes-Based Practice

Outcomes-Based Practice (OBP):
A multidisciplinary practice method that supports achievement of both cost and quality outcomes with the patient and family as the unifying concern. OBP includes collaborative practice behaviors, a continuum view, uses tools and systems, gets data, and focuses on intentional, proactive practice.

OBP IS NOT:
Crisis, task focused, fragmented, small picture.

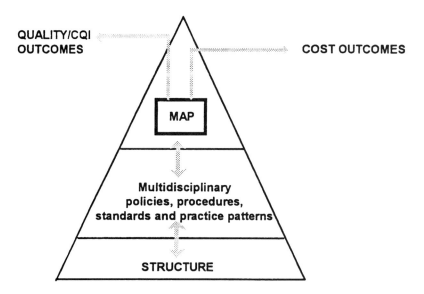

FIGURE 15-1. The critical path/CareMap® is the access point to all levels of information. Reprinted with permission from The Center for Case Management. Copyright, The Center for Case Management.

or panic. Meaningful operational restructuring will occur based on data acquired through real-time use of proactively designed care systems. It is the difference between going forward in care with a plan and going forward in care without one. All models using an outcomes approach will rely on specific, practical strategies, such as restructured roles or critical path/CareMap® systems.

Strategies for Outcomes Practice: Critical Path/CareMap® Tools

Critical pathways are grids that define categories of care and interventions and plot these across time. The expected interventions are written for a case type population (homogeneously defined group, procedure, or condition) and can be tracked through a process called variance analysis. Variance from the path is analyzed to determine reasons or strategies for managing the departures from expected care or progress. The timeline allows for the opportunity to preplan key care events such as collaborative team meetings, assessments, teaching, and family interventions. Timelines are described in anything from minutes (as in emergency department paths), to around-the-clock shifts, to weeks, to visits.

A CareMap® tool is the enhanced version of the critical path. The CareMap® tool adds the problems or focus areas and intermediate and discharge outcomes. The outcomes are plotted across time and correlate with the interventions stated in those time frames (Bower, 1993; Zander 1993). Critical path/CareMap® strategies have evolved from a need to care for patients within complex organizations and manage their needs tightly from the moment they enter systems to the moment they exit. However, as stand-alone strategies or single-discipline dominated projects (Zander, 1993), they would only partially succeed or perhaps fail. The best results are achieved when the strategies are used in the context of a system commitment to an outcomes management initiative.

Critical path/CareMap® tools emphasize the element of task and outcome timing. When the individual patient departs or differs from the predicted plan of care, variance occurs. When variance is detected, caregivers analyze the reason for the variance, make care management decisions, and intervene when appropriate to do so (Fig. 15-2). Variance analysis, then, becomes critical to clinical decision making by emphasizing evaluation of care, both at the bedside and through providing data about the case type issues in aggregate (retrospective analysis).

Critical path/CareMap® tools are used to support multidisciplinary communication and are a central point from which all disciplines can view the most recent snapshot of the patient condition. In addition, critical path/ CareMap® tools, when developed by multidisciplinary teams, (1) incorporate standards, (2) clarify accountabilities, and (3) signal specific tasks and outcomes to track as sources for data analysis and continuous quality improvement. Since their inception in 1989, CareMap® tools and systems have emerged as a method that supports continuity of plan and in many agencies are a core component of a medical record, incorporating many other doc-

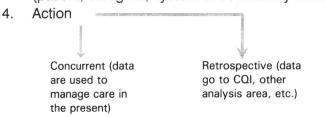

1. Detection
2. Analysis (met/not met?, done/not done?)
3. Assigning (coding) the reason for the variance (patient, caregiver, system or community factors)
4. Action

Concurrent (data are used to manage care in the present)

Retrospective (data go to CQI, other analysis area, etc.)

FIGURE 15-2. Variance from outcomes is detected, analyzed, coded, and acted on either concurrently or retrospectively. Reprinted with permission from The Center for Case Mangement. Copyright, The Center for Case Management.

umentation and information management tasks. In many instances, maps and pathways have helped turn patient medical records into what they were originally designed for: records of clinical process and results, communication tools, databases, and a device that protects patients, caregivers, and healthcare agencies (Nolin and Lang, 1994; Pozgar, 1990).

Automation of the Critical Path/CareMap®

When a complex process can be sorted into its respective elements, relationships, patterns, and directions, it is a process that lends itself to some automated assistance. Automation has the potential to support path/map strategies by getting caregivers the clinically meaningful information needed to manage care at both cost and quality levels.

What Is Clinically Meaningful Information?

Information obtained by caregivers has clinical relevance in two ways: It is either concurrent information that supports clinical decision making at the moment it is required or retrospective information—aggregated data used to review trends or issues in care management at the system and clinical care level. Making and keeping information meaningful (Table 15-3) demands that information have the characteristics discussed in the following subsections.

Accessible and Findable

Whether information is in the form of paper tools or computer terminals, caregivers require maximum access to it. Caregivers have long complained that time spent in searching for documentation or carrying out documentation is a major factor in inefficient care. For example, one attending physician attempting to manage short-stay chemotherapy patients described the daily ritual of searching out the following forms he had to locate before he was able to see the patient:

TABLE 15-3. What Is Clinically Meaningful Information?

- Accessible and Findable
- Timely
- Relevant
- Accurate
- Gives perspective
- Disciplined
- Communicates potential and actual problems

Reprinted with permission from The Center for Case Management. Copyright, The Center for Case Management

- Temperature, Pulse, Respiration (TPR) sheet (not available in any single place)
- Nursing admission note
- Medication administration record
- Finger stick sheet
- Narcotics administration record.

This illustrates that information that is collected and available to one discipline must also be available to other disciplines if both rely on the information for care managing. Accessible information is in one place, easily located and open for access as appropriate. Another example is that "information gatekeepers" sometimes restrict access to data that can educate and inform caregivers and decision makers about cost and quality issues. Bower states that "the philosophy and approach to sharing data are vital to the functioning of the case management program and its evaluation. The most effective approach incorporates openness with data and a willingness to share the data with the clinicians involved with case types" (Bower, 1993, p. 64).

Access is one issue, but finding information is another. Findable information is crucial to clinical reasoning. If the information is cluttered, unrecognizable, or lost, it is impossible to rely on it to form clinical opinions and use it as the basis for actions. As in the preceding example, caregivers are spending time searching for, reobtaining, or documenting lost information. Information must first be findable for the purposes of concurrent care management. Following this, clinicians or case managers can designate information to be collected, stored, retrieved, tabulated, and analyzed for retrospective detection of trends and issues. In automatic systems, information that is recordable in one place could be distributed automatically to several related places. For example, if blood pressure was entered via a keyboard or direct entry, so that it displayed as a value on the computer screen, it would also be imported to a screen and graphically displayed at the touch of a keystroke (or mouse). Being able to locate information consistently is important. Online directories and information maps are useful in assisting caregivers to locate information consistently.

Timely

For information to be meaningful, it must be timely. Having timely information means that it is, first, easy to record closest to the time of discovery and, second, is available to query (read) on demand. An example of this is the ability to view the history of how a variance issue progressed within 8-hour, 24-hour, and 48-hour time frames.

Relevant

Caregivers require complete access to relevant information—in other words, information that is pertinent to the problem or focus at hand. This may include pieces (rather than entire data sheets) of known patient history, most recent clinical data and measurements, results of the latest multidisciplinary assessments, and status of current treatments, as well as where the patient is geographically in the system. For example, an MD making rounds of his patients would need to know the present clinical status, a comparative status (such as how the patient was doing the day before), problems (or indications of problems), and whether or not the patient is able to be seen (is the patient at a test or procedure?). Relevant information takes on a different focus for case managers and clinicians concerned with managing care from the context of the big-picture view. They ask, "Is this a complex discharge? If so, when do we start evaluating placement issues? Will this likely result in an extended length of stay? Who will need to be informed?" and so on.

Accurate

Clinical information that is reliable, accurate, and trustable is meaningful. For example, mechanical monitoring of blood pressure, pulse, and temperature, although used for years in critical care settings, does not necessarily record the information in the medical record. Thus, while automation solves the measurement issue on one hand, it does not solve the entry issue on the other. When sensors that directly interface with what they are to measure record and route it to the proper place (all with impeccable accuracy), then clinical management of information can move to the next level—analysis.

For retrospective use of data, it is important to have sound formulas about combining cost and quality data in ways that will yield accurate results. For example, length-of-stay information can be skewed by not excluding outliers. Measuring mortality outcomes for cardiac surgeons can likewise be skewed if one does control for severity. The manner in which data are analyzed will take on greater importance as indicators are looked at in relation to each other. Barnes Hospital in St. Louis, Missouri believes that a "comprehensive clinical and financial evaluation system provides the information necessary for the organization to determine whether clinical standards of care successfully meet desired patient outcomes and whether these standards can be delivered in a cost-effective manner" (Weilitz and Potter, 1993, p. 52).

Gives Perspective

The ability to evaluate progressions in care (e.g., progress on pain control, ambulation distances, self-management) gives caregivers important information on the success of their interventions. In addition, it is important to be able to visualize and identify care areas and prepare patients and their families for what to expect next. Although caregivers evaluate the effect of their actions, they have often been handicapped by the short-term nature of their contact with patients and have been denied a full perspective on total outcome over the long run. With newer clinical management systems like case management systems and CareMap® tools, the progressions are visible on the grid and illustrate the relation of one phase of care to another. Clinical knowledge of relevant, well-planned interventions that produce predictable outcomes is emerging as a result of coordinated outcomes practice. For example, facilities using maps offer reports that correlate use of maps with stabilized lengths of stay, lowered complication rates, and improved precision of interventions. With accurate perspective on the effect and influence of specific interventions over the course of care, caregivers can be accountable for managing those actions that will produce the predicted results.

Disciplined

Added information that is irrelevant to care should be kept to a minimum so that information clutter is avoided. To do this effectively, caregivers must sharpen documentation skills to limit descriptions to the purpose of the entry. In addition, a disciplined medical record system that emphasizes clarity, relevancy, and communication and has written guidelines for use is a system that supports clinicians, healthcare facilities, and patients in getting the most out of their medical record.

Communicates Potential and Actual Problems

One method for assuring that information is clinically meaningful is to have a system that flags or quickly identifies problems crucial for caregivers to be aware of. Often that first line of defense is the observant nurse or other caregiver, who detects problems. The difficulty lies in what happens after that information is detected. At times, reaching caregivers for orders, consultation, or intervention is the only important thing that matters. In automated systems, critical information must be differentiated as that which is timely and requires urgent routing to the proper caregiver or department. Automated systems can manage critical information in two ways: Alert caregivers in the present and store data for analysis later.

Incorporating Critical Path/CareMap® Tools in an Automated Information System

Automated Information Systems

Information systems (IS) are systems that connect all technology to meet the needs of clinical management. Broadly defined, IS can include anything from change-of-shift report to voice mail, automated order entry to facsimile machines in the pharmacy, automated CareMap® tools to decision sup-

TABLE 15-4. Automated Modules Available for Healthcare Facilities

- Clinical data management
- Discharge barrier management
- Assessment
- Automated monitoring of follow-up activities
- Electronic record
- Order automation/entry
- Clinical alerts and reminders
- Quality assurance
- Admission, discharge, and transfer automation (ADT)
- Scheduling
- Acuity
- Expert systems
- Materials management
- Utilization management
- Decision support

port software, and so on. Healthcare facilities are challenged to meet the increasing demand for timely and accurate information by taking a second look at all communication strategies within a facility. Automated systems take advantage of powerful computer processing to facilitate IS requirements. The increased attention to this area by both clinicians and automated vendors has already resulted in the availability of a variety of automated modules capable of addressing almost any process (Table 15-4). So why the delay? There are a number of reasons for the delay, some having to do with expense, integration with preexisting information systems, hardware platforms, and technology maturity. But the biggest reason relates to the ability of clinicians, executives, and vendors to merge their interests into a clear vision for automation. Effective clinician, executive, and vendor partnerships that will produce the best automated solutions will be organized around the following beliefs (Table 15-5):

1. Clinicians are capable of managing both cost and quality. Clinicians who are already demonstrating tighter outcomes management are able to do

TABLE 15-5. Partnership Guidelines for Producing and Purchasing Effective Automated Systems

1. Clinicians are capable of managing both cost and quality.
2. Both clinical and financial automated systems have value.
3. Automated vendors will require input from clinicians at the earliest point of design.
4. Facility-based IS experts, in partnership with clinicians, are key to evaluating automated products.
5. Automated designs must informate, not automate staff.
6. Interim automated strategies can help stabilize care.
7. Collaborative strategies are key to resolving potential partnership barriers.

so when given good information about costs/quality results, work effectively as teams, and stay focused on the patient/family outcomes.

2. Both clinical and financial automated systems have value. Administrative managers are moving from purchasing technology that is strictly related to cost accounting to packages that have clinical and cost applications.

3. Automation vendors will require input from clinicians at the earliest point of design. Involving caregivers in defining the structure of care and how they are able to do what they do is important, and automated developers should do so. Likewise, if clinicians can "flowchart" their clinical processes, this allows for IS developers to architect an appropriate solution.

4. Facility-based IS experts, in partnership with clinicians, are key to evaluating automated products. Because there are many hardware and software solutions coming onto clinical markets, there is increased pressure on executives and caregivers to assess the field properly and progress with the best automation plan possible for the facility. This reflects a need for both executives and caregivers to upgrade their technology assessment skills, something they often find themselves having to do on the run. Choices become less problematic when caregivers and executives can describe and understand the structure of their care and what is needed. If the who, what, when, where, why, and how of clinical care can be communicated structurally and differentiated by clinical needs and environment, then IS people can represent the facilities' technical status and better determine what is required to complement, replace, or integrate with preexisting systems.

5. Automated designs need to "informate," not automate staff. There is a tendency in organizations to overemploy information technology to automate tasks and processes but underemploy it to informate employees (Zuboff, 1988, pp. 10–11). Informated staff, as opposed to automated staff, will use information to make judgments about care and outcomes management. Automating work processes (such as scheduling and order entry) will be a part of technological support in the healthcare setting of the future, but informating will be necessary to produce effective collaborations, key to systems of outcomes-based practice.

6. Interim automated strategies can help stabilize care. The present challenge for facilities is to find an interim solution to a long-term automation strategy. Two approaches that offer possibilities as intermediate strategies to stabilizing care are bridging and niching. Bridging refers to both the bridging of mature technology (financials/operations/decision support) to the clinical side of care as well as connecting information across disparate care areas and geographical locations. Niching refers to short-term solutions to care management, such as stand-alone automated systems that perform specific functions and can be integrated into larger system uses later.

7. Collaborative strategies are key to resolving potential partnership barriers. To get an effective system, information system experts and vendors need to become part of the equation. Facility-based IS personnel are hired to coordinate information, interpret vendor capabilities, match these to system needs, and assist in making IS purchase and implementation decisions. IS employees, however, require education and consultation about clinical management needs. This is also true for external technology vendor companies. A formidable partnership barrier exists when all the players are at different levels of understanding regarding care structure and process. Vendors often have a limited understanding of how to pursue clinical information development when it involves mapping and case management technology. Healthcare agencies will require expertise in defining the parameters for a vendor contract that will need to resolve issues such as technology licensing, source code agreements, confidentiality, development method, implementation, and reselling. It will be important for clinicians and executives to address these key issues in the context of a collaborative approach with vendors to focus on obtaining the best automated system and to derive maximum benefits from it.

Critical path/CareMap® methods affect all levels of healthcare workers and will require comprehensive systems of information management to support their functions. Clinicians and executives will need each other to define the mandate for automation. They will work together to form a strategy for clarifying the information demands, sorting out the technology, and focusing the financial investment. Following the facility lead, automation vendors will design and build systems that achieve facility purposes.

Pathway/Map Functions That Automated Systems Will Support

Automated systems for pathways/maps and case management will need to support the following functions (Table 15-6):

TABLE 15-6. Critical Path/CareMap® Tools: Functions That Automated Systems Will Be Required to Support

1. Collaboration, coordination and communication
2. Display of planning grid
3. Monitoring, care planning, and variance analysis
4. Fast, relevant, and focused documentation
5. Automatic sorting of data for multiple uses
6. Obtains data for continuous quality improvement.

Reprinted with permission from The Center for Case Management. Copyright, The Center for Case Management

1. Handle collaboration, coordination, and communication. Multidisciplinary and multidepartmental collaboration can be supported by automated systems in several ways: multidisciplinary access to the same
information, patient scheduling, planning care, and predefining the minimum number of times that the team should meet to discuss key evaluations in care. CareMap® tools have the advantage of clarifying caregiver
roles and utilization while at the same time illustrating how one caregiver
relates to another. Automated systems would need to maintain this function. Yet despite the presence of a path or map, the urge to differentiate
roles is powerful. For example, recently when discussing the possibility
of automating a CareMap® tool on a computer system, a physician stated
that he thought that was all just fine, but was he going to be able to have
his own view of the data? Clinician differentiation within systems is important, especially where accountability is concerned, but if overused it
results in isolated practice and fragmentation. It seems that to avoid
building yet another system that will repeat the mistakes of the past
(recall charts where everyone has their own section), it will be important
to stay focused on what information clinicians need that is both similar
and different and build options into these automated systems.

Communicating is and is not difficult to automate. Although E-mail,
facsimiles, and voice mail go a long way, unless the communication is
two-way it is difficult to guarantee that the messages sent are received
accurately. Nothing should replace the value of face-to-face communications where complex systems are involved. Pathways/maps and case
management can formalize communication by describing standards for
communication activities for the case type. Formalizing communication
has the advantage of defining minimum communication expectations as
well as clarifying when communication would be expected to occur, between whom, and when. For example, a case management team using a
CareMap® tool for coordinating care of cardiovascular accident (CVA)
patients prescribed a healthcare team meeting to occur by day 4 post-
CVA. The CVA CareMap® tool prompted the caregivers to meet and
specified what questions about prognosis and family communication
were to be the focus at that time.

A full range of systems of clinical information could benefit caregivers
using paths/maps and/or case management. For example, software packages that provide opportunities for accessing, planning, documenting,
monitoring, intervening, and evaluating care would assist caregivers and
case managers in achieving the purpose of their roles (Table 15-7).
Communication with the Patient/Family:
Maps often specify what type of teaching or communications should
be taking place between caregivers and patients and their families. Automated information support would be valuable in continuing to prompt
caregiver attention to this. This would include not only prompts to review teaching content but a place for recording patient/family response

TABLE 15-7. Access to a Full Range of Systems of Clinical Information Will Benefit Multidisciplinary Caregivers Using Paths/Maps or Case Management

- Assessment tools and clinical data bases
- Clinical data measurements (blood results, vital signs, height, weight, etc.)
- Medications: orders, given, taken, side-effects
- Orders: treatments, tests, activities, diets, etc.
- Plans: intended direction of care, including predicted outcomes
- Schedules: appointments, completion of tests, activities
- Team participants: the multidisciplinary caregivers and how to reach them
- Multidisciplinary evaluations of the patient/family status

Reprinted with permission from The Center for Case Management. Copyright, The Center for Case Management

at the moment and then in relation to the outcomes. In addition, outcomes of the patient/family interactions need to be documented, especially if these communications have everything to do with proceeding to the next level of care (i.e., informed consents, evidence of discussions of risk, benefits and alternatives, demonstrated patient competency in self-care, etc.). It may not be too far off to expect that in the future, patients and their families may directly document (or log on) and enter their own assessment of outcomes.

2. Display the planning grid for coordinating services and resources across the episode of care. The ability to see more than one day at a time assists caregivers in viewing the larger picture of care, anticipating care needs, and seeing where care is going and where it has been.

3. Handle monitoring, care planning, and variance analysis. CareMap® tools are the multidisciplinary plans of care. Comparing the actual patient to the predicted plan of care (path or map) involves analysis of the real versus the predicted and often generates variance information. Figure 15-3 illustrates how one automated system responds to the detection of a variance by displaying a series of windows that guide the caregiver through a series of "forced-choice" options and support the critical thinking process all the way through evaluation of outcome.

Automated systems record the data learned at each step in variance analysis, aggregate it, and report it in facility-defined reports and at specified time intervals. For example, if clinicians wanted to know how well postoperative pain was managed in surgical case types, variance from an outcome stated as "postop pain adequately managed/states levels 1–2 on pain scale" is detected when pain is unrelieved. A simple variance analysis strategy would be to document the reason for pain (inadequate medication dosage), the corrective actions taken (increased dose), and the effect on outcome (pain relieved within 2 hours postoperative). This could be tabulated for occurrences within a single time frame on a map (i.e., postoperative) or trended in the aggregate to evaluate how many surgical patients had unrelieved pain across case types for the past year.

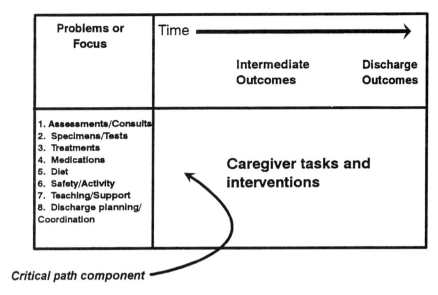

FIGURE 15-3. The CareMap® tool. (CareMap® is a registered trademark and concept of The Center for Case Management.) Reprinted with permission from The Center for Case Management.

Tracking variance by hand or even on simple spreadsheets does not necessarily capture anything more than the reasons for the variance from outcome. The other information about corrective actions and ultimate resolution of the outcomes, though documented, may not be measured. Hand tabulation of variance often stops short of measuring corrective actions or resolutions to outcomes because the amount of information to sort and interpret becomes unwieldy. Automated variance, on the other hand, can tell caregivers and administrators more and in much faster turnaround times.

4. Provide fast, relevant, and focused documentation. Documentation has long been a difficult part of care managing. Cumbersome and rarely informative documentation systems are under scrutiny again. Part of the difficulty with documentation has been the historical perception that more was better. Documentation is being revisited to evaluate specifically when more is better (about patient outcomes and the interventions) and when it is not (documenting tasks and facility-based routines that have little to do with necessary care). Pathways and maps support streamlined documentation methods such as documentation by exception or focused charting because they present a standard of care to document against. Automated systems make documentation of outcomes, tasks, and significant variances as easy as a series of single keystrokes.

5. Automatically sort data in multiple ways. Tagged data entered at one point in the automated system can be used at other multiple points for

analysis. For example, when a patient is discharged late by one day, that information is retrieved for analysis on a number of levels: overall performance by diagnostic related groupings (DRG), relation to complications, relation to physician/team/location, relation to patient/family variances, and so on. Sorting and analysis are strengths of computer processing systems and allow the caregiver to focus energy instead on determining precisely what variables he or she wishes to look at and in what sequence or relationship to view them.

6. Obtain data for continuous quality improvement.

Critical Path/CareMap® Precision and Development:

Statements on a map evolve as practice and knowledge of care evolves. At Barnes Hospital, Care Path Project Manager Pamela Weilitz has described how maps improve and reflect increasing precision in care as caregivers develop them over time. Weilitz states that current practice represents the first development effort and captures care as practiced in the present. Next comes best practice, whereby maps make the best use of knowledge and resources, and finally ideal practice, a state of maximum care effectiveness and efficiency. Automation that yields data about map efficacy assists caregivers in progressing toward the ideal practice level. In addition, automated map systems with storage can provide an archive record for practice development and evolution.

Continuous Quality Improvement for Programs of Care:

Clinical information that can be pooled from similar case types (e.g., cardiac surgical or orthopedic surgery case types) has great value in understanding the impact of outcomes on whole programs of care. This aggregate data can be used to analyze costs, detect quality issues across similar case types, improve related processes, and keep caregivers focused not only on improving but on sustaining high-quality, efficient programs.

Variance Data for Quality Improvement Activities:

Critical path/CareMap® tools yield data about reasons for variance from outcomes. Sometimes the reasons are patient related and sometimes clinician and facility (process) related. The data, whether on paper or computer, can provide comprehensive quality information. But providing information is one thing, how information is used is another. Paying attention, interpreting data, and using data to augment change cannot be automated.

The New Skyscrapers

There are other levels of information required to manage the patient through complex systems of care. Many computer software vendors are fast developing entire clinical information packages that address the expressed needs of their clients. Critical path/CareMap® tool methods represent strategies for progressing to outcome-based practice. Automating outcome-based practice represents a formidable challenge for automation vendors, clinicians, and executives. As clinicians gain expertise in using these map and case management strategies, they will be in a better position to speak authoritatively about where such strategies fit and under what circumstances they are used. As automation vendors better understand how clinicians use these strategies in actual practice, they will be in a better position to architect useful designs. If "form follows function" (Sullivan, 1896) was true for building skyscrapers at the turn of the century, then it is even more true now, as clinicians seek the skyscraper for automation solutions that suit the cost/quality management functions required of them.

With today's technology, any configuration for automated systems is possible. However, the effort it will take to make it all work will not be a solitary but a collaborative one. Clinicians, executives, and vendors who respond together to the challenge of building outcomes-based practice and the automated support for it will see results that profit both industry and patient. The promise of patient-centered outcomes practice will only be realized through unprecedented collaborations along with a deep understanding of the structure of care.

References

Bower KA: Case management: Work redesign with patient outcomes in mind. In: McDonagh KJ, ed. *Patient-Centered Hospital Care: Reform from Within.* Ann Arbor, MI: Health Administration Press, 1993; 47–69.

Nolin CE, Lang CG: *An Analysis of the Use and Effect of CareMap® Tools in Medical Malpractice Litigation.* Expert Library, Vol. 1. South Natick, MA: The Center for Case Management, 1994.

Pozgar GD: *Legal Aspects of Health Care Administration.* 4th ed. Rockville, MD: Aspen, 1990.

Sullivan HL: The tall office building artistically considered. *Lippincott Magazine,* 1896; March.

Weilitz PB, Potter P: A managed care system: Financial and clinical evaluation. *Journal of Nursing Administration* 1993; 23(11): 51–57.

Zander K: Nurses and case management: To control or to collaborate? In: *Changing Practice* 1993; 254–260.

Zuboff S: *In the Age of the Smart Machine: The Future of Work and Power.* New York: Basic Books, 1988; 10–11.

16
Clinical Imaging: Applications and Implications for Nursing

KAREN LAFFERTY ZIMMERMAN

Problem Definition

For many clinicians, one of the most frustrating aspects of the traditional Hospital Information System (HIS) is that it has not served as a single source of patient information. Explanations abound, but one of the most common is that the nature, format, and source of the information did not lend themselves to the traditional coded (bits and bytes) and structured (field-oriented and contained within a database file) information type that the HIS was developed to capture and store. Examples of nonconforming data are electrocardiogram (EKG) rhythm strips and radiology films. Other more frustrating examples, based on the comprehensiveness of the respective HIS, include histories and physicals, physicians' and nurses' progress notes, vital signs, medication administration records, and discharge instructions. The result is that the clinician must rely on multiple sources for data, often in widely disparate locations, to obtain a comprehensive patient profile. Obviously, this results in inefficiency.

Problem Resolution

Simply stated, what the clinician wants and needs to provide optimal patient care is access to a terminal to find, quickly and easily, any piece of information within the clinician's security ranking. One interesting and exciting approach to resolving the problem is the introduction of imaging technology to the clinical environment. To use a simplistic analogy, imaging is like an electronic photograph. Instead of the traditional camera and film as the source of the image, though, this technology uses a scanner to digitalize documents (known as document-based imaging). Conversely, image-ready equipment—such as the latest EKG management systems, magnetic resonance imaging (MRI) scanners, and picture archiving and communication systems (PACs)—are also used in radiology (known as image-based imaging). There is a wide variety of other employable input devices for an imaging system, such as facsimile machines, microfilm image scanners, and computer output to laser disk (COLD), which is a direct link from the HIS host to the imaging system. In addition, computer assisted design (CAD) and some innovative companies are making available multimedia input for voice and video.

Hospitals across the country already have one or more of these imaging technologies installed and operational. Again, the solution has been piece-meal. Many of the hospitals that have entered the world of imaging have done so through the back door, in the financial and billing areas. Others have gone the additional step of scanning parts of the entire medical record and making it available to clinicians on specialized devices throughout the organization.

Most imaging systems store information on optical disks. In larger applications, optical disks are stored in jukeboxes. The benefit of this storage medium is easy accessibility to a large volume of information with relative speed by an end user. There is one important caveat: Accessibility is limited to the indexes predefined and attached to each record at the time of storage. Often these indexes are manually applied to the record. Typical indexes may be patient medical record number, social security number, date of service, and physician name. The more indexes, the more potential for manual intervention.

There are assistive technologies available that limit the manual indexing requirement. Such technologies include optical character recognition (OCR), bar coding, and programmed indexing. Programmed indexing is most useful in COLD applications or when larger batches of similar documents are being scanned and the index profile can be input directly into the scanner.

This massive amount of readily accessible data is managed by the database management system (DBMS) and the jukebox management system for control of the platters that require access for the information requested. The DBMS is responsible for version control, security-based access, and the functionality that the user can employ while reviewing a record, such as applying "sticky notes," reviewing two records (such as EKG strips) on the screen simultaneously, accessing electronic signatures (especially important for radiologists' and cardiologists' verification of interpretations), and routing and reporting, to name a few.

In the specialized departments that use imaging, such as Hospital Information Management (HIM), Radiology, and Cardiology, one of the most important tools the system offers is work flow management. The functionality of the work flow application within an imaging solution can provide a primary cost justification for the system. Work flow basically provides the user and the department with tools such as sophisticated routing options, scheduling of work in process, deadline control, reminders, work status, and sorting and prioritization, to name a few. All the functionality can be user defined to meet specific needs.

Another exciting application of imaging is in conjunction with a broad category of technology known as telemedicine. Telemedicine utilizes interactive audiovisual technology between patients, doctors, and nurses in physically separated locations. Telemedicine utilizes voice, facsimile, pictures, video, and even specialized examination/diagnostic equipment such as electronic microscopes, laryngoscopes, colposcopes, otoscopes, and stethoscopes. The data are transmitted over an integrated services digital network (ISDN), which is commonly referred to as the information highway of the 1990s because of its ability to transmit voice, data, and images simultaneously.

Telemedicine applications include transmission of computerized or imaged medical records, teleradiology, telecardiology, videoed surgical procedures, and interactive patient examinations. All of these applications and others encourage consultative practices, educational opportunities, and referral networks between remote locations and regional medical centers. Health maintenance organizations (HMOs) and managed care organizations are particularly supportive of these developments due to the aspect of eliminating unnecessary patient transport, hospital admissions, and duplication of diagnostic procedures. The aforementioned telemedicine applications are all potential input sources for optical storage and retrieval.

Challenges

The future of image-enabled health care is tremendously exciting. However, as already mentioned, finding a way to integrate the piecemeal solutions into a total solution to solve the same old problem of accessing all the patient data when and where the clinician needs it remains a significant challenge. The challenges include standardization of the multitude of components (document transfer, network, data exchange, display devices, interfaces, etc.) required in a diverse environment such as a hospital. Purchasing compatible, image-ready equipment across departments within a single hospital is alone a tremendous challenge, much less selecting from the vast array of specialized equipment with its respective technologies from the overall vendor market. There are significant efforts to provide international standards in imaging technology, and vendors have partially adopted many of these to the extent of their current state of completeness.

Other challenges are the initial and ongoing costs of imaging technology and the potential for return on investment. These are concerns across industries, but they are of particular concern to the healthcare industry in a time of major transition, as we see today with managed care. The cost of these technologies will decrease over time, but the impact on an organization of implementing imaging and the resulting reengineering process will remain a high-cost, high-commitment item in terms of time, internal resources, vendor and consultant support, and the ongoing integration of additional equipment and applications.

Additional challenges involve security and confidentiality of data (which are not exclusively, or even particularly, technological issues as much as cultural or behavioral issues); rapidly evolving technology, to the point of the newly purchased imaging system being obsolete by the time it is installed; and reimbursement. As of this writing, the federal government has reversed an earlier decision to reimburse telemedicine charges for Medicare patients. The impact of this decision on the advancement of telemedicine applications remains to be seen.

Opportunities for Nursing

In a healthcare environment where traditional clinical nursing positions are increasingly difficult to find, nurses have the opportunity to become involved in clinical imaging in a variety of ways. Involvement and/or sponsorship of clinical imaging projects is particularly important because this technology typically has to be "sold" to administration. Involvement in developing a methodology to ensure purchasing practices of image-ready and compatible equipment across all domains of the organization is of fundamental importance, especially if a multitude of uncoordinated imaging projects spring up throughout the organization, which is typically the case. Nursing involvement is especially needed for input in a prioritization process for clinical imaging projects. Finally, direct positions will be required for staffing remote transmission sites for telemedicine applications.

Questions

1. What are some areas and/or functions in your organization that could benefit from the use of imaging technology?
2. What role could a nurse play in the selection and implementation of imaging technology?

17
Usability Concepts and the Clinical Workstation

Nancy Staggers

Nothing is more apparent than the need for usability concepts in clinical systems, a need made immediately obvious to anyone attending vendor demonstrations. Recently, authors advocated usability principles in health-care systems (Fralic, 1992; Lowery and Martin, 1990; Zielstorff, Hudgings, and Grobe, 1993). The National Center for Nursing Research expert panel was more emphatic about the importance of usability: "The quality of patient care is determined in part by how accurately and easily the nurse can enter, retrieve, interpret, and comprehend data" (National Center for Nursing Research, 1993, p. 65). To date, these calls for action about system usability have seemingly been ignored. The evidence for usability in software exists outside health care, yet our industry is virtually untouched by these concepts. Why do we need usability concepts in healthcare computing? What is usability? How are usability concepts useful in clinical workstation design? These questions are discussed in this chapter. Specific usability solutions are recommended as fundamental techniques for clinical workstation development.

Usability Problems in Healthcare Computing

The world is full of useless and frustrating software (Nielsen, 1992). In healthcare computing, the evidence for usability problems is ubiquitous. We need usability concepts in healthcare computing because we still have systems with screens like the one shown in Figure 17-1. Not only is the text hard to read because it is in all capital letters, but there are more fundamental problems. The display is categorized by order type in chronological order within the categories. The entire order is in conflict with the way clinicians think about patient care. Clinicians, of course, need orders displayed in reverse chronological order with the most current orders displayed as a set. Additionally, the syntax is unfamiliar to clinicians, who find the structure within sentences odd and the stilted language more suitable

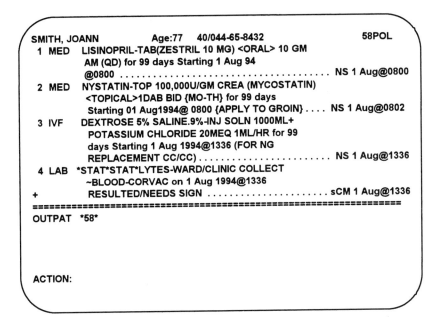

SMITH, JOANN   Age:77   40/044-65-8432   58POL
 1 MED   LISINOPRIL-TAB(ZESTRIL 10 MG) <ORAL> 10 GM
          AM (QD) for 99 days Starting 1 Aug 94
          @0800 . . . . NS 1 Aug@0800
 2 MED   NYSTATIN-TOP 100,000U/GM CREA (MYCOSTATIN)
          <TOPICAL>1DAB BID {MO-TH} for 99 days
          Starting 01 Aug1994@ 0800 {APPLY TO GROIN} . . . . NS 1 Aug@0802
 3 IVF   DEXTROSE 5% SALINE.9%-INJ SOLN 1000ML+
          POTASSIUM CHLORIDE 20MEQ 1ML/HR for 99
          days Starting 1 Aug 1994@1336 (FOR NG
          REPLACEMENT CC/CC) . . . . NS 1 Aug@1336
 4 LAB   *STAT*STAT*LYTES-WARD/CLINIC COLLECT
          ~BLOOD-CORVAC on 1 Aug 1994@1336
 +   RESULTED/NEEDS SIGN . . . . sCM 1 Aug@1336
==
OUTPAT *58*

ACTION:

FIGURE 17-1. Sample screen.

for computer files than for human understanding. These are elementary
usability problems.

In another example, one site trains new users on its clinical information
system for 3 hours, producing users who require little follow-on assistance.
Another system requires 40 hours of training for users; even then, users
need a preceptor to help with system interactions during the first week or
two. The difference relates to required memorization of commands, unusual language, nonintuitiveness of interactions, and buried functions—all
usability issues.

On the personal computer (PC) side, we have for years admonished our
healthcare PC users to back up their files to avoid disaster. As Thimbleby
(1990) noted, the blame was in the wrong direction. Usable systems ought
to back up their own files.

Probably the most vivid example comes from a bewildering electronic
mail message meant to be helpful to a new user of an existing hospital
information system (HIS). The new user asked how to enter a patient problem list so that it displays on all pertinent screens and forms in the system.
The response was as follows:

The PROBLEM LIST is a Patient Text topic in Desktop. Place your cursor next to
the patient you want to enter and press F9. This is a shortcut into Patient Text.
Enter the Patient Text topic as PROBLEM LIST (two words, all caps). Make the
PROBLEM LIST "public." Enter the problem list as you like. The PROBLEM

LIST automatically prints on the PBL and TXT options as with TEL. You could also set up a UDK.

Is there any wonder why we need to incorporate usability concepts into healthcare computing when we have systems like this one in use today? The costs to individuals and organizations for poorly designed systems range across these dimensions: decreases in productivity, extreme user frustration, underutilization of expensive systems, understated errors, extra personnel to train cumbersome systems, open resistance to awkward applications, and millions of dollars for system redesign. Incorporating usability concepts can help defray these costs.

What Is Usability?

Usability concerns the effectiveness of interactions between users, tasks, and systems in a particular environment. Computer usability is, then, an estimation of the degree to which task requirements are met by system use (Lindgaard, 1992). Usability factors are multidimensional, including

- Ease to learn
- Ease to use
- Ease to remember
- User satisfaction with system interactions
- Efficiency of use
- Error-free/error-forgiving interactions
- Seamless fit to the task(s) at hand.

All of these are applicable criteria for successful clinical workstations. Usability begins with systems that require a minimum of learning so that users may begin work quickly (Nielsen, 1993). Ease of use implies an optimized computer interface and easy navigation about the system. If systems are easy to remember, intermittent usage or returning after a lapse in use will not require relearning the entire system. Users should find interactions suitable, unobtrusive, and agreeable, facilitating desired tasks and leading to overall user satisfaction (Opaluch and Tsao, 1993). The system should be efficient for all levels of users from naive to expert by allowing high productivity and shortcuts for adapted users. Usability implies error-trapping to prevent catastrophic errors (Nielsen, 1993) and the facility to undo most actions where and when reasonable. The incorporation of usability concepts means that the dyad of user and system are compatible in completing the task at hand.

Usability goals for clinical workstations include optimizing productivity and protecting patient safety. These are not modest goals. If a system is designed well, the computer interface can effectively disappear, allowing users to focus only on the task at hand. This unobtrusiveness occurs not because the interface between humans and computer does not exist (Norman, 1990) but because it blends seamlessly among user, task, system, and environment.

Vision for the Usable Clinical Workstation

Probably the ultimate usable system is the computer portrayed in the television show "Star Trek: The Next Generation." Users merely address the system by saying, "Computer" . . . and speak a command. In usability terms, this system requires virtually no learning, is very easy to use, and, while available everywhere, it is obtrusive nowhere. Of course, we know little about its error-trapping capabilities, but from surface evaluations, any clinical user would welcome this computer based on its convenience and natural language interface. Our own experience with federal computer users indicates that physicians would be comfortable with a speech interface once the technology is more advanced. Nurses, on the other hand, currently find pen-pad technology more appealing. At any rate, clinical users will need to wait a few versions until a "Next Generation" computer appears. In the meantime, an intermediate solution for a usable clinical workstation is possible.

The clinical workstation will be predicated on comprehensive functions, integrating communications, knowledge bases, and clinical applications. Workstations will accommodate images, notes, letters, test results, critical paths, guidelines, protocols, and research information. However, few of these comprehensive functions will be utilized fully unless usability concepts are considered. Clinical workstations will need to adhere to the aforementioned general usability factors. In addition, they will need to be convenient and at least as quick to use as manual methods. In fact, for physicians, the target to beat for data input is preprinted orders and a pen. For nurses, a similar target is preprinted plans of care and a pen. The clinical workstation must fit easily into the culture and work practices of current environments. Finally, the system must be flexible and customizable to sites and users. As can be seen, usability concepts go well beyond screen design into a deep understanding of users, tasks, and user-system interactions. By discussing these three topics, the translation from abstract concepts into beginning operational level concepts is begun and workstation design can proceed.

The Foundation of Usability: Users, Tasks, and User-System Interactions

Users

One of the most often repeated axioms of usability is to "know the user." But how do system designers know users? Knowing users involves understanding at least these characteristics of system users: ages, computer experience, work experience, general visual acuity, and language skills (Nielsen, 1992). If designers are unfamiliar with clinicians' work settings, they must come to understand users' characteristics by observing users during site visits.

Shared Values

In the case of clinicians, knowing users also means understanding shared clinical values. Unlike informatics specialists, typical clinical system users are apt to view computers as tools, not captivating hobbies. Their first interest is patient care and expediting the care process. While there are pockets of computer enthusiasts in clinical settings, many outside informatics do not have a penetrating interest in computers. Computers merely facilitate work. More important, time is one of the most valued assets for clinicians. Anything that wastes time is an anathema and intolerable.

There are several implications of these observations. The problems with systems that technicians view as interesting clinicians will view as frustrating. Normal "bugs" in new software will not be seen as challenges to fix (a technical view) but impediments to work. Many clinical users have little patience for system reliability problems. They will quickly reject slow systems. Therefore, screen changes that take less than a second are mandatory. Clinicians may tolerate several-second delays if complex data such as images are being retrieved, however. Interestingly, clinicians are reasonably tolerant of poor screen designs and multiple screen changes as long as the system is blindingly quick. Clinicians will use nearly any system if the perceived value of the product is more than the cost of using the system. That is, clinicians may tolerate an inelegant results retrieval menu that takes longer than needed as long as the information they get in return is worth the extra time spent navigating the system.

Although much of the literature in the United States emphasizes physician applications in workstations, the clinical workstation must serve a range of disciplines. This integrated approach to clinical workstation development is articulated by a British effort called an "integrated clinical workstation programme" (National Health Service, 1994). This national program has been developed to address information needs of all healthcare professionals. Moving away from discipline-specific design to a patient-centered focus would mean facilitating views of data in care processes and designing for integrated interactions. Designing for a range of users means that the system will need to be customized by both site and user. The caveat is that if the time to customize to specific preferences is great, clinicians will not use preference options or they will find creative solutions to save time (e.g., borrowing another clinician's setup). To facilitate time savings, presetting sample preferences such as order sets or using default options is desirable.

Most clinicians will probably tend not to explore options in computers after the first few days. They will quickly adapt to a familiar subset of options and expend little cognitive energy on system options after that. Therefore, if good applications are not readily apparent, many clinicians will miss opportunities to use them. Once users find options that they value, they will adapt quickly. In fact, many of our federal system users know options so well that they do not look at screens as they chart. They have long since memorized the key sequences. If new releases change the key sequence and users are unaware, the outcome will be angry users.

The majority of clinical users want only essential, system survival training. Some of the users will have competing time commitments and may not be able to attend much training, especially new release training. The system must be designed to accommodate these users as well as intermittent users, such as per diem or agency nurses. Many users, including clinical users, would rather not read user documentation. An informative help desk, super users, or contextual online help may be better options.

Mental Models

An essential element of usability in clinical workstations is the congruence between the way information is presented to users and the way clinicians process information cognitively. These concepts concern users' mental models of the workstation.

While interacting with systems, users form internal representations or mental models of the system at hand. The notion of users' mental models is a widely accepted concept in the human-computer interaction literature, but authors use various terms to describe the concept. A target system is a particular system a user is learning or using. A design or conceptual model is invented by designers or educators as an accurate, consistent, and complete representation of the target system. The system image is the impression the device portrays to users (Norman, 1983). The problem is that the conceptual model of the system may or may not be consistent with the system image. In fact, designers may not be cognizant of their models. However, even if they are implicit, models are projected to users.

Mental models, on the other hand, are created by users as they interact with the target system and system image and may or may not be equivalent to conceptual models. Mental models are "what people really have in their heads and guide their use of things" (Norman, 1983, p. 12). The basic dilemma between designers and users is summarized by Norman (1986, p. 46–47):

The problem is to design a system so that, first, it follows a consistent, coherent conceptualization—a design model and, second so that the user can develop a mental model of that system—a user model, consistent with the design model. . . . The user model is not formed from the design model: It results from the way the user interprets the system image. Thus, in many ways, the primary task of the designer is to construct an appropriate system image, realizing that everything the user interacts with helps to form that image.

Mental models can range from fairly impoverished models to rich, visual images of systems and are important for system learning, performance, and design (Staggers and Norcio, 1993). Many authors propose that giving individuals a conceptual model of a system before instruction enhances user learning (Carroll and Mack, 1985). The model may then function as a knowledge organizer to promote understanding of the system. Mental models and user-system performance are intimately linked. Overall, even impoverished mental models assist users in system problem solving and allow more efficient and accurate user interactions. Therefore, designers must create a clear conceptual model and system image of a clinical workstation to allow users to create appropriate mental models.

User Metaphor

User metaphor follows closely on the concept of mental models. The purpose of a user metaphor is to provide users with a useful and easily recognizable model around which system functions are organized. This model is then portrayed as part of the system image. A good user metaphor will allow users to build a more complete mental model of the system in an efficient manner.

Typically, designers look for real-world objects or events that will allow users to relate to the system. For instance, current Windows™ user interface presentations use an office or desktop metaphor around which all user interactions proceed. The system has symbols and icons for file cabinets, folders, documents, and files. Users interact with familiar objects in a familiar order. More critically, users are able to predict the sequence of interactions by translating real-world experiences with the model into interactions with the system. This is why the office metaphor has been so successful for business applications. The same metaphor is useful for business transactions in patient care. However, the metaphor does not extend well into patient-centered clinical activities because the notion of an office, files, and documents does not depict realistic expectations of what happens with patient care processes.

Good metaphors are essential for ease of use in systems (Erickson, 1990). For patient care activities, finding a suitable metaphor is somewhat of an enigma. As Esterhay (1994) suggests, new metaphors are needed, and one metaphor may not be enough to encompass all clinical activities. Clinical workstations may have to use several metaphors to afford a comprehensive model of all activities.

Only a small amount of work has been done in this arena. Esterhay (1994) provides an excellent discussion of potential user metaphors for an oncologist's workstation. He suggests using flowsheets as a way of examining categories of patient data. For other activities, the use of rooms may be helpful in modeling users' work. Each room would contain tasks and interactive objects. Doors provide access to other rooms of activities.

A few current systems use a paper chart metaphor. There are tabs at the bottom or side of the chart much like dividers in the paper chart. Users interact with the system by clicking on the tabs and jumping to applications. This metaphor requires little training and is immediately familiar, but it ignores process redesign and leaves little room for growth in the future. Perhaps its best use is as a transitional model until better metaphors can be extrapolated and tested.

Usability Solution: User-Centered Design

Probably the most critical usability solution is user-centered software design. This software development method is used effectively outside our discipline but little within health care. User-centered design has as its decree that users' needs are central to software design. Besides conceptually knowing users, user-centered design is operationalized either by having an end user as part of a project team or having users as participants in an iterative software design process (Nielsen, 1993; Opaluch and Tsao, 1993). When designing a clinical workstation, including informatics clinicians on a project team is a step in the right direction; however, true end users must also be included in the process as well. User-centered design focuses on feedback from end users at every level of an iterative product design. Users' comments about the product are then given utmost credence in redesign.

Tasks

Norman (1990) makes a strong case for understanding tasks users need to accomplish. According to him, tasks should dominate and the tool should become invisible. Both the user interface and the computer should be subservient to the task. Designers, then, must pay special attention to the tasks to understand how the job can best be done. Focused questions include "What is the task(s) to be done?" "What data/information do clinicians need?" "How is the task done now?" "How can the task be computerized for maximum efficacy?" Throughout the process, the fundamental question is "What does the user want to do?" (Laurel and Mountford, 1990).

For clinical system users, tasks are complex. Clinicians, especially nurses, are information integrators. Information processing spans across sources—patients, medicine, nutrition, families, pharmacy, laboratory, radiology, social work, and occupational/physical therapy. Information processing occurs in a variety of contexts from hospital ships to shock-trauma units to living rooms. Yet little is known about how nurses and other clinicians integrate information from disparate sources and make clinical decisions, and much less is known about how to support integration in a computerized fashion.

Clinical workstation design must begin with an understanding of tasks users perform most frequently. Frequently performed tasks must be easily accessible and quickly executable; less frequently used tasks can be less visible. Beyond that, basic research is needed to understand clinical tasks and users' information processing. In particular, the following information integration tasks should be studied: nurses' change-of-shift activities, physicians' rounds report, and clinicians' preparation to write plans of care and progress notes. It is during these times that the most information-intense activities occur.

Considering work design and contexts is imperative. Work in clinical settings is frequently accomplished through a team approach. A team of nursing personnel may be organized for inpatient care. In medical centers, a separate team of physicians, from interns to attending staff, may care for patients. In other settings, an integrated team of providers may be organized around a clinical product line. The clinical workstation must facilitate a team approach to patient care that crosses the inpatient/ambulatory care continuum. In addition to supporting integrated and separate provider views, information must be linked to team members. For example, the workstation must automatically make laboratory results available to the entire team and notify the primary provider about abnormal results. If the primary provider is on vacation, the system must alert the covering provider about abnormal results.

Usability Solution: Understanding Tasks

Understanding clinical tasks is pivotal to creating usable workstations. A number of techniques are available to help with understanding tasks, including think-aloud protocols, task analysis, ethnographic studies, semantic network representations (Tang and Patel, 1994), and focus groups.

High-level task analysis was helpful in designing laboratory and radiology results retrieval for clinicians using a federal computer system. A team of software analysts, programmers, and clinicians analyzed the task by understanding the cognitive flow of information during manual processing of laboratory slips. Using the information processing model in Jonassen, Hannum, and Tessmer (1989), a high-level task analysis was performed to understand how providers cognitively process paper lab slips. Analysts listened to clinicians describe getting a pile of inpatient/outpatient lab slips and sorting them into typical categories (more action required, discard, file). From that understanding, analysts created a computerized flow of information that was compatible with this model. All tests ordered by a particular provider were presented in a format allowing quick, visual identification of the set of results to be processed. Abnormal results were made visually distinct by highlighting. Quick access to the actual results was provided by circumventing the usual menu paths and allowing users to jump from the highlighted test name directly to the test results. An "action bar" allowed quick discarding or forwarding of listed results either individually or in groups. By understanding the task at hand, software was designed to complement that process. Workstation design should be similar to this process: Understand the task and emulate cognitive information processing.

User-System Interactions

Once the fundamental analyses of users and tasks are completed, the knowledge can be used in iterative software design for clinical workstations. Iterative software design involves a series of system designs presented to users for evaluation. With each set of screens, designers assess user-system interactions and identify problems. These specific problems are the basis for software redesign and subsequent reassessment of user-system interaction. In this manner, designers effect steady refinements of the software. During iterative software design, systems are typically presented to users as prototypes rather than fully coded products. Severe design problems may then be corrected before the system is completely coded, a more economical technique than waiting until later in the software design cycle.

The principal precept of iterative software design includes systematic user-system interaction evaluations. Empirical testing includes traditional quantitative research methods and objective criteria, such as online task metrics, captured user keystrokes, or controlled user task performance measured in seconds with the numbers of errors committed per task. These data are useful in many instances for baseline usability data and determining optimal screen design methods (Staggers, 1993).

Designers must also ask focused questions about design preferences and explore the reasons underlying quicker interactions. Determining why one design or another is optimal is the key to effective design. The point is to determine where and why users trip in navigating systems, where language is inconsistent, where interactions are inconsistent, where functions are not intuitive, and where catastrophic errors occur. To capture these data, other research techniques may be useful for subjective but rich data: think-aloud protocols, videotaping interactions, and interviewing subjects. The prime notion in using any technique is that systematic methods are used to capture interaction information. The information is then fed directly into redesign— in this case, clinical workstation design.

Usability Solutions: Usability Labs

Usability laboratories provide a place to study users systematically as they interact with workstation hardware and software. Usability labs have been used effectively by Bellcore (Bell Communications) and Microsoft to assure system usability. As of this writing, no healthcare vendors or agencies have published information about healthcare usability labs. Yet these laboratories would be invaluable in creating usable clinical workstations as well as other healthcare products.

Typically, usability labs provide a controlled setting for monitoring users' interactions with systems. They can be as informal as several personal computers in a quiet room with a solo trained observer or as formal as a room with a one-way mirror, videotaping equipment, eye-movement tracking equipment, and a staff of trained analysts and researchers. A spectrum of research methods could be used. A lab might concentrate on a particular interest area, such as determining users' mental models for the clinical workstation or designing and testing applications for subspecialty system users. Other labs might focus on testing hardware for clinical personnel (for instance, whether portable technology, trackballs, or mice are preferable given scarce counter space in many settings).

Summary

This chapter is a call to action: We need usable clinical workstations. Usability concepts must be imported from human-computer interaction literature and the computer industry and translated into usefulness in health care. Healthcare usability labs must become a part of healthcare software design for the clinical workstation as well as other healthcare products. User-centered design, usability testing, and iterative software design should be commonplace. A usable clinical workstation will only be realized with these usability solutions. Donald Norman (1993) summarizes the usability issue well with his motto: "People propose, science studies, technology conforms."

Questions

1. Why do we need usability concepts in healthcare computing?
2. What is usability?
3. How are usability concepts useful in clinical workstation design?

References

Carroll JM, Mack RL: Metaphor, computing systems, and active learning. *International Journal of Man-Machine Studies* 1985; 22: 39–57.

Erickson TD: Creativity and design—Introduction. In: Laurel B, ed. *The Art of Human-Computer Interface Design.* Reading, MA: Addison-Wesley, 1990; 1–4.

Esterhay RJ: User metaphors of health care professional workstations. *International Journal of Bio-Medical Computing* 1994; 34: 95–113.

Fralic MF: Into the future: Nurse executives and the world of information technology. *Journal of Nursing Administration* 1992; 22: 11–12.

Jonassen DH, Hannum WH, Tessmer M: *Handbook of Task Analysis.* New York: Praeger, 1989.

Laurel B, Mountford SJ: Introduction. In: Laurel B, ed. *The Art of Human-Computer Interface Design.* Reading, MA: Addison-Wesley, 1990; xi–xvi.

Lindgaard G: Evaluating user interfaces in context: The ecological value of time-and-motion studies. *Applied Ergonomics* 1992; 23(2): 105–114.

Lowery JC, Martin JB: Evaluation of healthcare software from a usability perspective. *Journal of Medical Systems* 1990; 14(1): 17–29.

National Center for Nursing Research: *Nursing Informatics: Enhancing Patient Care* (NIH publication No. 93–2419). Bethesda, MD: National Institutes of Health, 1993.

National Health Service: *Clinical Workstations: Focus for the Future.* Information Management Group of the NHS Management Executive, Department of Health. England: Author, 1994.

Nielsen J: The usability engineering life cycle. *Computer* 1992; 25(3): 12–22.

Nielsen J: Iterative user-interface design. *Computer* 1993; 26(11): 32–41.

Norman DA: Some observations on mental models. In: Gentner D, Stevens AL, eds. *Mental Models.* Hillsdale, NJ: Erlbaum, 1983; 15–34.

Norman DA: Cognitive engineering. In: Norman DA, Draper SW, eds. *User Centered Systems Design.* Hillsdale, NJ: Erlbaum, 1986; 31–61.

Norman DA: Why interfaces don't work. In: Laurel B, ed. *The Art of Human-Computer Interface Design.* Reading, MA: Addison-Wesley, 1990; 201–219.

Norman DA: *Things That Make Us Smart: Defining Human Attributes in the Age of the Machine.* Reading, MA: Addison-Wesley, 1993.

Opaluch RE, Tsao YC: Ten ways to improve usability engineering-designing user interfaces for ease of use. *AT&T Technical Journal* 1993; 72(3): 75–88.

Staggers N: Impact of screen density on clinical nurses' computer task performance and subjective screen satisfaction. *International Journal of Man-Machine Studies* 1993, 39: 775–792.

Staggers N, Norcio A: Mental models: Concepts for human-computer interaction research. *International Journal of Man-Machine Studies* 1993; 38: 587–605.

Tang PC, Patel VL: Major issues in user interface design for health professional workstations: Summary and recommendations. *International Journal of Bio-Medical Computing* 1994; 34(1): 139–148.

Thimbleby H: *User Interface Design.* New York: ACM Press, 1990.

Zielstorff RD, Hudgings CI, Grobe SJ: *Next Generation Nursing Information Systems.* Washington, DC: American Nurses Association, 1993.

Unit 4
Administration and Nursing Informatics

Unit Introduction

Administration systems are a critical component in providing clinical care. Shamian and Hannah begin this unit by discussing management information systems for the nurse executive. They include an explanation of the nursing management minimum data set. Harsanyi, Wilson, Daniels, Allan, and Anderson provide a vendor viewpoint on healthcare information systems. They relate how the traditional Hospital Information System is changing to provide for the management and processing of patient-centered data, information, and knowledge across the healthcare continuum. Mills reinforces the nursing role in the selection process and gives a sample of a request for proposal (included in detail in Appendix C). In the next chapter, Jenkins indentifies three roles nursing must play in implementing an information system. She details key factors to ensure a successful implementation. Edmunds, who has much experience in the design of information systems, offers tips, techniques, and examples of good design concepts. In her chapter on business process reengineering, Happ delineates an action plan for nursing so that nurses may participate in changing how patient care is delivered and managed.

18
Management Information Systems for the Nurse Executive[1]

Judith Shamian and Kathryn J. Hannah

Ensuring effective as well as efficient care became a central function of the chief nurse executive during the late 1980s and the current decade. Concomitantly, the public is demanding more accountability, more involvement, and more information about healthcare services. The public wants evidence that care is delivered when it is necessary, in the most competent and cost-effective manner, and with interventions that lead to the desired outcomes. Access to information is considered a corporate strategic resource and key to making appropriate allocation decisions as well as the source of required evaluative data for the public.

Financial applications were the first computer-based management information systems available in healthcare organizations and, thus, accessible to chief nursing officers. Although the benefits of financial systems are easily observable and measurable, the usefulness of other management information systems to nurse executives continues to increase. Nurse executives are recognizing the value of information and the necessity to make data-based resource decisions. The spiraling complexity of patient care problems, the shift from the hospital to the community as the base of care, and the pressures for quality care that is fiscally responsible have prompted nurse executives to require timely access to useful and reliable information.

To meet these challenges, new management methods and automated tools are required. Manual data processing has become increasingly ineffective in supporting management decision making. The advantages of automation extend beyond its number crunching capabilities and great speed and include enhanced accuracy, increased detail, and flexibility and standardization in reporting.

Nurse executives generally have a variety of automated tools for examining and monitoring components of expense and clinical data. They get

[1]Parts of this chapter are used with permission from the following: M. Peterson and K. J. Hannah (1988). Nursing management information systems. In M. J. Ball, K. J. Hannah, U. Gerdin-Jelger, and H. Peterson (eds.). *Nursing Informatics: Where Caring and Technology Meet* (pp. 190–202). New York: Springer-Verlag; K. J. Hannah, M. J. Ball, and M. J. A. Edwards (1994). *Introduction to Nursing Informatics*. New York: Springer-Verlag.

salary and supply budget reports, workload measurement reports, length-of-stay data, resource utilization and quality management data, patient demographics, and other staff and financial documents. The difficulty with these indicators is that little is revealed about the level, quality, appropriateness, cost, or clinical outcomes of care delivered to a specific patient. Information about ambulatory care is either not available or in a format incompatible for comparison with inpatient information. The materials are presented and viewed linearly and singularly. There is a lack of standardization of indicators and terminology across institutions; this makes benchmarking and identifying best practices difficult or impossible. Additionally, the data often are outdated because of the time lag between the episodes of care and the processing of the information. Overall, nurse executives are left to cope with management information systems that are data rich and information poor.

In this chapter, we examine how automation and computers can assist nursing administration leadership in decision making. We discuss the definition of management information systems and a variety of management information systems and other computer applications that may be valuable to the nurse executive. Following a review of these applications, we present some considerations to ensure that information is useful and relevant as well as challenging to the nurse executive in the development and use of new applications.

Management Information Systems: A Definition

Management information systems have been developed largely in the business and industrial sectors by management scientists but are relevant to nursing and all other health professions. A management information system is an array of components designed to transform a collective set of data into knowledge that is directly useful and applicable in the process of directing and controlling resources and their application to the achievement of specific management objectives (Hanson, 1982). Austin (1992) defines a management information system as a "set of formalized procedures designed to provide current information for management planning and control" (p. 327). More simply, a management information system is a system that provides information to assist the manager and administrator in the decision-making process and would broadly include financial, clinical, and human resources information. The level of involvement in the decision making varies. In some instances, the management information system is limited to processing, storing, and retrieving of information. Other systems allow the user to estimate the outcomes of alternative decisions through modeling. Finally, one group of applications allows networking with personnel within one's own work setting as well as with colleagues globally. These applications, which include office automation, local access networks, and the Internet, allow the chief nurse executive to communicate interactively, to ask for information, or to announce a decision once it has been reached.

From the nurse executive's perspective, the primary intent of a nursing management information system is the provision of information to make decisions about the effective and efficient allocation of resources for the highest quality of patient care (Hannah and Shamian, 1992). Although this description could apply to both manual and automated systems, the following review will be limited to the most common automated management information systems.

Management Information Systems Applications

Increasingly, the nurse executive's role in resource allocation and management is being facilitated by the use of management information systems. With recent advances in computer software, nursing management applications support decision making and strategic planning and provide a mechanism for communicating decisions. Automated systems now play a critical part in fiscal, clinical, human resources, and office management. Specific systems include fiscal resource management, patient care services costs, quality and patient care process management, workload measurement, personnel management, staff scheduling, and inter- and intraoffice networking.

Fiscal Management

Operating Budgets

Nurse executives may have access to information about both the expenses and revenues of their institutions. Computers can easily store and manipulate the range of data required for budgetary purposes. In most healthcare institutions, nursing personnel costs are a major portion of the institution's operating costs. Examples of other budgets within the purview of the nurse executive, either indirectly or in collaboration with other departments, are supply, capital equipment, renovation, and information technology budgets. Management information systems collect, summarize, and format data for use in administrative decision making related to the nursing and nursing-influenced budgets. Periodically produced reports allow the monitoring of budgets, identification of budget variances (difference in actual versus planned expenses), and assistance with planning future budgets. The reports can be numerical or graphic displays and can include trending of specific budget information. An advantage of the use of automated financial systems is the speed with which data can be retrieved, compiled, summarized, and presented in a consistent, meaningful, and comprehensive form. Another benefit is the ability to design reports for individual needs and situations. This facilitates the ongoing monitoring of activities within the institution and preparation of reports to other corporate staff or departments, the board of trustees, or outside agencies.

Costing Systems

"The most basic function of cost accounting is the determination of the costs of running the organization" (Finkler, 1991). Cost accounting systems assist in understanding the costs and cost behaviors of a defined unit. In health care, these systems primarily have generated retrospective cost information with the department as the unit of analysis. Although these historical data are still important, there is a shift in the use of these systems to project what costs should be and to establish cost standards. In addition, there is a movement toward costing out nursing care for specific patient care groups as well as determining the cost of an entire episode of care for a designated patient group.

Given the increasing emphasis on cost control, nurse executives understand that they must be able to cost out nursing services as well as nursing's contribution to defined patient care processes to compete for limited resources (Johnson, 1989). There are many cost accounting systems used to determine nursing's contribution. These include using per diem, diagnosis or diagnostic-related groups, or workload measurement and patient classification systems to determine cost. As in other components of management information systems, the actual costs associated with collecting the cost data and access to usable and valid data are issues in determining the costs of nursing and patient care processes. Integrated management information systems are critical to the ability of a nurse executive, and the entire organization, to obtain and use cost information for decision making about the allocation of resources.

Human Resources Management

At the most basic level, computer applications can be used to accumulate data regarding the employment and educational history of each staff member. Information stored may include absenteeism rate, sick and vacation time status, as well as highest degree obtained, certifications, contact hours, and performance appraisals. Personnel databases are useful for accreditation purposes, to locate a staff member with special skills, or to monitor adherence to institutional requirements for annual educational endeavors. Moreover, an automated system allows ease in retrieving personnel information to determine staffing assignments via a workload measurement system.

Workload Measurement

Nurses' salaries and benefits generally are a significant portion of the overall institutional budget. The challenge for the nurse executive is to ensure that nursing staff is available at a level sufficient to meet patient needs yet be cost effective. Patient census data were used in the past to forecast the appropriate level of staffing. However, as patient care needs have increased in complexity, this single measure has become inadequate. Other factors such as personnel mix, ancillary support, environmental factors, physician practices, and care delivery system must be considered in determining effective staffing requirements.

Workload measurement systems have been developed to address the multivariate indicators of patient complexity. The workload systems provide both direct and indirect estimates of nursing care within a particular medical case type by day and over time. The ability of the computer to store, manipulate, and retrieve large volumes of data rapidly is essential.

Examples of systems include GRASP, Medicus, and PRN 80. The various systems differ in their theoretical basis and approach. For example, in the GRASP system, time standards for nursing activities carried out for and with patients are measured; nursing hours of care are defined as the sum of all activities. The Medicus system defines a patient type through the application of indicators, and nursing hours of care are developed for each patient type. There is no standard within nursing for workload measurement, and comparative differences have been found among the different systems (O'Brien-Pallas, Cockerill, and Leatt, 1992).

Staffing Systems

Immeasurable time has been spent in healthcare institutions generating staffing schedules. Even with the use of master rotation plans, manual scheduling does not seem to eliminate all the problems related to perceived biases in assignments, balancing adequate staffing with cost, and integrating special requests. Thus, automated staff scheduling is a potentially useful component of a nursing management system. The types of systems range from the use of the computer to print what is essentially a manual rotation schedule to adjusting staff on a shift-by-shift basis by considering patient acuity, workload levels, and the expertise of the staff. The more sophisticated scheduling systems require an upfront investment of intense planning and data gathering. Necessary information includes identification of levels of staff expertise, and criteria for determining patient acuity and nursing workload must be established. Personnel policies, including elements of union contracts, must be defined. A computer program is then designed that integrates all the information and schedules nursing staff by units.

The ability of the computer to manipulate large numbers of variables consistently and quickly makes personnel time assignments an excellent use of this technology. Advantages of the use of automated scheduling include less time spent on scheduling, unbiased assignments, and advance notice of staff shortages. Of most interest to the nurse executive is the availability of information about the relationship between staff size and characteristics regarding quality of care.

Clinical Management

Quality Management

Total quality management and continuous quality improvement have superseded the previous quality assurance movement. Nurse executives use these processes to assess the overall quality of patient care within their institution and to receive and communicate opportunities that enhance patient care and organizational effectiveness. Additionally, external agencies, such as the Joint Commission on Accreditation for Healthcare Organizations, Medicare, and the Canadian Council on Hospital Facilities Accreditation, require the monitoring of specific quality indicators.

Institutions use a variety of approaches to gather information to evaluate the quality of patient care. For quality assessment, information needs might include patient care data, patients' evaluations of and satisfaction with care provided, chart documentation, care plans or care paths, performance appraisals, and incident reports. Audit reviews are a major tool for any quality program, and audits of these potential information sources are reviewed either concurrently or retrospectively.

Nurse executives have found integrated hospital information systems very useful in the retrieving, summarizing, and comparing large volumes of data necessary for quality improvement initiatives. Unfortunately, only a few healthcare institutions have systems that provide the capacity for on-line (computerized) integrated data retrieval, particularly concurrent data, for audit purposes. Costly and timely manual systems or reports from isolated systems are used for much of the data collection for quality initiatives. It is difficult to identify and analyze utilization patterns and outcomes in clinically meaningful groups of patients or phases of care using either a manual approach or unrelated reports. Certainly, the scarcity of integrated hospital systems is one of the obstacles to the use of computers to support total quality management and continuous quality improvement programs.

Other obstacles include the lack of a widely accepted method for coding patient care activities and interventions and the focus on the process aspects of quality management rather than the product. The quality of the tools used to provide input is another problem with computerized quality management programs. Most tools lack relevant patient outcome indicators, and the validity of even the most widely used audit tools and criteria is largely unsubstantiated.

Patient Care Process Management

Nurse executives usually receive reports of patient census data, volume determination, patient acuity data, and admission, discharge, and transfer data. Often, this information can be accessed via a personal computer connection to the healthcare institution's mainframe. Some institutions are automating their clinical process management tools, known as care paths or critical pathways. Care paths are discussed in Chapter 15 of this book, and these pathways can be important tools for the nurse executive in determining the cost of nursing care related to a designated patient group or planning resource allocations.

Other Applications

Office Automation

Office automation is the application of computer and communications technology to office activities. The purposes of such automation are to improve effectiveness, improve efficiency, and control office operations.

Computerization and communication technologies are changing the work environments of all workers in health care, including administrative, clinical, and clerical staff. Office technology has the potential to affect most aspects of a nursing department's work, such as text processing, filing, meeting planning, and distributing meeting agendas and minutes.

Word processing via a single computer is a simple example of office automation. It involves the automated manipulation of text to produce office communications in a printed medium. Word processing offers many advantages. It reduces the time and expense invested in correcting or retyping text material and shortens the time needed to produce a finished document. Storage and retrieval of documents can be handled quickly and efficiently. It is possible to search for documents by key words, titles, or date of preparation.

A local area network (LAN) allows the grouping of freestanding personal computers into a coordinated, multiuser computer system. Users of a LAN can communicate via computers between multiple sites, share information easily, and send a complete document electronically. Rather than the usual "telephone tag," ease in scheduling appointments, planning meetings, and asking and responding to questions via the LAN electronic mail (E-mail) is beneficial. Widespread distribution of agendas and minutes and database and software sharing are all possible via the LAN. Other advantages include ease in accessing information and increased accuracy, timeliness, and efficiency of information for decision making. It is important for the nurse executive to understand that implementation of a LAN requires ongoing support in both the technical and the educational realms. Moreover, the nurse executive's use of the LAN will model, and thus encourage, the use of the system (Chapman et al., 1994).

Internet

The Internet is a network of networks that circles the globe. It is a "vast, sprawling network that reaches into computer sites worldwide . . . [and] this interlinked web of networks defies attempts at quantification" (Gilster, 1994, p. 15). This international network provides an opportunity for the nurse executive to network widely and to gather information easily and quickly from colleagues across town, country, and world.

One of the most basic and used services of the Internet is electronic mail (E-mail). Via this function, nurse executives can ask questions, request or share information, or simply communicate and network with colleagues about common interests.

Other opportunities on the Internet for the nurse executive include broadcasting messages and questions to colleagues who belong to online groups regarding specific topic areas and receiving responses from around the world, accessing external databases for clinical and cost data from other institutions, obtaining sharable software, performing literature searches, and conducting electronic meetings. Nurse executives may access the Internet through an organizational LAN, university connection, commercial service, or free service (Free-Net) that some cities provide (Nicoll, 1994).

Nursing Management Information Systems: Issues and Challenges for the Nurse Executive

With the proliferation of computers, acquiring information has been influenced in many aspects, including the speed with which information is obtained, ease of access, availability of new information or information in different forms, and timeliness of information (Danziger and Kraemer, 1986). All of these contribute to the nurse executive's ability to use information to make swift decisions. The advantage of automated management information systems is their ability to process more timely data at a greater speed. This statement suggests that more is equated with better in the realm of management information. However, a distinction must be made between data and information. Data are simply a string of characters, whereas information acts as a signal that predisposes a person to take action. The role of the computer, therefore, is to process data so they take a useful and relevant form, called information. Unfortunately, because of the lack of integration of the multiple information systems in healthcare institutions, much of the output of computers is data rather than information. There is not the technology to bring all the pieces of data together to do the kind of analysis that gives the nurse executive confidence that planning and action are based on information and not just gut reactions to data. A more desirable approach is an integrated system that defines the healthcare institution's output in relation to the number and types of patients who are receiving care. Once the output is defined in a more meaningful way (i.e., patients versus departments), the cost or resources used to produce the outputs and healthcare outcomes achieved via the outputs can be explored in an integrated manner. Cost effectiveness rather than cost containment will be the focus. Cost, quality, and outcome data all contribute to the wise decision making related to resource allocation.

Nursing must become the key figure, not the key target, in shaping the interface between cost and quality. Nurse executives must be bilingual, understanding the outputs from both cost and quality information systems. Nurses can be active participants in ensuring that organizations assimilate and incorporate a philosophy of balancing cost and quality. Integrated information systems can certainly advance or strengthen this balance. Clinically accurate decision making that achieves a balance of cost and quality will be dependent on the integration of these fiscal, clinical, and personnel information components.

In a recent survey of hospitals of various sizes, an overwhelming majority (93% of 688 hospitals) reported that they planned to increase their spending on information systems by an average of 10% on operations and approximately 12% on capital projects over the next 3 years (Morrissey, 1994). It seems timely for nurse executives to be active players in these information systems decisions. To support this role for the nurse executive, selected issues and challenges, with relevant strategies, are discussed.

Data Issues

The concern about reliability and validity of data is a significant and widespread issue for all components of nursing management information systems (see Table 18-1). The quality of what one gets as output is dependent on the quality of the input. The quality of the input can be influenced by the accuracy, compliance, and completeness of the input. A thorough initial assessment followed by ongoing assessment of the quality is critical. The nurse executive needs to ask questions, such as "Are the data sufficient?" "Are accurate (versus biased) data being collected and used for decision making?" For example, regular monthly screening to document the consistent application of indicators and patient types is essential to valid and reliable workload measures. Nursing costs have never been projected reliably because fluctuating patient acuity levels and the related needs for nursing care have not been incorporated. With the integration of fiscal, human resources, and clinical data, costs for nursing care of individual patients will be available.

The availability of real-time rather than only retrospective data is closely related to the issues of validity and reliability. Historical data are important for understanding overtime events (trending). However, in the frenetic environment of health care today, nurse executives need management information systems that provide timely data for resource allocation as well as clinical decisions. Some management information systems, such as the financial components, can only provide data that are weeks or even months old. This lag leads to missed opportunities for timely decisions. The use of

TABLE 18-1. Management Information Data Issues, Challenges, and Strategies for the Nurse Executive

Issues/Challenges	Strategies
Data Issues	
Reliability and validity	1. Conduct regular checks for accuracy and completeness of data sets 2. Monitor compliance of data input
Real time versus retrospective	1. Document differences in decisions made when using real-time rather than retrospective data 2. Advocate for purchase/upgrade of systems that provide real-time data
Availability of necessary data to capture entire episode of care	1. Educate information services and fiscal personnel about the need to include outpatient data in all systems 2. When new systems are being purchased and/or developed, support systems that can integrate financial, human resources, and clinical data for both inpatient and outpatient care 3. Have nursing actively participate in the definition of cost, quality, and outcome components

real-time data to determine staffing requirements or to adjust a care path based on a patient's clinical profile is vital to ensuring high-quality care that is efficient (i.e., to ensuring the quality/cost balance). Nurse executives are in a position to document the differences in the financial, human resources, and/or clinical decisions made when using real-time versus retrospective data.

One final issue relates to the availability of necessary data and the responsiveness of organizations in providing these data. Of particular challenge in today's environment is the capacity of information systems to integrate data across the continuum of care. The core business of health care is shifting from the acute, inpatient setting to primary care and wellness (Shortell, Gillies, Anderson, Mitchell, and Morgan, 1993), and management information systems need to be better equipped to provide nurse executives with quality and cost information about a patient's entire episode of care. The challenge will be the definition of the cost, quality, and outcome components as well as the availability of the data for processing.

Collaboration/Relationship Issues

Strategic alliances are critical to the development of useful management information systems (see Table 18-2). No longer can the nurse executive make decisions about resources in isolation. There is a need for dialogue, collaboration, and working agreements among all senior administrators regarding identification and management of resources. Additionally, these

TABLE 18-2. Relationship and Collaboration Issues, Challenges, and Strategies for Management Information Systems

Issues/Challenges	Strategies
Nurse administrator working with data and information in isolation	1. Form a strong partnership among nursing, other care providers, finance, human resources, and information services senior administrators to create integrated systems and information 2. Initiate dialogue and collaboration with all senior administrators regarding the identification and management of resources 3. Establish a solid nursing informatics expertise in the nursing department to drive nursing information needs 4. Educate nonclinical administrators about clinical care 5. Take and make the opportunities to learn the language and detail of the data requirements of the finance, human resources, and information services departments 6. Ensure that nursing is an active participant in the selection, installation, and evaluation of any financial, human resources, and/or clinical system 7. Articulate the benefits of merging financial, human resources, and clinical databases
Nurse executive as role model in use of data for decision making	1. Explicitly use data to illustrate how resource decision was made 2. Require nurse managers to use data to substantiate resource and clinical decisions
Sharing data across Institutions	1. Support a nursing management minimum data set, including pursuing Institutional backing for standardized data collection and processing 2. Access Internet to network and give and receive information from other nurse executives throughout the world

partnerships must extend to the priority-setting and decision-making processes surrounding management information systems. Nurse executives can be champions for implementing user-friendly management information systems and leaders in articulating the potential benefits of merging financial, human resources, and clinical components of an institution's information systems so that resource allocation decisions are made based on information rather than simply on unsubstantiated data, history, or feelings.

Nursing administrators may serve as role models for the use of data to make decisions. When making presentations to other senior managers or to nurse managers, the nurse executive should illustrate explicitly how data were used to arrive at a particular decision related to resource allocation. Similarly, the nurse executive might reinforce the significance of management information systems and the available data by requiring nurse managers to use data to substantiate resource and clinical decisions.

It is useful to have nurses with informatics expertise within the nursing department or access to this expertise through agreements with university faculty or consultants. Along with the nurse executive, these experts can educate others in the organization about clinical care, the value and meaning of data, and clinical systems requirements. Moreover, the nurse executive and nursing informatics experts must learn the data sources and requirements in other departments so that they can use all existing data and are knowledgeable contributors to decisions about creating integrated systems and information.

Nursing is a major stakeholder in a healthcare organization and thus needs to be "at the table" and an active participant in all components of the selection and installation of management information systems. A strong nursing presence is required in all phases. These include the needs and feasibility assessment, the request for proposals, the system design and software development, implementation, and evaluation and maintenance.

In addition to within organization collaboration, interaction is needed across institutions. The ability to identify best practices and/or benchmark via shared databases would be of great benefit to nurse executives and, ultimately, patient care. Huber and associates (Huber, Delaney, Crossley, Mehmert, and Ellerbe, 1992) have proposed a nursing management minimum data set.

This data set is a collection of core data elements that would assist nurse managers and executives in decision making about care effectiveness. The data set would include uniform elements so that comparisons could be made within as well as across healthcare institutions. Elements of interest include four dimensions: structure, process, resources; outcomes; personnel; and relational database links. Nursing unit characteristics, Medicare case mix cost, staff resources, budget, patient and provider satisfaction, and average intensity of nursing care are examples of potential data elements. Computerization would provide the opportunity for ease in processing, sharing, and comparing the nursing management minimum data set, but issues related to its implementation are significant. Critical to the success of such a venture is the determination of common terminology and definitions of data elements and a uniform method for collecting and reporting data elements.

The issue of knowing the data, using them, and maximizing them is essential. Nurse executives and members of an institution and a nursing department could enhance their decision-making abilities by using systems and processes recommended in this chapter. The relationship between management information systems and nurse executives must be a dynamic one. Continuous development and changes in both the area of information systems and technology and health care and nursing provide an ongoing fertile ground for development. Current and future innovations in information systems and technology could further empower nurse executives to achieve a quality and cost balance in health care.

As the core business of health care shifts from the acute, inpatient setting to primary care and wellness (Shortell et al., 1993), management information systems need to be better equipped to provide nurse executives with the quality and cost information about a patient's entire episode of care. The challenge will be the definition of cost, quality, and outcome components as well as the availability of the data for processing.

Questions

1. How are management information systems defined in this chapter? Would you change this definition in any way?
2. What are some of the advantages of using a computer system for staffing and scheduling?
3. What obstacles are there to using computers for quality management?
4. How are computers changing the work environment of healthcare workers?
5. What are some of the elements you would propose be included in a nursing management minimum data set? Think about the information needs in your organization as a start.

References

Austin CJ: *Information Systems for Health Services Administration.* 4th ed. Ann Arbor, MI: Health Administration Press, 1992.

Chapman RH, Reiley P, McKinney J, Welch K, Toomey B, McCausland M: Implementing a local area network for nursing in a large teaching hospital. *Computers in Nursing* 1994; 12: 82–88.

Danziger JN, Kraemer KL: *People and Computers: The Impacts of Computing on End Users in Organizations.* New York: Columbia University Press, 1986.

Finkler S: *Finance & Accounting for Nonfinancial Managers.* Englewood Cliffs, NJ: Prentice Hall, 1991.

Gilster P: *The Internet Navigator.* 2nd ed. New York: Wiley, 1994.

Hannah K, Shamian J: Integrating a nursing professional practice model and nursing informatics in a collective bargaining environment. *Nursing Clinics of North America* 1992; 27: 31–45.

Hanson R: Applying management information systems to staffing. *Journal of Nursing Administration* 1982; 12(10): 5–9.

Huber DG, Delaney C, Crossley J, Mehmert M, Ellerbe S: A nursing management minimum data set. *Journal of Nursing Administration* 1992; 22(7/8): 35–40.

Johnson M: Perspectives on costing nursing. *Nursing Administration Quarterly* 1989; 14(1): 65–71.

Morrissey J: Spending more on computers to help keep costs in line. *Modern Healthcare* 1994; February 14: 63–70.

Nicoll LH: An introduction to the Internet. Part I: History, structure, and access. *Journal of Nursing Administration* 1994; 24(3): 9–11.

O'Brien-Pallas L, Cockerill R. Leatt P: Different systems, different costs? *Journal of Nursing Administration* 1992; 22(12): 17–22.

Shortell SM, Gillies RR, Anderson DA, Mitchell JB, Morgan KL: Creating organized delivery systems: The barriers and facilitators. *Hospital & Health Services Administration* 1993; 38: 447–466.

19
Healthcare Information Systems

BENNIE E. HARSANYI, DAVID H. WILSON,
MARGUERITE A. DANIELS, KATHLEEN C. ALLAN,
AND JOHN ANDERSON

Introduction

Healthcare reform arising from the consumer's demand for cost-effective health access, services, and quality requires a new, previously unimagined health delivery system. The healthcare industry, administrators, and care providers are challenging traditional approaches, structures, roles, practices, and information system technology. Healthcare organizations are exploring such avenues as continuous quality improvement, managed care, patient-centered reengineering, integrated health networks, and a computer-based patient record. The traditional hospital information system is changing to provide for the management and processing of patient-centered data, information, and knowledge across the healthcare continuum, patient's life span, windows of time, and diffuse organizational and geographical boundaries. The traditional hospital information system has now become a healthcare information system.

Patient-Centered Collaborative Care Delivery Framework

A traditional hospital information system "is a communication network linking terminals and output devices in key patient care or service areas to a central processing unit that coordinates all essential patient care activities" (Hannah, Ball, and Edwards, 1994, p. 45). The traditional hospital information system typically includes financial, administrative, clinical, and stand-alone systems and a communications network (Hannah et al., 1994). This view also requires interface engine technology for complex and numerous interfaces to coordinate applications and databases from diverse and disparate information systems. In an era of reform, a key requirement is an integrated, patient-centered information management system distributed over a network. In this type of system, clinical, financial, internal data, external data, information, and knowledge are integrated. In addition, there is the need for intuitive, common, seamless access to data by expanded and diverse user groups, thus also expanding the purpose of the traditional hospital information system.

The patient-centered collaborative care delivery framework (Fig. 19-1) illustrates a healthcare perspective and the requirements for integration. Patient-centered care, at the core of the framework, cannot be achieved without considering the ever-changing healthcare system, environment, and informatics technology. All of these impact the access, cost/value, quality/outcomes, and services provided to the educated consumer. These integrated components, especially informatics technology, require consideration in the design, implementation, and evaluation of systems managing and processing patient-centered data across the healthcare continuum. Healthcare informatics is an avenue for the definition, measurement, and evaluation of the healthcare delivery process.

A dynamic and cyclical process is reflected in the circular nature of this framework. The managed reengineering of healthcare delivery structures, processes, resources, treatment patterns, outcomes, and technology requires the ongoing exchange of information, as reflected by the arrows in each of the circles in Figure 19-1. Just as the integration of patient-centered data, information, and knowledge is necessary, framework component integration is necessary for healthcare information systems today and in the future. The goal of this patient-centered collaborative care delivery framework is to facilitate cost-efficient quality care and outcomes valued by the

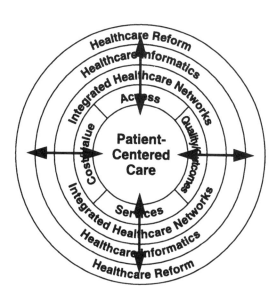

FIGURE 19-1. Patient-centered collaborative care delivery framework.

consumer (Harsanyi, 1993; Harsanyi, Lehmkuhl, Hott, Myers, and Mc-Geehan, 1994).

The healthcare challenges today are to ensure a healthy population and to treat illness using the most cost-effective therapeutic options affording minimal risk and predictable outcomes. Today, healthcare delivery is expanding beyond the walls of the hospital and the acute care inpatient episode. Hospitals are uniting with the community to offer expanded services focusing on care, wellness, and prevention. Hospitals are networking with clinics, physicians' offices, wellness centers, and affiliated remote satellite healthcare facilities.

The care provider's need for integrated patient-centered data, information, and knowledge is a driving force in the expansion of healthcare information systems applications and functionality. At the core of the healthcare continuum are the individual patient, families, and community. Information systems technology enhances the integrated collaborative health care provided by diverse care providers in the acute care setting as well as the extended community care setting.

Technology Perspective

As a result of healthcare reform, healthcare information systems (HISs) have shifted from billing to the management and coordination of health care. As health care continues to be delivered in nontraditional settings for consumer convenience, the purpose of healthcare information systems will continue to be redefined. At the heart of the healthcare information system is the computer-based patient record. The purpose of the computer-based patient record is to provide user accessibility to comprehensive and accurate data, including alerts and reminders. It also provides integration with clinical decision support systems, knowledge bases, and other aids for enhancing quality care delivery (Ball and Collen, 1992; Dick and Steen, 1991; McDonald, Tierney, Overhage, Martin, and Wilson, 1992).

Three major components of the computer-based patient record are collection, storage, and retrieval of patient-centered data. In the evolution of the computer-based patient record, the sources of patient data are first automated and integrated. Second, clinical workstations for information retrieval and data entry functions for care providers are implemented. Third, knowledge-based functions are phased into the computer-based patient record. Finally, this record is linked with the institutions in the community and ultimately linked into a national and global network (Johnson, 1994).

Although numerous barriers to achieving a computer-based patient record are being identified, the most salient ones are legality, confidentiality, and security (Ball and Collen, 1992; Fishman, 1994). New and evolving technologies provide for the automation and integration of diverse data types across the healthcare continuum and a future global network. Diagnostic images, waveform signals, motion video, voice, and document images are examples of data types for inclusion in the computer-based patient record (Abdelhak, Firouzan, and Ullman, 1993; Ball and Collen, 1992; Johnson, 1994).

A good example of distributed computing is an architecture known as client server. Client server technology can extend and enhance the healthcare information system by distributing computing services between a "requester" and a "provider." The requester, or "client," could be a PC, whether a laptop, handheld, pen-based, or standard desktop model. The provider, or "server," could be another PC, a Reduced Instruction Set Computer (RISC), a minicomputer, a mainframe or microframe computer. Both the client and the server assume certain responsibilities for processing. For example, the client handles presentation services, so the user can interact with sophisticated graphical user interfaces like Microsoft Windows, integrating common services such as electronic mail, medical dictionaries, and external system linkages. The server or servers then handle such things as application execution, database services, and even some network services. The point is that each component is configured to achieve the best possible result.

Client-server technology provides ease of use through its presentation of information in graphical formats and multimedia capabilities, such as imaging support. Client-server technology also offers the ability to tailor solutions around the care provider's needs instead of changing his or her work patterns to fit the computer's requirements. Information access is greatly enhanced by graphical presentations, integration of desktop packages, medical dictionaries, electronic mail, and external database linkages. Client-server capabilities offer the care provider access to advanced graphical user interfaces, integration tools, multimedia, and end user tailoring tools. Security in this type of environment typically includes network, application, and database security.

Network infrastructures provide the conduit for the sharing and integration of applications using open system standards. Local area networks and wide area networks using fiber optic technology provide the avenue for the high-speed transmission required for today's environment. In the past, retrieved data took the form of approximately 600 characters per screen blip. Today, the care provider receives 50,000 characters of information for a document image, 1,000,000 characters for a server application, and up to 8,000,000 characters for a medical image. For example, the transmission of a medical image over a typical 19.2 kilobytes per second analog line will take 55.5 minutes to reach the diagnostician. Today's answer is fiber optic cabling using glass fibers, not subject to interference, with the transmission capability of the speed of light. Speeds of 100,000,000 characters per second can be reached using this technology. This means that the aforementioned diagnostic image can be transmitted in approximately six-tenths of a second as opposed to nearly 1 hour.

Applications written for the client-server environment employ languages that are portable in nature, such as C++; therefore, the applications can run on different platforms without having to be rewritten. Languages such as C++ use "objects" to describe things like a patient, a visit, or an order. These objects can then be modified, assembled, and reused in other applications. The net effect of this approach is that systems become easier to build and adapt. Systems can then employ a layer of software known as middleware to make the application relatively database independent. For example, a clinical repository could reside in a number of industry standard database management products.

Client-server systems may also use different desktop operating systems and graphical user interfaces to improve the care provider's ability to format the data. Open systems are used to allow any system to communicate with any other system, using any communications protocol, transferring data in any format regardless of the sending or receiving system's hardware, software, or communications architecture. Messaging standards such as Health Level Seven (HL7) are used to build a common structure for exchanging information between disparate systems. Industry standard reporting options also provide the care provider ease of use.

Access

To illustrate the use of healthcare information systems for access, cost/ value, quality/outcomes, and services, significant technological components and examples will be highlighted. This discussion is not meant to be all-inclusive.

Healthcare reform calls for universal consumer access to standardized essential services delivered in convenient, familiar, and nontraditional settings familiar to the consumer. This care is delivered by transdisciplinary care providers using cost-efficient options for the prevention, restoration, and maintenance of health and wellness (American Nurses Association, 1991). The care provider also requires access to patient-centered data across the patient's life span, care continuum, and diverse delivery settings.

The initial healthcare information system venture into clinical information systems began with the design of patient management capabilities to support inpatient and outpatient registration. This same patient management functionality can also be interfaced with a physician practice system to address the financial, clinical, and administrative needs of academic practice plans, freestanding clinics, and hospital-based physicians.

Using an integrated and client-server-based HIS, a nurse practitioner could sign on from home to all systems for his practicing environment via a network access password and sign-on. At this time, the nurse could check his or her personal and professional schedule for the day, including clinical information regarding her first patient, Mrs. Jordan, pregnant with her first child. At the primary care clinic, a patient care representative could quickly identify and reregister Mrs. Jordan while also surveying past encounters. Health coverage could also be identified and initiated. The ob/gyn physician, using a clinical workstation, could access existing clinical data while also scheduling the appropriate tests, examinations, consultations, referrals, and treatments. Concurrently, as the resources are scheduled, costs are determined. Once the care, charges, and billing are completed, an electronic claim is sent to the insurance company. The care provider can check on the status of this claim, and payment can automatically be transmitted and posted to the billing system. Communication to colleagues or notification to Mrs. Jordan that her annual physical is due can also occur.

One technological component in this scenario is the ability to use point-of-care technologies to access the common, seamless presentation of patient-centered data. Diverse technologies are necessary to support a continuum of care. The physician might use a PC-based clinical workstation, whereas an ICU nurse might use a stationary bedside device. Additional devices used by an ambulatory care or home health nurse could include a laptop PC workstation, portable tablet, and handheld devices using radio frequency technology.

A second technological component regarding access in this scenario is a patient/member repository of demographic data shared by all users across the healthcare organization. A patient/member repository, using relational database technology, includes key identification, demographic, and event information. Admission clerks and caregivers access this repository regarding information about patients/members, guarantors, employees, physicians, and insurance carriers. This repository facilitates the management of numerous business functions, such as fiscal management, continuous quality improvement, patient satisfaction, and care provider management. For example, fiscal management provides reporting across member populations. The demographic repository streamlines the registration process by initially providing comprehensive, complete, and accurate member information. Consumer satisfaction is improved by care provider knowledge of the member and his or her encounters with the healthcare organization. Care provider management is enhanced by a common, seamless access to this and other portions of the computer-based patient record.

As illustrated in Figure 19-2, a third technological component regarding access is an electronic data interchange service and applications that provide an information conduit outside of the healthcare organization to other hospitals, payors, suppliers, external case managers, and employers. Bidirectional transmission and data translation into a format that all information systems can use are also provided by this conduit. Using open system standards, services such as eligibility, financial settlement, capitated membership, care support, care authorization, utilization monitoring, and coordination of benefits and services can be integrated easily.

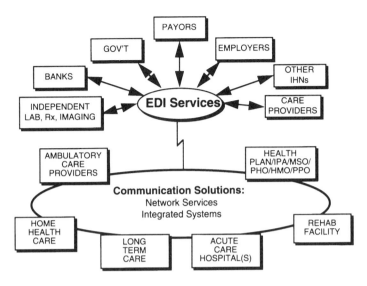

FIGURE 19-2. Electronic data interchange.

Care support services enable payors to communicate patient-specific information at the time care is provided. This can include details of benefit plan coverage, copayment requirements, managed care rules, coordination of benefits rules, status of deductibles, and clinical guidelines. A by-product of this communication process is a database, enhanced by intelligent processing, that adds value and perspective beyond that which can be obtained using traditional individual operational systems. When integrated with a clinical repository encompassing comprehensive security measures, the care provider has an integrated view of financial and clinical information.

Quality/Outcomes

The definitions of quality care and quality of life are changing. This change has resulted in continuous quality improvement initiatives, a consumer satisfaction focus, increasing care provider accountability, and outcomes management. It also requires the availability of cost-effective therapeutic options with predictable outcomes for the consumer's quality of life across the life span. Concomitantly, the comparison with comparable institutions and care providers regarding quality, lengths of stay, resource allocation, mortality, morbidity, and consumer satisfaction is resulting in the need for outcome analysis (American Nurses Association, 1991).

A fourth technological component, a clinical repository, provides for the tracking of consumer compliance to protocols for the preservation, restoration, and maintenance of health. The value of a clinical repository is the availability of consistent standardized data for outcome research regarding prevention, treatment, and education of the consumer. The ability to aggregate like patient population data for comparing clinical variances and outcomes improves care standards and treatment practices. For example, one research study using a database comparing 15 hospitals over a designated time period concluded that the mortality rate of patients with AIDS was related to the hospital's experience or lack of experience in treating AIDS patients with pneumocystis carinii pneumonia (Bennett et al., 1989). Clinical and institutional performance benchmarks can also be determined using a clinical repository. The development of standardized algorithms, statistical analysis, and evaluation tools also can be derived. Research activities using local, regional, national, and future global databases resulting in strategies for the refinement of health science, delivery, policies, and reform are essential (Joint Commission on Accreditation of Healthcare Organizations, 1994; Vibbert and Reichard, 1993).

A clinical repository, consisting of a relational database, provides patient-centered data for a 71-year-old patient, Mrs. Bloom, from across the patient's life span, care continuum, windows of time, organizational boundaries, and episodes of care (see Fig. 19-3). The care provider needs patient-specific data such as assessments and discharge plans as well as agency-specific data and domain-specific data such as policies and procedures and efficacy of various treatments for specific diagnoses (Zielstorff, Hudgings, and Grobe, 1993). Data collection of atomic-level data is necessary for this clinical repository, a key component of the computer-based patient record. "Essential, precise, and discrete elements captured at the point of care represent the atomic level data necessary for a clinical repository" (Graves and Corcoran, 1989).

The data in the clinical repository require the constancy and standardization of data elements. For nursing care delivery, the Nursing Minimum Data Set (NMDS) is an example affording comparability of aggregate populations across the care continuum, institutions, and time (Werley and Lang, 1988; Zielstorff et al., 1993). Numerous theoretical frameworks, data dictionaries, and lexicons are being proposed for care provider usage. A major effort is the development of a unified nursing language system for bridging numerous lexicons and the unified medical language system for medical terminology (Zielstorff et al., 1993). The American Nurses Association's Data Base Steering Committee recommended four research and practice classification systems: North American Nursing Diagnosis Association (NANDA), Georgetown Intervention Classification (also known as the Home Health Care Classification), the Omaha System, and the Iowa Nursing Interventions Classification (Hays, Norris, Martin, and Androwich, 1994; Martin and Scheet, 1992; McCloskey and Bulechek, 1992; North American Nursing Diagnosis Association, 1992; Saba et al., 1991).

Two additional technological components are an electronic flowsheet and a clinical decision-support system. The electronic flowsheet, supporting in-

CLINICAL REPOSITORY FLOW SHEET
FROM 03/01/87 TO 1/14/92   Page 1

BLOOM, VALERIE   MR#: 1030527   BDATE: 12/12/19   SEX: F

Active Problems	11/20/91 10:00	Medications	11/20/91 10:00	Allergies	11/20/91 10:00
Renal Artery Stenosis		Nephrocaps 1 tab/day		Penicillin	
Chronic Renal Failure		NPH Insulin 70U q am		Sulfa	
Coronary Artery Disease		Atenolol 25mg po hs			
Congestive Heart Failure		Tenex 1mg po bid			
Chronic Hypertension		Catapres 1 mg po bid			
Diabetes (IDDM) 7/88		Procardia 20mg po bid			
Peripheral Neuropathy		Coumadin 1mg po daily			

LABORATORY

	11/18/91 18:00	08/01/91 11:30	07/29/91 07:00	07/29/91 06:00	07/29/91 00:30	07/28/91 22:00	02/02/90 16:00	03/04/91 06:30	03/03/87 21:00
Chemistry									
Sodium	133*L	130*L	129*L	132*L	120*L		128*L	130*L	132*L
Potass	4.7	5.6*H	5.0	6.6*H			5.8*H	5.2*L	5.0
Chloride	90*L	96*L	91*L	94*L	92*L		102	96*L	102
Bicarbon	19*L	21*L	25	22	25				
BUN	86*H			61*H			75*H	50*H	35*H
Creatinine	8.2*HH	7.8*HH	6.7*H	8.8*H			8.2*H	6.5*H	3.5*H
Glucose	154*H	130*H	108	154*H			91	145*H	140*H
CPK	84			45		30			
CPK-MB	3.3			3.0		3.6			
LOH	255*H			182		153			
LDH1	74			40		38			
LDH2	102*H			70		61			
LDH1/LDH	0.73	4.60		0.57		0.61			
Glucose	154*H	130*H	108	154*H			91	145*H	140*H
Urea N		79*HH		74*HH					
Creatinine	8.2*HH	7.8*HH	6.7*H	8.8*HH			8.2*H	6.5*H	3.5*H
BUN/Crea		10		9			9	8	10
Sodium	133*L	130*L	129*L	132*L	120*L		128*L	130	132*L
Potass	4.7	5.6*H	5.0	6.6*H			5.8*H	5.2*L	5.0
Chloride	90*L	96*L	91*L	94*L	92*L		102	96*L	102
Bicarb	19*L	21*L	25	22	25				
Calcium		8.8		9.0			9.0	8.5	8.9
Hematology									
WBC	14.9*H			17.5				10.0	10.5*H
RBC	4.18*L			2.84*L				3.10*L	3.30*L
Hcrt%	37.0			26.2*L				30.0*L	34.0*L
Hgb	12.0			8.7*L				10.0*L	11.0*L
MCV	88.5			92.2			93.0	88.0	88.0

DISCHARGE SUMMARY
Disposition   11/20/91 10:00
She is on a low potassium diet, no activity restrictions. She is to see Dr. Morehouse in about 10 days and the phone number was given. Visiting nurse will be seeing her to review the diet and medications.

Adam Martelli, M.D.

This was one of several admissions for this patient, a 71 yr. old female with severe systolic hypertension and hyperkalemia. She was admitted the night prior to admission because of uncontrolled blood pressure, chest discomfort. She has a past history of renal artery stenosis, several admissions for congestive heart failure, esophageal ulcers, aortic stenosis, coronary artery disease, and diabetes. She is dialysed 3x/week and she recently had an episode of bradycardia for which she was seen by Dr. Morehouse as an outpatient.

FIGURE 19-3. Clinical repository flowsheet.

teractive charting, provides access to both current and historical data while using tailoring tools for user-defined formats to enhance clinical decision making. An electronic chart running on a PC clinical workstation can provide access to user-defined menu items, PC programs, HIS functions, PC-based applications, and external databases, including CD-ROM capability.

The care provider can also index large volumes of data similar to creating folders in a file cabinet. Graphical displays of user-defined data, including flowsheets, worklists, reports, graphs, waveforms, and images, are retrieved instantly from a clinical repository. For example, a case manager could tailor a list of patients for review and access integrated data comparing diverse variables. In the example of Mrs. Bloom, she is also an insulin-dependent diabetic, which can complicate her care. The case manager can access the electronic flowsheet and compare the administered insulin against the laboratory glucose values as well as the vital signs (see Fig. 19-4). Formats can include lists, tables, abstracts, bar/line graphs, and columnar trending by date ranges, occurrences, type of observations, and display sequences. All data ranging from a longitudinal problem list to waveforms such as electrocardiogram (EKG) strips are retrievable via this electronic flowsheet and a common clinical repository.

Documentation integration and compliance with quality improvement initiatives can be streamlined with interactive flowsheet charting. Various documentation models and formats, including standard and predefined charting selections, can be used with interactive charting. For example,

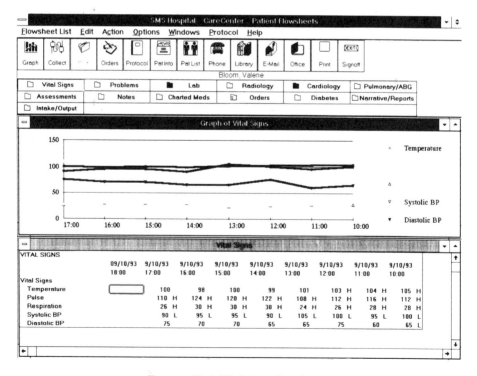

FIGURE 19-4. Vital signs flowsheet.

when documenting data for a patient whose condition has not changed, redundant data entry is eliminated with copy forward capability. The care provider can quickly highlight the text from the previous entry and copy it directly into the next entry as well as use legends and symbols as illustrated in Figure 19-5.

Another major technological component is a clinical decision-support system. Knowledge repository types that must be accommodated are reference, algorithmic, diagnostic inferences, treatment and care process logic, and outcomes and results information. Rules engines, acting on all data, and patterns of care recognition capability are integral components of patient-centered care delivery and evaluation. Clinician-defined rules provide alerts and reminders to clinicians, interactive feedback regarding physician order entry, and assistance in the assignment and adjustment of protocols of care. For example, Mrs. Jordan is also taking an antibiotic, Gentamicin, and her serum creatinine increases. A message would be sent to the care provider stating that, "creatinine is increased, consider renal insufficiency due to Gentamicin and diabetes diagnosis." Clinical decision-support integration provides complex logic and math, incorporates new knowledge from clinical research, and enhances quality improvement and cost containment for patient care management.

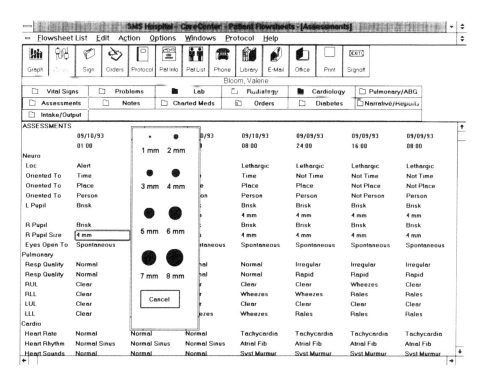

FIGURE 19-5. Assessment documentation.

Cost/Value

By the year 2000, virtually all Americans will be covered under a managed care plan. In determining the cost/value of healthcare delivery, the concept of integrated healthcare information systems is critical in a managed care environment. In support of a continuum of care, physician practice management, financial/accounting, managed care, and decision support are examples of the type of integrated software used. For example, a vice president of nursing is evaluating the feasibility of merging services to develop a women's health program. By using the daily information tracked in a decision-support module, the administrator studies inpatient and outpatient women's health encounters, compares the level of service to other hospitals in the region, and examines community demand for such services.

The administrator also wishes to evaluate clinical effectiveness and utilization of services while analyzing value and costs. Performance is measured by using cost, efficiency, and treatment profiles for the analysis of the care process. For example, a continuous quality improvement team uses the knowledge gained from the analysis of treatment patterns by physician, diagnosis, and outcomes to develop standards and protocols for a maternal and child health program.

By comparing outcomes and resource utilization to user-defined standards, differences in results are identified and the causes are isolated; therefore, problems and opportunities are immediately known. The vice president of nursing selects one button on her clinical workstation and accesses colored graphs and alerts regarding staffing, productivity, and profitability, thus enhancing the management team's focus on immediate needs. Detailed operational data stored in an integrated relational database provide the administrator with access to structured, exception, and custom reports while also providing "drill-down" capabilities for performance analysis. The vice president of nursing notices that patient volume in the maternal and child health program is decreasing. Decision-support payor information indicates that there is a decline in patients from two large health maintenance organizations (HMOs) that offer enrollees hospital choices. Using product line information, it is determined that preventive care and outpatient follow-up after the acute episode are components affording the greatest opportunity for improved quality and profitability. The maternal and child health services are repackaged as a comprehensive outreach program, including consumer education, preventive care, inpatient services, outpatient follow-up, and home care, thus revising an ineffective marketing strategy.

Upon reviewing a net income by payor contract, the vice president of nursing and chief executive officer observe that the profitability of one HMO contract, covering routine and low-volume work-related injuries, is decreasing. Drill-down reveals that an increase in volume and severity of case mix requiring comprehensive rehabilitation services is occurring. The reason for a profitability decrease is that the negotiated rate structure does not anticipate the case mix changes. Resource consumption is analyzed and decision support recalculates a new suggested rate. The vice president of nursing and the chief executive officer now have objective facts to propose that a split rate approach is necessary for quality care delivery to severely injured HMO enrollees.

Services

Case management, rooted in the client-provider relationship, is used to facilitate the consumer's lifelong access to services across the care continuum (American Nurses Association, 1991; Kongstvedt, 1993). While the major emphasis in patient assessment has been directed toward the diagnosis of disease and disease processes, one of the advantages of the computer-based patient record is the ability to monitor the health of the consumer as well.

To achieve this, the clinician needs rapid access to all patient-centered data, information, and knowledge at the point of care (thus the requirement for a clinical and demographic repository). Productivity tools, such as hand-held devices, physiological monitoring, and voice recognition, are also required at the point of care. Automated patient assessment supports the setting up of default values, displaying of the most recent values, and charting by exception for the diverse types of services delivered. Logic-based access to multiple views of data based on specific patient, clinician, specialty, and situation needs is also needed (thus the electronic flowsheet and clinical decision support). It is not the unique configuration of the data display as much as it is the breadth, flexibility, and power of the review and analysis functionality that creates value for the clinician.

A technological component to delivering services across the care continuum is the automation of integrated clinical standards/protocols, with orders, results, quality improvement initiatives, assessments, documentation, and clinical decision support. Automated clinical protocols support the definition and documentation of standards of care, associated variance management, and outcomes measurement across the continuum of care. To automate changing care delivery models, technological requirements include the capability to user-define protocols, tailor protocols based on the patient's clinical profile, use a critical path/map to identify and sequence the care and services, and evaluate the outcomes based on the standards/protocols.

Automated clinical protocols provide the framework for organizing the treatment, identifying the outcomes, and structuring the evaluation of care. As illustrated in Figure 19-6, an automated critical path shows the exact timing of key events and patient activities that must occur for the

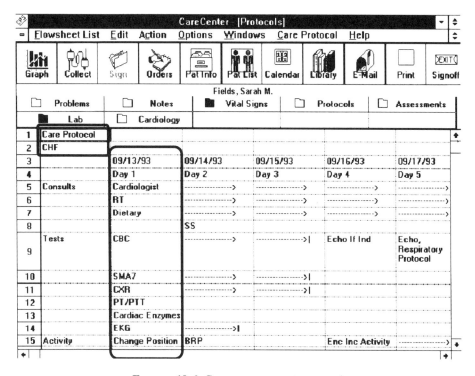

FIGURE 19-6. Case management protocol.

patient to achieve the defined outcomes within the designated time frames. Technological requirements also include the ability to define time-based, event-driven, and merged protocols such as the merging of Mrs. Jordan's pregnancy and diabetic protocols. To support consumer responsibility for the prevention, restoration, and maintenance of health, the use of computer-based interactive instruction and patient and family education adhering to the same defined standards enhances consumer compliance and satisfaction.

Summary

As is illustrated in Figure 19-7, the healthcare information system is expanding beyond the walls of the hospital and the acute care inpatient episode into an integrated health network. The goal is to promote, restore, and maintain health and wellness of the patient, family, and community. The care provider must assume a leadership role in the design, implementation, and evaluation of healthcare information systems for clinical practice, education, administration, and research.

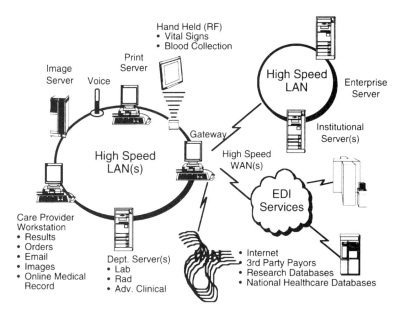

FIGURE 19-7. Integrated health network.

Questions

1. Discuss the barriers to achieving a computer-based patient record: legality, confidentiality, and security.
2. How does the patient-centered collaborative care delivery framework differ from the traditional hospital information system? How does the information system in your organization compare to the patient-centered collaborative system?

References

Abdelhak M, Firouzan PA, Ullman L: Hospital information systems applications and potential: A literature review revisited, 1982–1992. *Topics in Health Information Management* 1993; 13: 1–14.

American Nurses Association: *Nursing's Agenda for Health Care Reform.* Washington, DC: American Nurses Publishing, 1991.

Ball MJ, Collen MF: *Aspects of the Computer-Based Patient Record.* New York: Springer-Verlag, 1992.

Bennett CH, Garfinkle JB, Grumfield S, Druper D, Rogers W, Matthews WC, Kansuge DE: The relationship between hospital experience and in-hospital mortality for patients with AIDS-related PCP. *Journal of the American Medical Association* 1989; 261: 2975–2979.

Dick RS, Steen EB eds: *The Computer-Based Patient Record: An Essential Technology for Health Care.* Washington, DC: National Academy Press, 1991.

Fishman D: Confidentiality. *Computers in Nursing* 1994; 12(2): 73–77.

Graves JR, Corcoran S: The study of nursing informatics. *Image: Journal of Nursing Scholarship* 1989; 21(4): 227–231.

Hannah KJ, Ball MJ, Edwards MJA: *Introduction to Nursing Informatics.* New York: Springer-Verlag, 1994.

Harsanyi BE: Use of information systems to facilitate collaborative health care delivery. In: American Hospital Association, ed. *Proceedings of the 1993 Annual HIMSS Conference.* Chicago: Healthcare Information and Management Systems Society of the American Hospital Association, 1993; 229–240.

Harsanyi BE, Lehmkuhl D, Hott R, Myers S, McGeehan L: Nursing informatics: The key to managing and evaluating quality. In: Grobe SJ, Pluyter-Wenting ESP, eds. *Nursing Informatics: An International Overview for Nursing in a Technological Era.* Amsterdam: Elsevier, 1994; 655–659.

Hays BJ, Norris J, Martin KS, Androwich I: Informatics issues for nursing's future. *Advances in Nursing Science* 1994; 16: 71–81.

Johnson G: Computer-based patient record systems—a planned evolution. *Healthcare Informatics* 1994; 1(1): 42–51.

Joint Commission on Accreditation of Healthcare Organizations: *1994 Accreditation Manual for Health Care Networks (AMHCN) Volume 1, Standards.* Chicago: Joint Commission on Accreditation of Healthcare Organizations, 1994.

Kongstvedt PR: *The Managed Health Care Handbook.* 2nd ed. Rockville, MD: Aspen, 1993.

Martin KS, Scheet NJ: *The Omaha System: Applications for Community Health Nursing.* Philadelphia: W.B. Saunders, 1992.

McCloskey JC, Bulechek M, eds: *Nursing Interventions Classification.* St. Louis, MO: Mosby, 1992.

McDonald CJ, Tierney WM, Overhage JM, Martin DK, Wilson GA: The Regenstrief medical record system: 20 years of experience in hospitals, clinics, and neighborhood health centers. *Computing* 1992; 9: 206–217.

North American Nursing Diagnosis Association: *NANDA Nursing Diagnoses: Definitions and Classifications.* St. Louis, MO: NANDA, 1992.

Saba VK, O'Hare PA, Zuckerman AE, Boondas J, Levine E, Oatway, DM: A nursing intervention taxonomy for home health care. *Nursing Health Care* 1991; 12: 296–299.

Vibbert S, Reichard J, eds: *The 1993–1994 Medical Outcomes and Guidelines Sourcebook.* Washington, DC: Faulkner and Gray, 1993.

Werley HH, Lang NM, eds: *Identification of the Nursing Minimum Data Set.* New York: Springer Publishing, 1988.

Zielstorff RD, Hudgings CI, Grobe SJ: *Next-Generation Nursing Information Systems: Essential Characteristics for Professional Practice.* Washington, DC: American Nurses Publishing, 1993.

20
Nursing Participation in the Selection of Healthcare Information Systems

MARY ETTA MILLS

The changing nature of healthcare delivery systems has brought new significance to the selection and application of computer-based information systems. A paradigm shift toward the management of patient care and related costs across a continuum of service needs and over the life span of each individual is focusing increased attention on how best to define, represent, and communicate healthcare data. Nursing has key responsibility and accountability in planning, evaluating, and delivering patient care services within this new framework. Consequently, participation in the selection of healthcare information systems that will support clinical and managerial decision making is critical.

External Requirements for Information Management

It is important that any information management system facilitates the organization's ability to satisfy external regulatory requirements and uniform standards of practice. Among the sources of these standards are the Joint Commission for Accreditation of Healthcare Organizations (JCAHO), the Computer-Based Patient Record Institute (CPRI), and the Federal Health Reform Act. Efforts directed by each of these sources focus on the ability of healthcare organizations to coordinate and integrate information necessary to the provision of efficient and effective patient care at a reasonable cost.

Joint Commission for Accreditation of Healthcare Organizations

The 1994 JCAHO *Accreditation Manual for Hospitals* provides a separate chapter that addresses the management of information (pp. 35–44). Within this framework of standards, the goal of information management is to "obtain, manage, and use information to enhance and improve individual and organizational performance in patient care, governance, management, and support processes" (p. 35). While not requiring computerization, the standards are "compatible with current, cutting-edge technologies" (p. 35). As outlined, the standards address the identification, design, capture, analysis, communication, and use of information. Organizational achievement of the standards is expected to take up to 5 years.

Within the standards, criteria impacting on information system selection include expectations for

- Information confidentiality and security
- Uniform data definitions (such as minimum data sets and standardized classifications)
- Standard format for transmitting data
- Combining of data and information
- Sharing of information between systems
- Linkage of patient care and nonpatient care data (i.e., clinical and fiscal) over time and among the organizational elements
- Linkage to external databases (e.g., professional library, practice guidelines, comparative data)
- Patient-specific data (e.g., demographic, assessment, treatment plan, advance directives, informed consent, therapeutic orders, procedures performed, clinical observations, medications ordered and administered, etc.)
- Management of verbal orders and authentication of record entries
- Aggregation of data (e.g., for use in risk management, quality improvement, operational decision making, and planning).

Nursing often is the network by which patient care is not only delivered but coordinated. Thus, the ability of an information system to support the coordination and integration of information necessary to clinical and managerial decision making is a concept central to guiding the selection process.

The development of accreditation standards for healthcare networks further emphasizes the need for system-level interface and integration of information. Networks in this regard are viewed as systems composed of multiple healthcare delivery organizations. Guiding principles involve continuity of care and coordination of services supported by one-time data entry and immediate data availability to all users. Given that nursing care, facilitated through such modalities as critical paths, will eventually extend across care settings, information system selection must incorporate the possibility of data sharing across care delivery sites. In the future, technology such as an "integration hub" will support "multiple information systems links, including one-to-many and many-to-one transactions" (Corum, 1994, p. 26). This approach would eliminate the need to develop point-to-point system interfaces. The hub would thus serve as a clearinghouse to route information.

Computer-Based Patient Record Institute

The Institute of Medicine's (IOM) Vision 2000 supported the development of a computer-based patient record (CPR) and led to the creation of the Computer-Based Patient Record Institute (Dick and Steen, 1991). Among the goals of this project is the development of coordinated vendor standards and a uniform single patient record. Progress to achieve a standardized approach to the collection of nursing information at the level of individual healthcare organizations and networks will ensure that information appropriate to providing informed nursing care will be included in this process.

Federal Health Reform

The American Health Security Act of 1993 provided a working draft of a national framework for health information. Among its features were provisions for standard forms, uniform health data sets, electronic networks, and national standards for data transmission and confidentiality. The information system proposed was mandated to support consumer information, measurement of health status, health security cards, links among healthcare records, analysis of patterns of health care, health system evaluation, and data confidentiality and security.

The infrastructure of this thrust is supported by the Federal Coordinating Council for Science, Engineering, and Technology (1994, p. 88) through initiatives in high-performance computing and communications. Work to date has, in part, focused on

* Applications for improved healthcare delivery, including networks for linking hospitals, clinics, doctors' offices, libraries, and universities to enable healthcare providers and researchers to share medical data and imagery
* Database technology to provide healthcare providers with access to relevant medical information and literature
* Database technology for storing, accessing, and transmitting patients' medical records while protecting the accuracy and privacy of those records.

These initiatives serve to emphasize the importance of nursing's involvement in setting the strategic direction that healthcare information systems take at the local level. Knowing what future regulations are likely to require will facilitate informed selection and development of information systems that will meet nursing needs within an organizational context.

Information Systems Selection—Technical Details

The initial evaluation and selection of an information management system is critical to identifying a system that will best meet the needs of the institution it is to serve. Criteria on which an overall evaluation is based will generally include system function and features, functional architecture, references, quality of documentation, system design, risk, vendor support, vendor background, hardware and system software, and cost. Nursing is key to this evaluation process. Data systems personnel and financial analysts can assess the technical, mechanical, and cost feasibility of various systems, but nursing has the broad clinical and administrative perspective by which to critique the systems' programs and information.

System Selection Criteria

Evaluation of information systems should include consideration of some broad-based requirements as well as the ability to deliver specific information management functions.

Identify the Information Needed Most

Without trying to specify every data interaction that is currently performed, it is important to determine key categories of information that must be included in the information management system. Examples of priority nursing management information might include budget, patient acuity, reimbursement modeling, patient outcomes, case mix, and staffing. Clinical information priorities might include nursing diagnosis/problems/assessments, order communications and results reporting, care planning/mapping, medication documentation, patient care flowsheets, patient education, discharge planning, and procedure directory.

Establish Data Requirements

The second step is to consider the most useful way of visualizing data and converting it into information supportive of clinical and managerial decision making. For example, various forms of data might better be shown in one of the following formats: charts, graphs, tables, variance reporting, highlighting or colors, and trend tracking or forecasting.

Identify Type of System Capability Desired

System capability refers to the broad ability of the information system to meet departmental needs and organizational goals. Considerations might include the ability of the system to draw relationships between data coming from divergent sources, provide a unified patient record across care sites, enable prediction and simulation of "what if" scenarios, and adjust the format of information. These are support areas of data management that expand the possible uses of recorded data. For example, data may have multiple uses as "system drivers," in which clinical assessment data may feed automatically into the calculation of patient acuity and determination of staffing levels. Another example might involve "information drivers," in which relationships are drawn between critical path variance and cost of care.

Usability Principles

Unless nursing staff can use the information system easily to support their activities in patient care, the system will lead to frustration, additional requests for customization, and delayed or ineffective system use. A series of "usability principles" was suggested by Nielsen (1990). These review criteria include the system's ability to provide relevant information; speak the user's language; minimize what the user must remember; be consistent; offer feedback; and provide clearly marked exits, shortcuts, good error messages, and internal systems to help prevent errors.

Information Systems Selection—Administrative Process

The knowledge that nursing brings to the administrative selection process includes detail relevant to the interaction of departments participating in patient care management, the degree of systems enhancement that will or will not be necessary, the ease or difficulty of implementation based on system complexity, the expense of educational preparation of staff, and the potential for fully integrating system components. Most importantly, nursing can ascertain the system's potential to improve patient care. In this role, nursing provides a critical balance in facilitating the selection of a technically capable system that also yields maximum utility in a patient care environment.

The decision to implement an information management system represents a major financial commitment on the part of any institution. The potential of an information system to meet the unique needs of a specific healthcare facility is an essential ingredient for its long-term success in that environment. Nursing can be an invaluable component both formally and informally in structuring the evaluation process, making recommendations for mandatory and desirable components, assessing a system's potential relative to the needs of practicing professionals, and making a selection with both the present and the future in mind.

Representation

Most importantly, nursing must be represented on the information system selection committee or participate on the committee advising on this process. It is the responsibility of the chief nursing officer to make this expectation known and to facilitate the identification of appropriate clinical and management staff who can represent nursing knowledge important to be included in the information system. The development of information system selection criteria and the evaluation of vendors are time consuming, and the individuals who participate in the process must be able to spend the necessary time.

Preparation

Before entering into formal committee discussions, nursing should determine current system availability, capability, and design. In 1993, the Center for Healthcare Information Management (Simpson, 1993) published a guide to directing and managing nursing information systems. This guide provides a convenient action plan to facilitate systems inventory, assessment of multidisciplinary systems in relation to their benefit to nursing, consideration of the nursing information system in relation to the healthcare organization's strategic plan and to nursing's strategic plan, and the development of a business plan for a nursing information system.

Having information available specific to current resources and future needs will serve to provide informed nursing representation in the organizational selection process. Furthermore, a detailed understanding of need will ensure that critical nursing information elements are included in any system selected.

Request for Proposal

The request for proposal (RFP) is a document that invites vendors to demonstrate how they might meet the needs of the organization in consideration of a specified set of requirements determined by the selection committee. The RFP is developed by the selection committee and states the information management requirements expected to be included in any proposed system as well as other requirements the vendor is expected to fulfill. These might include features such as financing, equipment demonstration, staff training, system troubleshooting, and future software updates. Specific evaluation criteria are normally included in the RFP so that vendors understand the basis for system selection.

Sample nursing content that might be included in a request for proposal is included in Appendix C. To the extent that the RFP is completely understood by selection committee members, the process of discriminating between proposed systems and reaching an optimum decision will be more effective.

Decision Making

Nursing must participate in the information system selection decision. If the system does not meet nursing needs, there should be a right of veto. Computer-based information systems will revolutionize communications in health care and markedly impact nursing practice. The context of communications must be structured to define and facilitate the documentation of the nursing process; to streamline the clarity, availability, and integration of essential information; and to conserve nursing time so that it can be spent with the patient. The only way nursing can ensure that the system selected will facilitate these goals is to participate actively in the administrative selection process. A priority role for nursing will serve the best interests of the healthcare facility and the nursing profession. When that role has been a reality, information system selection has proven to be farsighted and positive. Implementation likewise has proceeded in a productive way when nurses work closely with other technical and professional members of the healthcare system. Nursing is critical to the selection, design, and implementation of an optimum clinical information system.

Summary

Nursing has a distinct and important role in the selection of healthcare information systems. External standards from the Joint Commission for Accreditation of Healthcare Organizations, emphasis on a computer-based patient record by the Institute of Medicine, and federal healthcare reform initiatives provide important considerations for the identification of nursing computing requirements and eventual system selection.

System selection requirements should be based on the identification of the information most needed to support clinical and managerial decisions. Data display requirements, system capability to transform and communicate data, and usability principles should be considered in developing RFPs and in evaluating proposed information systems. Key to the selection of an information system that will support nursing is the preparation and involvement of appropriate nursing staff on the system selection committee.

Questions

1. What are the major requirements for future information systems as guided by accreditation, standards, and regulation?
2. What are the four key considerations for information systems selection supportive of clinical and managerial decisions?
3. When and how should nursing be involved in the information system selection process?

References

Corum W: JCAHO standards and systems integration. *Healthcare Informatics* 1994; 1:22–28.
Dick RS, Steen EB, eds.: *The Computer-Based Patient Record: An Essential Technology for Health Care.* Washington, DC: National Academy Press, 1991.

Federal Coordinating Council for Science, Engineering, and Technology: *High Performance Computing and Communications: Toward a National Information Infrastructure.* Washington, DC: Office of Science and Technology Policy, 1994.

Joint Commission for Accreditation of Healthcare Organizations: Management of information. In: *Accreditation Manual for Hospitals, 1994.* Chicago, IL: JCAHO, 1994; 35–44.

Nielsen J: Traditional dialogue design applied to modern user interfaces. *Communications of the Association for Computing Machinery* 1990; 33(10): 109–118.

Simpson RL: *The Nurse Executive's Guide to Directing and Managing Nursing Information Systems.* Ann Arbor, MI: Center for Healthcare Information Management, 1993.

21
Nurses' Responsibilities in the Implementation of Information Systems

SUZANNE JENKINS

Selecting Hospital Information Systems

The influence of nursing on the decision-making process of selecting health-care information systems (HISs) is increasing. Systems planning and implementation are based not only on the capabilities of information technology but also on forces in the environment that impact health care. Computer decisions in the 1970s were primarily financially oriented. Hospitals saw the need to automate their patient billing process and other key systems, such as general ledger and accounts payable. Advanced technology led to increased sophistication of hardware and software capabilities, and concurrently the information needs of the hospital increased. More extensive reporting requirements, as well as the need for management reporting on productivity, became the norm.

The decisions in the early 1980s focused primarily on ancillary systems. Many of them were not integrated with the rest of the system and were categorized as stand-alone systems. As a result, redundant patient information had to be entered into each system. The laboratory, pharmacy, and radiology generally had their own systems, including an order entry function typically done by their departmental staff. If terminals were placed on the nursing unit, clerks or nursing staff could enter the orders.

The trend for the 1990s and beyond is taking patient care back to the bedside. Although terminals at each bedside can be an expensive venture, many vendors are claiming both reduced nursing costs and increased quality of patient care. Terminals provide online flowcharting, vital signs monitoring, and nursing care plans. The vendors claim that nurses can spend more time delivering care and less time charting. Nursing has now defined additional needs and requirements for information systems. For many institutions, the ultimate goal is to have a paperless system. The entire medical record can be stored and accessed online from a terminal device. This concept allows consolidated, accurate information to be available at the user's fingertips. Patient charts from previous visits need not be tracked down. Laboratory slips need not be filled out. Patient medication records can be easily accessed online. Online order entry means no more order/charge slips; all information can be captured automatically.

Also influencing the computer systems of the 1990s is the need for quality management and utilization management modules. Expedient, timely information about the patient is critical. Healthcare reform and managed care contracts are having a major impact on the financial arena and the patient's length of stay. This ultimately impacts the type and quality of care provided.

Meeting the Challenges

The implementation of any HIS—from selection through installation—is never 100% problem free. Problems to solve and challenges to face are what make every implementation unique and exciting. Unforeseen issues can occur at any stage of the implementation cycle, beginning with the selection of a system and moving through the next phases (i.e., installation, training, parallel testing, "going live") and even into postimplementation evaluation. The key to resolution is the identification of existing resistance factors. Once they are identified, plans can then be made to eliminate them through teamwork, transitional strategies, and educational offerings. The acquisition of a complete HIS is an expensive venture for a hospital to undertake and requires a large commitment from administration to support and guide the installation. Common barriers to overcome range from general mistrust of a computer system to misgivings regarding a specific system. Potential users may fear that implementation of a system will result in an increased workload without tangible benefits. These fears and inhibitions are some of the most difficult barriers to overcome. Together, they elongate the normal learning curve, increasing the time it takes to become familiar with the new system.

Often, the politics surrounding a major acquisition such as a computer system can slow or stall it. The idea of change is sometimes threatening and can delay the implementation process. Interestingly, though, the people most resistant to a new system often become its best promoters once they are knowledgeable about and comfortable with it. Changing from a manual mode to an automated system can generate insecurity and distrust, and even changing from one automated system to another automated system often elicits resistance. A common complaint is that "the old system didn't do it that way," regardless of comparative merit. It is sometimes easier to train people who have never used a system than to retrain people who are constantly making comparisons to previous systems.

An automated system should not only assist in expediting accurate patient information throughout the hospital but should somewhat reduce paper generation. Most of the necessary information can be viewed on a terminal, and only legal documents of the medical record must be printed. Yet for some people, seeing is believing. They derive a sense of security from the paper generated by the system. When they are no longer required to fill out manual requisitions and charge slips, they need the reassurance of the hard copy (paper) form before they believe that their orders have reached the designated department. During the implementation process, therefore, it is advisable to allow moderate amounts of paper printing to promote security that reliable information is being transmitted throughout the system. A postimplementation evaluation should expose unused printed reports. This indicates that either the information is not displayed in a usable format or, more commonly, the information can be accessed adequately online and may no longer need to be printed. Throughout the process, teamwork and cooperation among decision makers are essential to a smooth implementation. Otherwise, in-house politics can have the largest negative impact on system implementation. Power plays among people and/ or departments can bring an implementation to a virtual standstill. If one person on a committee of decision makers is following a different agenda from everyone else, all will experience frustration. Education and communication can prevent many of the negative perceptions.

There is a great sense of satisfaction and accomplishment at the completion of a successful implementation. The request for proposal (RFP) is one of the preliminary steps a hospital takes when selecting a computerized information system. The hospital produces a checklist of needs for each department, or alternatively employs a consultant to assist in succinctly defining and communicating those needs to many vendors. In either case, nursing defines the requirements to support the philosophy and practice of the nursing department. It is vital that nurses are involved in the definition process of requirements necessary to meet the needs of the nursing department as information input comes from ancillaries and other hospital departments (Table 21-1).

Nursing's involvement in defining requirements reflects its critical role as a key integrator in the provision of patient care. When patients are admitted to a hospital, they are deluged with questions, many of which are asked and documented more than once. It is the nurse who must integrate and collate all the information in a logical format and develop a comprehensive plan of care for the individual patient. Information the nurse collates is captured by registration, medical records, physicians, laboratory, pharmacy, radiology, physical therapy, dietary, and many other departments. The same information is fundamental to the utilization and quality management functions.

Integrating Systems

An integrated system should capture information once, sort it, and generate output in a readable, cohesive format. The point of information capture is most logically determined by nurses; they know what type of information should be captured at registration and what information should be captured

TABLE 21-1. Sample Specifications for RFPs by Area

Registration

1. Automatically utilize outpatient and emergency room data for inpatient registration.
2. Automatically utilize patient information from a previous visit recorded in the system.
3. Allow in the admission/discharge/transfer (ADT) system for the following fields: patient name, patient street address, city, state, zip code, home phone, birthday, sex, marital status, social security number, financial class, occupation, employer, employer address, and guarantor information.
4. Have a bed-hold feature for a specific time period for patients on leave of absence.
5. Provide the ability to add and delete beds and medical service units.
6. Allow placement of outpatients (i.e., same-day surgery) in inpatient beds, maintaining accurate statistics.

Order Entry

1. Provide online ordering and result reporting.
2. Provide online real-time, patient-centered scheduling.
3. Access status of tests/procedures ordered.
4. Change/cancel patient orders with audit trail.
5. Display possible conflicts between any current orders and those previously entered.
6. Charge orders at any given status (e.g., entered, complete, resulted).
7. Print results to appropriate and multiple locations (patient's current location, doctor's office, consulting physician's office, etc.).
8. List all orders not yet completed: Sort for nursing unit, caregiver, room number.

Nursing Management

1. Provide library of nursing care plans to which care items can be added, deleted, or otherwise made more specific.
2. Provide a predefined format for individualized care plans developed at the unit level.
3. Allow users to enter free text into the nursing care plan.
4. Provide worksheets for day-to-day and shift-to-shift planning of individual patient care.
5. Schedule nursing staff at the unit level and centrally.
6. Accommodate multiple versions of patient classification systems (e.g., obstetrics, critical care, and medical/surgical) and generate acuity values as a byproduct of charting.
7. Generate reports in terms of specific nursing care hours per day and per shift.
8. Maintain records for each employee, including credentials, competence verification, continuing education units, illness and absence profile.
9. Store, update, and print nursing policies and procedures.

Medication Charting

1. Display medications that are due both presently and at any time in the future.
2. Document medication administration online.
3. Provide online notification of overdue medications.
4. Calculate required dosage based on patient-specific data such as weight, age.

Quality Management

1. Set up defined criteria to which patient treatment can be compared.
2. Generate a list of exceptions when patient data fall outside the established range.
3. Override previously defined criteria for the purpose of performing projects or reviews.
4. Log incident reports, including patient information, type of incident, place, etc.

TABLE 21-1. *Continued*

Utilization Management

1. Identify on a daily basis those patients who have met hospital-defined criteria for concurrent admission review.
2. Allow online completion of utilization review worksheet, including discharge date, length of stay, number of reviews, physician referrals, denials, diagnosis, and disposition of patient.
3. Allow editing of utilization review data for accuracy and completeness.
4. Generate a monthly log of patient discharges and the number of patient-days denied, as specified by outside review agencies.
5. Maintain utilization review statistics reflecting monthly activity (e.g., total number of discharges denied, discharges with denials by insurance carrier, admissions and discharges, emergency and elective admissions).
6. Maintain a log of denials by third-party intermediaries.

by nursing. They can determine the critical points of integration that will improve the quality of information and eliminate duplication.

For example, many registration systems ask height and weight during the admission process. Regrettably, admissions personnel are not the most accurate source of this information and inaccurate information, once entered into the system, may be accessed throughout the entire hospital. It is the nurse who can best provide accurate information—information critical for the pharmacy to calculate drug dosages appropriate for the patient. All of the departments that make up a hospital are important and vital to the care of the patient, but they are generally focused on just one area (their own) and may tend to be myopic in their view of the patient. The nurse, on the other hand, is the focal point as caregiver for the patient, compiling all pertinent patient information and disseminating appropriate data to a department or person (Fig. 21-1). It is imperative that the nurse as the integrator of an HIS work with the ancillaries in determining their requirements for computer systems and make sure those requirements are met.

Ancillaries interact with the patient on an individual basis, but the nurse coordinates the activities to benefit the patient. Social service consultations are generally initiated by nursing based on the patient's need for financial assistance, postdischarge placement, or general counseling. Dietary consultations are also usually initiated by nursing. Nurses inform the laboratory of any pertinent medications prescribed for the patient that might affect normal results (e.g., Coumadin affects prothrombin times [PTTs]). Registration and medical records information is often corrected and/or updated by nursing personnel. Nursing also interacts with departments that indirectly affect the patient's care, such as central supply, housekeeping, and transportation. Physicians write orders that direct the care provided to the patient, but nurses play an interpretive role for the physician and ensure that care is coordinated and integrated. The nurse needs access to *all* this information to provide quality care and thus is the most logical person to function as the integrator of the system.

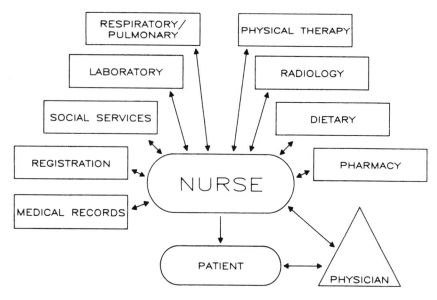

FIGURE 21-1. The nurse acts as the "hub" for patient information processing.

Implementing the System

The implementation of a hospital computer system begins almost immediately after a vendor has been selected. Nurses can play an extremely valuable part in the implementation, because nurses have more direct hands-on interaction with and knowledge of the different departments than perhaps any other member of the implementation team. Thus the nurse can be a direct source of information to facilitate the implementation of a system—whether a stand-alone single application or multiple applications—in ways that might not be intuitively obvious to implementation planners. Nurses also provide helpful input into the restatement of policy and procedures and work flow within hospital departments during a system implementation. By contributing in these two ways, nurses can move a step closer to their primary objective: making optimal use of resources to provide quality care to their patients.

These contributions of nursing begin in the selection process, when requirements are first established. They continue throughout the standard cycle of implementation once a selection is made.

Phase 1: Installation

During this phase, the software is loaded onto a computer and a complete system demonstration should be given by the vendor. The need to understand the system fully at this point cannot be overstressed. For the implementation to be successful, definition of software modifications to meet the hospital's needs should be undertaken at the same time (and through the same process) as the definition/redefinition of policies/procedures to meet the system requirements. Both serve as a basis for discussion with the vendor to determine the time frames for completion of implementation and to delineate vendor/client responsibilities.

Phase 2: Training

Once installation is complete or at least well under way, training begins. There are many approaches to training all the users of the system. Because nursing is generally the largest group of employees in a hospital to be trained and because accommodating multiple shifts is necessary, planning is of the utmost importance. Typically the vendor is responsible for training the trainer(s). Often a designee from each unit or department is responsible for making sure the training is complete and thorough. All future problems and issues as well as requests for changes in the system will be funneled through that designee. Training is most effective if taught in multiple short segments 2 to 4 hours long. Depending on the complexity of the application as well as previous user experience, the sessions can be shortened or lengthened. Videotape machines can record and replay standard training sessions for individual or group users. This method provides standardization and consistency for training. Trainers must assess individual users to determine additional or follow-up training requirements.

Phase 3: Parallel Testing

This involves a simulated dry run of what actually happens during the daily routine of a department. This phase is important to test the validity and reliability of the software as well as to ensure that new policies and procedures support the designed intent of the system. Information is sometimes duplicated during a parallel test. Patient orders may be entered into the system and may also be sent to the ancillary department for verification purposes. Parallel testing may last from a few days to a few weeks to test cumulative summaries thoroughly.

Phase 4: Going Live

This term is commonly used at the time the system goes into actual production. The parallel testing is complete and data are being communicated online, in real time. This step typically requires handholding support from the vendor. The users should be well trained and fairly comfortable with the system. This is the phase in which all the effort and hard work pay off.

Phase 5: Postimplementation Evaluation

There may be a temptation to shortchange the evaluation phase, but it is shortsighted to do so. If all is going well, this final phase will help to fine-tune the system just implemented. If problems exist, evaluation will prevent problems with implementing additional applications in the future. In either case, evaluation can provide valuable insights into the hospital and its many departments, especially nursing. Questions to be raised in evaluation include

- What reports are being printed and why? Is there a functional use for them?
- What problem areas are procedural? Who are the problem users and why? Is it because they do not understand the system? Do they need additional training? Do their problems result from not being involved in the implementation process?
- Is the system doing what the specifications say it is supposed to do? Is the work flow smoother? Is communication improved? Is there any increased efficiency in staff?

Nursing Involvement

In assisting throughout the entire process of implementing integrated hospital information systems, nurses can apply the familiar nursing model of assessment, planning, implementation, and evaluation.

Process Model

Assessment

The scope of the project, the players, the time frame, and the needs of the hospital are all analyzed and documented. Documenting the current work flow of any department will assist in determining the impact the computer system will have during and after the implementation. For example, it will show that because the system automatically notifies the nursing unit when a patient is admitted, a phone call from the admissions department can be eliminated. Similarly, orders entered into the system will eliminate the need for order requisitions to be manually completed and the need for the transport function to deliver the requisition to the respective ancillary department. These and many other time-consuming tasks are flowcharted during the analysis of the department work flow and identified as areas that will be eliminated with an automated system.

Planning

When the assessment phase is completed, roles and responsibilities are defined. The liaison nurse works closely with the vendor to identify checklists and checkpoints and to establish detailed training plans. The vendor will often suggest two or three options that best suit the hospital's resource situation. Another important step is establishing correct courses of action to follow when system problems arise. Nurses can help to determine who should be called when a problem has been identified as well as the chain of command. The vendor may be involved if the problem is software or hardware related. A solid plan is imperative to facilitate a smooth transition during any implementation.

Implementation

This is the third point at which nurses can contribute. Communication and coordination of scheduled activities within the hospital and with the vendor is the focus of this phase. Critical path activities must occur on schedule to ensure a timely and cost-effective implementation. Hospitals are responsible for more of the actual implementation activities than in years past, when the vendor performed many of the activities; thus this phase is key to the overall success of the implementation of a new system. A calm demeanor and problem-solving skills are an advantage during the actual implementation as last-minute issues arise.

Evaluation

Postimplementation analysis ensures that all defined requirements have been met. Comparing the specifications of a system provided by the vendor to the actual functioning of the system will identify any delinquent areas. For example, if the specifications indicate that the system will generate a certain report and the system clearly does not produce the report, the nurse must decide how important the report is to the overall functioning of the department. The identified areas must be assessed regarding the nature of the deficiency and prioritized. Plans must then be created and implemented to resolve any deficiencies. Often, a cost-benefit analysis is performed to identify improved areas of communication and reduced activities as they relate to cost, and an overall evaluation is carried out to determine improved productivity and quality care.

Roles Played

Nurses play a variety of roles during a system implementation, roles that can be accomplished without a programming or technical background: It is far more important that the nurse have a solid understanding of hospital policies and procedures and the ability to change those procedures to improve the work flow of the departments. Probably the two most important roles are communicator and coordinator. Other critical roles include mediator, decision maker, and politician/marketeer.

Communicator

The role of the nurse as communicator starts before the implementation begins and does not end until the postimplementation phase is completed to the satisfaction of all participants. Many different tasks occur simultaneously during the implementation phase. If one link is lost in the shuffle, it can cause great distress and distrust of the system as well as delay in implementation. The nurse can smooth the process and reduce confusion by identifying tasks and communicating with other involved hospital staff members. Many people need to be kept informed of the status of the project, but at varying levels.

Coordinator

Nurses spend much of their time prioritizing needs and coordinating the care of the patient. This experience lends itself to making nurses the focal coordinators of an HIS implementation. Responsibilities of coordination include conducting training and meetings with ancillaries, setting target dates, and defining a plan. It is important to keep issues focused and to observe priorities. The nurse/coordinator may delegate as needed to ensure timely implementation.

Mediator

Many decisions must be made during the implementation process of a computer system. When multiple departments are involved, many issues cross departmental boundaries. An individual should be designated to mediate and facilitate compromise. Because nurses interact with and understand so many of the hospital departments, they are the ideal choice for this role. A side benefit of this arrangement is that it gives nurses a chance to see what happens on the other side of a stat lab result or the process involved in dispensing therapeutic medications or transcribing radiology reports. Conversely, the arrangement allows the ancillary department to understand nursing responsibilities. The first few times all department representatives meet to discuss system needs may be like hungry lions sharing a meal. A mediator can be essential. An effective mediator can help create a spirit of cooperation and a vision of how the rest of the hospital operates, greatly facilitating the implementation process. Ultimately, one person should be responsible for seeing that decisions are made and are made appropriately.

Decision Maker

The role of decision maker during the implementation of a system is highly important. The input of many people must be considered because the outcome affects the entire institution. A nurse with authority to make decisions is essential to keep the project moving forward. Knowing hospital policies and procedures aids the nurse during the decision-making process. Questions to be answered in decision making center on access to information:

- Who are the authorized users?
- Who should print reports? Where? When?
- Will nursing enter orders or will ward clerks do so?
- What is the sign-off process of orders?
- Will orders be held in the system until an RN reviews them? Or will orders be automatically released to the ancillary department with verification taking place later?

These are just a few examples of questions that require decisions. Ultimately, one person should be responsible for ensuring that decisions are made and communicated to all affected personnel.

Politician/Marketeer

The nurse's role as marketeer of the system should be enjoyable. It is the responsibility of nursing to propagate positive information, solicit support, and promote the system. There are no hard-and-fast rules to follow to make this role successful. A feeling of ownership of the system clearly helps in establishing a positive attitude toward the system. Getting people involved is imperative but also difficult when considering the activity and workload that occur in a hospital. Videotapes, buttons, and coffee socials are all methods of encouraging staff participation and support of the system. Skepticism may be prevalent initially, but curiosity usually overcomes the skeptics when everyone gets involved.

Keys to a Successful Implementation

All the roles the nurse plays during a system implementation have an impact on how well the system is received and utilized by the entire hospital staff. For the implementation to be truly successful, six key factors must be in place:

1. Make sure nursing is involved in the decision-making process of the HIS selection. If hospital administration makes an independent decision without consulting nursing, system implementation can be greatly inhibited. The system will change how nurses' work flow takes place. The Joint Commission on Accreditation of Healthcare Organizations (JCAHO) now requires that nurse executives demonstrate input into a system selection.
2. Solicit upper-management support. Strong support from upper management positively impacts the implementation process. Nurses feel more confident and are more open to change if they know management is supporting their decision. A positive attitude at the top will generate a positive attitude throughout the institution.
3. Make sure that the time schedule is appropriate for success. Ask questions to determine whether adequate time has been allotted:

- What is the commitment of the hospital?
- Is staffing adequate for training and coverage?
- Does the hospital want to implement the system on one unit or multiple pilot units?
- Does the hospital want to implement the system in one ancillary at a time or in multiple ancillaries?

The action plan should be closely coordinated with the vendor. It is important to define the responsibilities of the hospital staff and the vendor up front.

4. Realize that mindset and attitudes can make or break a system. If the leaders of each unit are upbeat and enthusiastic, their positive attitudes will create a general feeling of security and support. No implementation is problem free. Every implementation presents different challenges, but all problems can be overcome by working as a team.

5. Designate a liaison person from the hospital. Nursing representatives are often the best candidates for this role. The selected nurse should be one who understands the hospital's policies and procedures and who has the authority to make decisions. Subcommittees and working committees are great but tend to drag out the decision-making process and can delay the installation of a system. Nurses can accurately define the requirements of a system to meet the needs of the nursing department. Nurses also add the valuable experience of interaction with ancillaries, administration, and physicians.

6. Highlight communication as an essential ingredient in the implementation process. Keeping the right people informed is a monumental task but one that should be addressed. Weekly or monthly newsletters and/or meetings can be instrumental in a successful implementation because misinterpretation of issues will be decreased and negative rumors will be squelched. The project will also be more focused on critical issues that need immediate attention and resolution.

New Opportunities for Nurses

The increasing involvement of nurses in the implementation of hospital information systems may be partially responsible for the current shortage of hospital nurses. Today, nurses are moving away from the bedside and into the boardroom. In some major metropolitan areas, per diem nurses are earning upward of $35 per hour. Certainly there are at least as many nurses graduating from school today as there were 10 years ago, and there are more professional working women than ever before. Where are these nurses going and why? Many nurses are choosing to use their hard-earned degrees and experience to move into the business side of the healthcare industry. They are putting away their uniforms, donning business suits, and entering the healthcare market through a different door. This seems to be a natural path for many nurses because they are familiar with the process, politics, and terminology that occur in a healthcare environment. This can be accomplished in many different ways and through many different roles.

Some are taking the experience they have gained from being part of an implementation team of an HIS, updating their résumés, and joining the corporate world. Others are part of the increasing enrollment in master's programs for computer sciences. It does not require technical brilliance to earn a degree in management information systems. This field is just what it implies—managing information—and it's making nurses marketable in the healthcare industry. New programs are emerging in the nursing informatics area as well. The computer industry is fast paced and forever changing—not an unfamiliar situation for nurses. Unlike nursing, it offers many opportunities for growth and promotion in a short period of time. Nurses associated with the computer industry can impact bedside nursing by facilitating the information processing relating to patient care. Nurses never give themselves credit for the multifaceted roles they play every day. They have marketable skills of which they are not even aware. They are analysts, consultants, politicians, and problem solvers. They are also logical thinkers and skilled communicators with experience in prioritization and organization. These roles that nurses fulfill in traditional patient care areas can be transferred effectively to the computer healthcare industry.

Analyst

Nurses are trained to observe, to make decisions, and to act on decisions. Nurses have trained eyes for clinical and psychosocial situations. They have been taught to analyze the situation thoroughly before making those critical decisions. They are adept in dealing with change—they do so every day. They have learned to be nonjudgmental and to ask critical questions to get to the heart of the matter. In short, nurses are analytical. Their skills translate well to the role an analyst plays in the implementation process. An analyst must look logically at how the system works and how the hospital will be impacted. Analyst positions are available in hospital information systems departments as well as in the vendor community.

Programmer

Nurses who enjoy the technical side of nursing—where things are concrete and planned actions produce anticipated results—may be interested in learning to program. Many of the analytical skills developed through bedside nursing can be transferred, but some structured training is usually required to become a programmer. This is a highly sought-after combination in the healthcare computer marketplace today. It is much easier to teach a nurse how to program than it is to teach a programmer about the inner workings of a hospital. Although nurses quickly lose their stereotype in this industry, they learn to keep an aspirin bottle handy for colleagues who come to them for a professional opinion on everyday maladies.

Consultant

The opportunities continue to grow for nursing in the consulting field. Almost every hospital purchasing an information system today is using a consultant to aid in the selection process. Consulting in health care is a multi-million-dollar business. The nurse is the best resource for determining a hospital's needs and deciding what vendor meets those needs. Consulting contracts range from remote question-and-answer support to extensive analysis of the current work flow and requirements of a hospital. Extended contracts may include long-range planning and marketing tactics for the hospital to employ in attracting patients. Nurses provide expert assistance in determining system requirements for a hospital. The nurse's ability to take a large amount of data and organize it into a big picture is a positive asset in the consulting field. A certain level of detail is required, but the key is to take all the pieces and assimilate them into a big-picture concept.

Developer

Experience gained from being part of an installation team (either the hospital side or the vendor side) provides credentials to develop new systems. The development of a system requires a healthy balance of technical expertise and practical user experience. The technical design by programmers is important to ensure efficiency of computer resources without degrading response time. Nurses can provide the work flow design and requirements of a system as well as contribute to the human factor by influencing design of the screens. Neither side can work in a vacuum. Teamwork is essential to ensure the success of a newly developed system.

Salesperson/Sales Support Person

Nurses provide a tremendous amount of credibility and knowledge of hospitals in the sales cycle of an HIS. Healthcare professionals feel more comfortable talking to peers who understand the issues facing hospitals today. Medical jargon can be overwhelming to a nonhospital person. Nurses provide the link of interpretation and communication between the non-hospital person (sales representative) and the hospital professional. Other sales skills that nurses possess include the ability to handle many different personalities and to use different approaches with people as the situation dictates. Product demonstrations require knowledge of that product as well as teaching skills that nurses have practiced and perfected over the years.

Marketeer

Nurses can apply their creative side to marketing special products or total healthcare information systems. The strengths of interpreting medical terminology and knowing what hospitals want to hear will assist any business in appealing to the marketplace. Having an inside track to the future of hospitals makes nurses a valuable commodity. Suggestions to help develop some background with computers include

- Attending healthcare computer trade shows
- Subscribing to journals (these will identify trade show dates and locations)
- Getting involved in a hospital system implementation as an insider
- Attending classes at a local community college or university
- Joining a local network group.

Summary

Nurses today have the opportunity to affect health care in many ways. They may choose to remain at the bedside, using handheld terminals to deliver better care. They may elect to enter the decision-making arena, working to integrate information systems. Or they may move into the corporate world and represent the interests of health care there. But wherever nurses go, the computer will not be far away. Nurses will become more and more involved with information management and with the technology that supports it.

Questions

1. Identify three roles the nurse can play during a system implementation.
2. Identify four key factors that ensure a successful implementation.
3. Assimilate the nursing process (assess, plan, implement, and evaluate) into the implementation of a computer system.

22
Evolution of the User Interface and Nursing's Role in Its Design

Linda Edmunds

Proper system design means achieving a patient record system that properly fits, interacts with, and communicates in the accepted manner of every user community the system supports. This kind of design is necessary if automated patient record systems are to be adopted by users. (Dick and Steen, 1991, p. 35)

This excerpt from the Institute of Medicine (IOM) report on the computerized patient record (CPR) clearly defines the objective of interface design—it is to provide clinicians with systems that they will willingly adopt. Interface design focuses on the cognitive, manual, and aesthetic response of the user to a software application. It addresses the manner in which the system will meet stated requirements, the appearance of the software, and how the user will interact with it.

This chapter describes (1) where interface design fits into the development process, (2) how evolving technology has increased the importance of the interface design process, and (3) the contributions that nurse informatics specialists and nurse clinicians can make to designing systems that will help to make the CPR a reality.

The Software Development Process

The software development process proceeds through at least three phases: planning, programming, and implementation (Fig. 22-1). In the planning phase, decisions about what to build are made. In the programming phase, the databases and application programs are written and tested. During implementation, users are trained, debugging continues, and the application is distributed throughout the facility. The time and effort committed to each phase are usually determined by the complexity of the project, the nature of the organization undertaking it, and the experience of the development team.

The planning phase can itself be divided into three distinct processes: strategic planning, requirements analysis, and user interface design (Fig.

FIGURE 22-1. Major phases in system development.

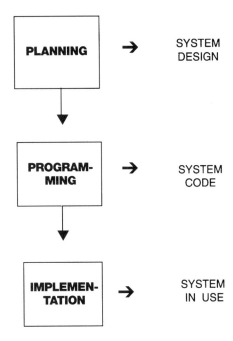

22-2). During strategic planning, institutional objectives are defined by identifying and prioritizing issues that the institution hopes to resolve by using technology.

In the analysis phase, these objectives are translated into detailed system requirements. The output may be of a list of functions the completed system will perform and/or a set of models that define system entities, their attributes and interrelationships, and how data flow between the entities and the external environment. The output of the analysis phase is abstract in the sense that the same requirements may be physically programmed in a variety of ways, all of which meet the requirements. In other words, if three programmers are given a requirements document or model set, the system built by each technician might accomplish the same functions but look and feel totally different to the user.

During the interface design phase, attention is directed to the way each function will be implemented, what the software will look like, and how the user will enter data and retrieve information. Windows, screens, reports, graphics, and flows are described, drawn, and/or prototyped in detail. User representatives are brought in to try out, evaluate, and eventually validate the proposed interface. The object is to ensure that the completed application will be in conformance with defined requirements and that the technology will not distract attention from the user's primary focus, which in this case is care delivery. This requires, among other things, that data input mirrors the clinician's way of collecting information and that data displays enhance the clinician's decision-making process.

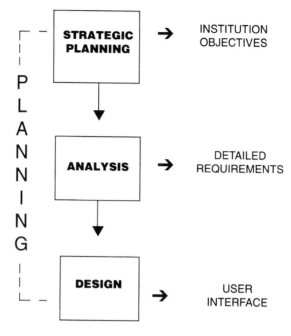

FIGURE 22-2. The planning process.

The Evolution of Interfaces

Attention to the interface design process has become increasingly important as technology has advanced. As the industry has moved from central mainframe and minicomputers to client-server networks, from dumb video terminals to powerful workstations, from procedure-driven to object-oriented programming languages, the technical options available to system developers have expanded considerably. Because there are multiple options for programming a set of system requirements, many more decisions are required during the design process. While technology now has the potential to support the type of systems that clinicians really want to use, lack of attention to interface design can result in unusual but unusable systems. In a world where graphic user interfaces (GUIs) and object-oriented interfaces (OOIs) are becoming the accepted standard for all types of business software, interface design has emerged as a distinct and growing discipline (Shneiderman, 1992, p. 6) that has important contributions to make to the development of clinical software.

Command-Driven Systems

Initially, most computer systems were command driven. DOS, for example, is a command-driven operating system. In a command-driven system, the user types in responses to a series of prompts or questions that the application displays on the terminal (Fig. 22-3). Interface design is focused on decisions about the number of prompts, their clarity, and the format of the required response. For example, if the user must remember numerous coded responses, the learning process will likely be slow and user frustration high. On the other hand, if normal words and sentences are acceptable responses, the problem of combining and manipulating inputted data becomes difficult if not impossible. Similarly, if a long series of yes/no or single-word responses are used to elicit data or decisions, the number of prompts required may try the patience of a busy practitioner, particularly when the same sequences are used frequently. While there are certainly user interface issues to be considered in building a command-driven application, these are confined for the most part to the use of language to elicit responses efficiently and without the user making unnecessary errors.

Menu-Driven Systems

Menu-driven systems consist of a series of lists or menus from which the user makes appropriate selections using the keyboard or a pointing device such as a light pen (Fig. 22-4). When the user makes a selection, another menu may be displayed. Menu-driven applications introduce a second set of issues for the designer. In addition to the use of language, the designer must also think about the visual organization and the density of selections on each menu as well the sequence in which the menus are shown. Does the designer, for example, put many or few selections on one menu? Many choices on a single menu often confuse the novice, but many menus, each with a few choices, can result in a lengthy sequence that frustrates the ex-

```
C:\RALPH HALES\VIEW OR DOCUMENT?> Document

C:\RALPH HALES\V/S OR NOTES OR I&O?> V/S

C:\RALPH HALES\TEMP PULSE RESP BP?> TEMP

C:\RALPH HALES\TEMP ?> 99.2

C:\RALPH HALES\TEMP MODIFIER ?> ARMPIT
INVALID ENTRY

C:\RALPH HALES\TEMP MODIFIER ?> AXILLERY
INVALID ENTRY

C:\RALPH HALES\TEMP MODIFIER ?> AXILLARY

C:\RALPH HALES\TEMPERATURE 99.2 AXILLARY OK (Y/N)?> Y
```

FIGURE 22-3. Command-driven vital sign entry.

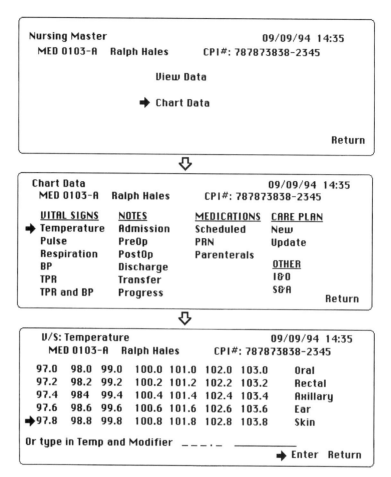

FIGURE 22-4. Menu-driven vital sign entry. A three-screen sequence is displayed for documenting temperature. The patient has already been selected from a previous menu. The light pen is used to select Chart Data on the first screen. The second screen lists selections for different types of charting. Note the organization of selections into categories and the various options for charting vital signs. The user selects Temperature with the light pen. On the temperature screen, the user can select the value for the temperature and a modifier. As selections are made, they appear in the same fields that can be used for typing in the temperature if the value is higher or lower than provided choices. In this type of design, if the user selected TPR instead of Temperature, three data collection screens would be shown sequentially. Are the temperature choices applicable to all clinical specialties? How could the flow be made more efficient? How would you modify the design so that the user could easily review previously entered data?

perienced user, particularly when the central computer is busy and response time is slow.

Menu-driven systems also require some data to be typed in response to prompts displayed on the terminal screen. The designer must decide when to use a menu and when to use the keyboard to collect information and how to switch between the two modalities so that it is not awkward for the user, who must pick up and put down the pointing device.

Mainframe or mini-based menu-driven systems using dumb terminals impose a set of virtual, if not actual, limitations on the interface design. For example, graphic displays of data are generally not practical in this environment because of the computing overhead required to produce them and the impact this overhead has on the user community as a whole. Similarly, many existing mainframe clinical systems use flat file or hierarchical databases, which limit the number of ways the same data can be indexed and displayed. Without graphics and with limited indexing options, the designer may have to find nontraditional ways to display data that are still satisfactory to the clinician.

Two other issues that must be considered in designing menu-driven systems are the use of color and the incorporation of screen standards. Color is useful to organize selections, highlight data, and indicate warning situations. When the hardware environment is mixed (i.e., it includes both color and monochrome terminals), the designer must make certain that information conveyed to the user is the same regardless of the display device.

The use of standard screen conventions in an interface facilitates ease of use. Unfortunately, in the world of menu-driven clinical systems, there are very few widely accepted standards. Each system tends to reflect a unique mixture of tool-related, vendor-related, and facility-related conventions. The best that the interface designer can hope to accomplish is consistency within the application and accommodation of any local standards.

In summary, menu-driven systems pose many of the same language-related design issues as do command-driven systems. They also introduce issues that are central to graphic interfaces. The primary focus of the interface designer, however, is on the visual organization of menu selections and the sequential organization of the menus into pathways.

GUI Applications

Most systems currently under development are being designed with a GUI. Applications with a GUI differ from menu-driven applications in several important ways. First, the number of objects or controls that the designer has to work with is much greater. Second, GUI systems are supposed to have flexible rather than fixed pathways. Third, the use of color, fonts, and graphics is integral, not peripheral, to a GUI design. Finally, the availability and wide use of platform-specific workstation standards introduces some unique problems that the designer must resolve.

Controls

The range of elements available to the interface designer for collecting and displaying data in a GUI environment is substantially greater than in a menu-driven system. In a menu-driven system, the designer works with a fixed size screen and three basic field types: the selectable menu item, the input field for typing data, and the display field. In a GUI environment, different window types are used for different purposes and a window can be any size as well as movable, scrollable, closable, or resizable. In addition to text input and display fields, the controls that can be used inside a window include, among others, pushbuttons, radio buttons, list boxes, combination boxes, check boxes, slide bars, pop-up menus, menu bars, drop-down lists, tool bars, and status bars (Fig. 22-5). Many of these window types and controls have overlapping uses, and the designer must learn when and where to use each one appropriately. Given so many choices, the learning curve is not insignificant.

Modality

In a menu-driven system, sequences of screens are set by the designer and the user proceeds through a sequence until its end or at minimum to a limited number of designer-defined branching points. A system with set pathways that forces the user to proceed along in a specific direction is termed modal. Well-designed GUI systems are supposed to be nonmodal. A nonmodal system is designed so that there are many branches and thus many alternate pathways through it. It is the user, rather than the designer, who determines how it will be navigated. For example, in a nonmodal documentation system, the user might be able to interrupt entry of vital signs to look up the last administration of a drug, retrieve the blood level results, check E-mail, enter a stat order for another patient, and then resume charting at the point that he or she left off. In a modal system, the user would either complete the vital sign entry or exit it before accessing another pathway, another patient, or another application.

Designing a nonmodal interface is difficult because the designer must make certain that the flexibility of the system will not contribute to user error. Obviously, this is particularly critical when clinical data are involved. In a nonmodal system, the designer must also ensure that the user does not feel lost when moving through the branches of the application. This is accomplished by providing landmarks, help, and ways to undo actions and backtrack. In short, the reason it is difficult to design safe, nonmodal software is that it is more complex to determine what a user might do with a flexible system than it is to define what he or she must do with an inflexible one.

Color and Fonts

Workstations that run GUI applications commonly have at least 16, often 256, and sometimes thousands of colors. In addition to a variety of colors,

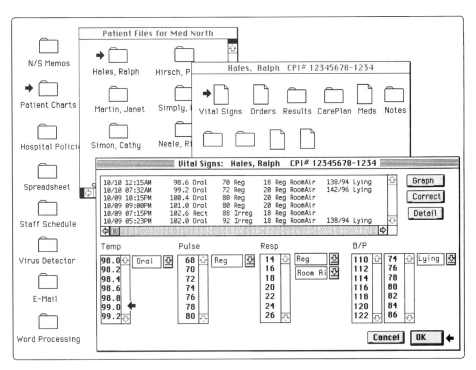

FIGURE 22-5. Graphic user interface vital sign entry. In this GUI design, the work-station desktop is shown as well as three open windows. There are eight folders on the desktop, three of which (Word Processing, Spread Sheets, and Virus Detection) are probably over-the-counter commercial applications. The E-Mail, Nursing Memo, Staff Scheduling, and Hospital Policy folders are more hospital oriented and may have been built in-house or purchased from a clinical software vendor and modified for the hospital. When the user selects Patient Charts, a window opens that displays a file for each patient on the nursing unit. Ralph Hales's file is selected with the mouse, and a third window opens that contains additional folders and file documents. Selecting Vital Signs opens a window that is used both to collect and to display data. Note the window controls: pushbuttons, scrollable list boxes, and drop-down list. When a drop-down next to the temperature values is picked, the temperature modifiers—oral, rectal, axillary, etc.—are displayed. If the user wants to see the data graphically, the Graph button can be used. Why do not the data display in graphic form when the user opens the window? Would it be better for the user to have separate windows for each of the vital signs? Note that the user can select another patient by bringing the Patient Files window forward. The user can look at E-Mail by clicking on the E-Mail folder visible on the desktop. The ability of the user to navigate around and among application software is the basis of a nonmodal design. Think how much easier it would be for a user to comment on the interface if he or she could try it out rather than looking at this black-and-white drawing.

a multitude of fonts are also available and each one can be made larger or smaller, italicized, bold, underlined, colored, etc. This is quite a contrast to mini or mainframe systems, which often limit the designer to a monochromatic or limited palette, one font type, and sometimes only uppercase.

The appropriate use of colors, fonts, and icons can do much to make systems aesthetically pleasing and easy to use. Colors and fonts can also help to organize data and highlight critical information. On the other hand, if used without restraint, they can disorient and tire the user. An enthusiastic interface designer who is a newcomer to the graphic environment has the potential to make as many visually glaring mistakes as a color-blind interior decorator with a large budget.

Standards

Each of the major workstation operating systems—Windows, OS/2, Apple, and UNIX—has introduced a set of user interface standards that define window types, controls, and the placement of other graphic elements such as tool bars. While there are many similarities between each platform's design standards, there are also differences, some subtle, some significant.

Whether you are using OS/2, Windows, UNIX, or a Mac, a pushbutton is a pushbutton. It may look slightly different on each platform, but clicking a mouse on any one of these platforms has essentially the same effect. Once the user is familiar with the interface conventions for a specific platform, learning new applications on that same platform is facilitated. Even when a user changes platforms, his or her learning curve on the new platform may be reduced because of the similarities among them. On the other hand, very experienced users for whom a platform's conventions are second nature often find the transition frustrating.

The most significant standard-related issue for the clinical interface designer is the varied workstation experience that clinicians bring with them when they are introduced to a new GUI clinical system. Not only are individual nurses used to varying standards, but there are many clinicians who are totally unfamiliar with personal computers or workstations. Despite what many computer pundits think, using a GUI interface is not intuitive. Learning to move a mouse and understanding what the controls and icons do take some time and practice.

Eventually, standard-related issues should diminish for two reasons. First, the integration of personal computers into educational curriculums at all levels will ensure that most clinicians will have some level of workstation proficiency. Second, the standards for the various platforms are growing more alike. For some time, however, because the range of computer experience among clinicians varies so widely, the clinical designer will have to create interfaces that are somewhat intuitive to the novice, use the conventions that are relatively consistent among different platforms, and do this while also providing the expert user with all of the shortcuts he or she is accustomed to.

OOI Applications

Object-oriented interfaces are graphic interfaces in which visual metaphors are employed. In an object-oriented interface, the user works with objects that are familiar from the real world. The object-oriented interface allows a user to incorporate what he or she already knows from the real world (Norman, 1988, p. 450) into his or her interactions with the software. For example, a patient chart may be used as a central metaphor for a clinical system. To open a section of the chart, the clinician clicks on a chart tab, knowing from real-world experience what data will be available (Fig. 22-6).

Using natural object metaphors is the key to creating intuitive interfaces for inexperienced users and to decreasing the amount of time necessary to train a new user. If the designer is not familiar with the user's world, however, he or she runs the risk of mixing metaphors and creating a system that in some ways parallels the user's experience and runs counter to it in others. When a metaphor does not follow the user's expectations, the resulting system can often be more confusing than when no metaphor is used at all.

Multimedia

A multimedia application is one in which sound, images, and other modalities are incorporated into the interface along with text and graphics. The use of sound may include voice commands, automatic conversion of the spoken word to text, and/or the recording and playback of clinically significant sounds. Image type technologies may include photos, videos, 3-D visualization, and handwriting recognition.

Clinical systems, with the exception of those used for specific diagnostic purposes, are only at the initial stages of incorporating multimedia into their interfaces. The primary challenge for the interface designer is to know when the introduction of one of these technologies is appropriate. At this time, the decision may be based solely on the maturity of the technology itself and ability of the system network to support it.

For example, if a voice translation product has a limited vocabulary and requires 5 hours of voice training per user, it may not be a good choice if the interface will be used by a staff of 1000. Similarly, the online availability of patient photographs may be useful to clinicians but not if it requires 2 minutes to transmit the image over the existing network infrastructure. The focus for the clinical interface designer should be to plan where multimedia

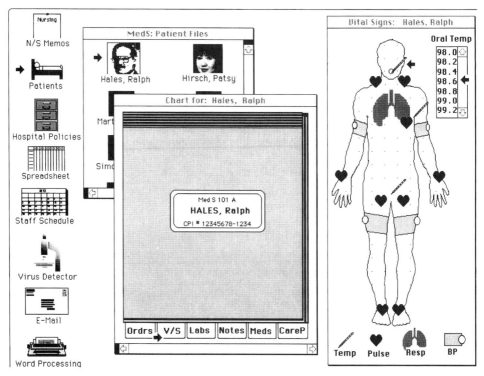

FIGURE 22-6. Object-oriented interface vital sign entry. The OOI design shown here is very similar to the GUI design displayed in Figure 22-5. Icons are used on the desktop, which helps users to locate a particular software application quickly. When the Patients icon is selected, a window opens that displays pictures of all the patients on the unit. Would it be helpful to have information in addition to the patient's name below the photo? When a patient is selected, his or her chart is opened. In this case, a chart metaphor is used. Even the inexperienced user would probably know what to do next to enter or obtain vitals signs. The Vital Signs window that opens uses another metaphor. An outline of the human body is marked with icons that indicate the usual places where temperature, pulse, respiration, and blood pressure are entered. To enter an oral temperature, the user selects the thermometer located at the patient's mouth. A scrollable list of values is displayed and the "oral" modifier is automatically captured. How could color be used in this design? What would be the best way of displaying past vital signs? Are the cuffs on the patient's thighs or the location of the rectal thermometer confusing? Should there be a separate window for each type of vital signs, or should additional ones be added (e.g., neurological signs)? Is it necessary to have a key to the vital signs icons?

components can be integrated into an interface so that when the technology is practical to use, the application can be expanded gracefully.

Nursing Participation in Design

Informatics Nurse Specialists

During the past 25 years, informatics nurse specialists often learned interface design on the job (Lafferty and Sheffield, 1988, p. 235) and honed their skills in response to feedback provided by team members and users. On-the-project training is, however, no longer a viable approach because most systems being designed today are workstation based, and designing workstation interfaces is more complicated than designing command- or menu-driven software.

Nurse informaticians who are playing or planning to play a role in software development need to be aware of what disciplines (such as human factors research, graphic design, and cognitive psychology) have contributed to the theory, mechanics, and art of interface design. For nurses currently in informatics programs, this exposure should logically be part of their master's or doctoral preparation. For those clinical analysts who are transitioning from menu-based to GUI or OOI design projects, there are many resources available to help them make the leap.

An essential introduction to the basic tenets of good design is *The Design of Everyday Things* by Donald A. Norman (1988). This thought-provoking and fun-to-read book addresses conceptual models, visible cues, standardization, error handling, and other topics that can be applied to the design of any product, not necessarily software. Ben Shneiderman's book *Designing the User Interface* (1992) addresses many practical and theoretical areas of interface design, and his first chapter includes an annotated list of classic and current books, journals, published standards, conference proceedings, videos, and special interest groups (pp. 39–49). *Graphic Design for Electronic Documents and User Interfaces,* by Aaron Marcus (1991), is an introduction to layout, color, typography, icons, and other physical aspects of design and includes a bibliography on each of these topics (pp. 221–250).

Requirements

The first responsibility of the nurse informatician is to make certain that an interface design addresses every one of the functional requirements defined during the analysis phase. It is assumed that any requirements for a nursing system will address the guidelines for data management, data security and integrity, flexibility, and accessibility outlined in the American Nurses Association's (ANA's) *Computer Design Criteria for Systems That Support the Nursing Process* (Zielstorff, McHugh, and Clinton, 1988). Satisfied that these criteria have been met, the focus of the informatician can be shifted to the usability of the interface design.

Prototypes

To test effectively for usability, there must be a specification or prototype that clinical users can easily understand, review in detail, and send back for revisions. Although an online prototype is optimal, interfaces for command- or menu-driven modal applications may be illustrated effectively using paper documents. The paper specification should include detailed drawings, with accompanying explanations, of each screen, screen sequence, and printout that will be available in the completed system. In a sense, a virtual user manual describing the entire system is created so it can be read by the users, modified, and validated before programming is started (Edmunds, 1992, pp. 17–32).

A paper specification is not sufficient when it comes to designing or eliciting user response to GUI, OOI, or multimedia applications. For these environments, an online prototype with which the designer and the user can interact is essential for many reasons. First, it is a cumbersome process for the designer to document completely on paper a nonmodal application that has many branching pathways. Even with such a document, it is difficult for the user to visualize how he or she will navigate through windows that can move, size, scroll, and close or how they will switch to other software products on the same workstation. It is also impractical for the designer to create an interface that relies on color and multiple fonts without using computerized drawing tools and seeing the graphics on a video display monitor. Most importantly, users cannot provide valid feedback about the usability of an interface until they use it. Neither can the designer identify the best solution to an interface problem without watching users try various options.

There are many tools for creating prototypes. Initial concepts can often be demonstrated using slide or presentation tools, such as Microsoft's *Power Point,* Lotus's *Freelance Graphics,* or Aldus's *Persuasion* in combination with clip art and drawing or painting software. Interactive prototypes can be built with some of the easier-to-user software tools, such as Apple's *Hypercard,* or with the simpler commands that are part of programming tools, such as Blyth's *Omnis,* Powersoft's *PowerBuilder,* or Microsoft's *Visual Basic.* If one of the more powerful toolkits is used to build the prototype, the one selected should be the one the programmers will use to build the final product.

It is advantageous for the nursing informatician to become facile with the prototyping tool and to contribute to the construction of the prototype. This gives the nurse a better understanding of the tool capabilities and may decrease the time required to make revisions based on user input. The essential objective, however, is that there be a prototype created in a reasonable time frame. Thus, if the learning curve for the prototyping tool is long, the nurse designer may be forced to work closely with a technician. This is often more of a challenge than learning simple programming. Working as the interface between technicians and users may require every nursing communication skill ever learned.

Interface Testing

Once the initial prototype is complete, it is time to bring in clinicians to try it out and critique it. A good deal has been written about the process and procedures of interface testing. Shneiderman (1992, p. 18) identifies five critical factors to be evaluated: time to learn, time to complete benchmark tasks, user error rates, retention over time, and individual satisfaction. For a pragmatic, step-by-step discussion of the techniques involved in user testing, including goal setting, task identification, selection of tools and subjects, review of results, scheduling, and the use of iteration, Penny Bauersfeld's (1994) book, *Software by Design: Creating People Friendly Software,* is recommended.

Standards

A nurse designer must be thoroughly familiar with the interface standards of the platform that will be the base of the proposed software. It is equally important that the designer be aware of other platform standards because the clinical user base is bound to have all types of platform experience. Becoming familiar with software built on a variety of platforms will help the designer to avoid design decisions that are confusing to a user subset.

Each of the major vendors publishes platform-specific detailed guidelines for designing user interfaces. The one published by Apple entitled *Macintosh Human Interface Guidelines* is an excellent introduction to window design and has many illustrations. It can be used in conjunction with an Apple-produced CD-ROM titled *Making It Macintosh,* which covers similar material but with interactive examples.

Nurse Clinicians

The participation of nurse informatics specialists in project teams responsible for designing and developing clinical software is critical but not sufficient if systems are to be built that nurses will adopt willingly. Nurse clinicians have a critical role to play in testing and evaluating interfaces. No matter how much previous clinical experience a nurse who specializes in informatics may have, clinical practice is changing too quickly and has too many specialties for the informatics nurse to be an expert in all areas. Nurses, or anyone else for that matter, who participate in software design are warned not to trust themselves to evaluate an interface for intuitiveness or ease of use. In addition to evaluating whether functionality is appropriate to the unique features of their own practice, nurse clinicians should consider the following when evaluating a prototype or paper specification.

Aesthetics

Visual aesthetics is certainly a subjective area in terms of user response to software. Essentially users ask themselves if they like the way the system looks: Are background colors restful; do highlighting colors stand out; are the fonts selected large enough to be readable but small enough so that displays are compact; is blank space used effectively to organize data; are objects within windows well organized and well proportioned? If multiple clinicians are involved in evaluating the interface and if the majority find it unattractive or displeasing, the designer must take a hard look at the design.

Intuitiveness

Intuitiveness is not as subjective an area as aesthetics, but it often depends on the familiarity of the user with the technology platform on which the application rests. Users with no platform experience should evaluate how far into the interface they can penetrate the application without help. The user experienced with a different platform should look for places in the design that are confusing because of their past experience. This information will be of particular importance to the designer if a large proportion of the user community also has the same background. Frequent users of the platform should serve as the "platform police" and identify any areas missed by the designer that do not conform to expected standards and conventions.

If a clinical metaphor is used, all users should evaluate the applicability of the metaphor and see if the software conforms to their expectations of the metaphor's operation. Clinicians should also determine if words, abbreviations, codes, messages, and other verbal forms are clinically accurate and free of technical jargon. In addition, as users go through this section of the analysis, they should attempt to estimate the amount and type of training time that would be required for the staff nurse. The number of resources necessary for user training is ultimately the most accurate measure of software intuitiveness.

Helpfulness

When the intuitiveness of a system breaks down, its helpfulness should kick in. The clinician reviewer should determine how easy it is to obtain help when he or she becomes confused. If online help is not part of the package, the system should at least provide the user with a phone number to call or direct them to an appropriate manual. If online help is part of the interface, the clinician should determine if answers to problems or questions that arise during testing are available, whether they are understandable, and if they could be located before frustration set in.

Forgiving

One of the most important features of any software application—whether it be command driven, menu driven, or a graphic interface—is its error-handling capabilities. The ability to "forgive" a user who makes an error by allowing for easy correction is particularly important in a clinical system, where incorrect patient data can be life threatening. Clinicians should be asking themselves the following as they test the software: How does the interface assist the user to avoid errors in data entry? If errors are made, how cumbersome is it to make a correction? Can corrections be made if the error is found at a later date and, if so, are these updates tracked so that audit can be performed if necessary? An interface should allow mistakes to be corrected, but it also must keep a record of these corrections for legal and safety reasons.

Customizability

The requirements analysis will identify where application flexibility is necessary so that the system can be used in a variety of clinical services and/or facilities. Individual users also differ in their likes and dislikes, and most commercial word processing, drawing, spreadsheet, and other applications allow users to modify some system features to suit their individual preferences. In evaluating a clinical interface, the nurse-user should review what features are customizable and whether the number of features and the options available for each will suit the majority of the users. It is often easier for the designer to build in these types of choices than to obtain consensus about a particular system feature.

Consistency

In addition to platform standards (if these are available), each application interface should be internally consistent in the way it uses design components such as window controls, icons, terminology, color, font, and functional sequences. For example, it is better to use the word "update" or the word "modify" to identify an error correction sequence than to use both words interchangeably. Similarly, the sequences for making modifications of data should be similar regardless of the data type. The clinician should be sensitive to and question anything in an interface that stands out as inconsistent or unexpected. Designers often introduce inconsistency inadvertently because they are too close to a design to be aware of its occurrence.

Navigation

As discussed earlier, an interface may be modal or nonmodal. In a modal interface, the designer makes most of the decisions on how the interface will be navigated, but the user still needs some elements of control, such as ways to get out of a flow or cues to let the user know where he or she is. Cues, such as the name of the patient on every screen, are particularly important in clinical applications because of the number of interruptions to which busy clinicians are subjected. When evaluating this element of the interface, the clinician should visualize the clinical work flow or thought process and then determine if the interface parallels it appropriately. Another element to be looked at is the availability of shortcuts, such as codes, fast keys, and user-defined macros. These will become in increasing demand as clinicians become experienced users and wish to cut down the time required to perform an action.

Transparency

The underlying goal of an interface designer is to make the interface transparent. What this means is that the user quickly forgets about the interface and can focus on what he or she is trying to do. For example, when you use a computer to write a paper, your focus should be on the paper's contents, not the keyboard. If, however, the keyboard has sticky keys, you will be distracted from the task at hand. Transparency is a characteristic of an interface that is best critiqued by a user already experienced in the platform.

Portability

If an application is going to be used on different platforms, the clinician should determine if the interface will appear the same and work identically on all of them. What is perceived as identical by the technician or nurse informatician may have enough subtle differences to confuse a clinician with limited workstation experience. This type of review is equally important if a single platform is to be deployed on hardware produced by different vendors or devices that are not configured identically.

Conclusion

Successful designers go beyond the vague notion of "user friendliness." . . . They must have a thorough understanding of the diverse community of users and the tasks that must be accomplished. Moreover, they must have a deep commitment to serving the users which strengthens their resolve when they face the pressures of short deadlines, tight budgets, and weak-willed compromisers." (Shneiderman, 1992, p. 8)

What difference does it make if the interface designer is a nurse or if nurses participate actively in the design process? Interface design requires, as Shneiderman points out, "a thorough understanding of the diverse community of users and the tasks that must be accomplished" (1992, p. 8). Similarly, the IOM report states that "proper system design means achieving a patient record system that properly fits with, interacts with and communicates in the accepted manner of every user community" (Dick and Steen, 1991, p. 35). When a nurse with a foundation in both health care and informatics makes design decisions in conjunction with nurses from a variety of clinical specialties, the resulting interface reflects the way nurses think and practice. For this reason, the software is more likely to be adopted willingly by the nursing community. Equally important, if a nonredundant, longitudinal CPR is to become a reality, nurses must also participate in the design of software that will be shared with other healthcare professions, such as medicine.

References

Bauersfeld P: *Software by Design: Creating People Friendly Software.* New York: M&T Books, Henry Holt, 1994.

Dick S, Steen E, eds: *The Computer-Based Patient Record: An Essential Technology for Health Care.* Washington, DC: National Academy Press, 1991.

Edmunds L: Methodologies for defining system requirements. In: Hughes S, ed. *Nursing Informatics: Today's Reality and Tomorrow's Potential.* Proceedings of a MedInfo 92 Workshop. Tempe, AZ: EMTEK Health Care Systems, Inc., 1992; 17–32.

Lafferty KD, Sheffield SD: The nursing function in designing health care information systems. In: Ball MJ, Hannah KJ, Gerdin Jelger U, Peterson H, eds. *Nursing Informatics: Where Caring and Technology Meet.* New York: Springer-Verlag, 1988, 235–242.

Marcus A: *Graphic Design for Electronic Documents and User Interfaces.* New York: ACM Press, 1991.

Norman DA: *The Design of Everyday Things.* New York: Doubleday, 1988.

Shneiderman B: *Designing the User Interface Strategies for Effective Human-Computer Interaction.* 2nd ed. Reading, MA: Addison-Wesley, 1992.

Zielstorff RD, McHugh ML, Clinton J: *Computer Design Criteria for Systems That Support the Nursing Process.* Kansas City, MO: American Nurses Association, 1988.

23
Business Process Reengineering

BARBARA A. HAPP

Introduction

There is a common vision in health care today: to provide affordable, high-quality care across the health continuum. However ideal, this is not what is happening. Neither the delivery systems in place nor the information available for decision making are adequate for today or the future. Healthcare reform and improved technologies are dramatically changing the systems and venues for health delivery. For example, when implemented broadly, telemedicine technology is said to reduce annual healthcare costs by at least $36 billion (Guterl, 1994). This includes home health electronic monitoring.

What are healthcare providers doing? Nursing has unlimited opportunities for reengineering care within the context of integrated delivery systems. The momentum for radical change is well underway. Results of the 1994 Hay Hospital Compensation Survey (Pierson and Williams, 1994) indicated that 60% of the 1036 hospitals surveyed are involved in some form of reengineering. Business process reengineering (BPR) is an important topic for all nurses because nurses are involved in planning, implementing, and evaluating this management strategy. Nurses should be on the team of architects reshaping healthcare systems because reengineering care means focusing on quality outcomes along with costs. The informatics nurse will be a major player in BPR because information technology is strategic to the success of BPR.

The metaphor that best describes business process reengineering in health care is the repair of an engine on a broken airplane in midflight, in a thunderstorm; the plane crashes, the pilot and mechanic parachute to safety, and a glider arises from the ashes (S. Kassam-Adams, personal communication, September 14, 1994). Keep this picture in mind as you read this chapter, in which BPR will be defined and described and healthcare examples will be cited. The critical success factors and benefits of BPR will be detailed and an action plan for nursing will be suggested.

What Is BPR?

There are many definitions of BPR. Klein (1994) defines BPR as a rapid and radical redesign of strategic, value-added business processes that include systems, policies, and organizational structures to optimize the work flows and productivity of the organization. Similarly, Hammer and Champy (1993) describe BPR as a fundamental rethinking and radical redesign of business processes to achieve dramatic improvement in measures of performance such as cost, quality, service, and speed.

Barrett (1994) says that dictionary definitions misguide BPR teams because BPR efforts provide unique opportunities for organizations to reconfigure themselves to become more effective, efficient, and humane. BPR is more than a vigorous analytic technique directed toward refining and streamlining an institution's operational process and data requirements. BPR is dramatic, transforming, and an agent of radical change in the healthcare organization. Information technology provides the infrastructure for organizational assessment, change management, implementation, and evaluation of BPR.

BPR in Health Care

What the aforementioned three authors and the metaphor are saying is that BPR facilitates dramatic change in how work is performed to improve organizational achievement. This change comes through drastic redesign of processes. Whetsell (cited in Bergman, 1994) applied Hammer's definition to health care to say that BPR is a radical redesign of the critical systems and processes used to produce, deliver, and support patient care to achieve dramatic improvement in organizational performance within a short period of time. If a process is a set of partially ordered steps intended to reach an objective (Curtis, Kellner, and Over, 1992), healthcare delivery is many administrative, clinical, and financial processes. Radical change in the business objectives and in the functional processes is needed to reap the benefits of reengineering. Benefits are measured as dramatic performance improvements in quality, service, and productivity with subsequent decline in expenditures and increase in return on investment.

Reengineering, transforming, or reinventing the healthcare business is about making fundamental changes in how a healthcare organization goes to market; provides services; deals with customers, suppliers, and competitors; and relates to and supports employees (Ryan, 1994). In other words, to accomplish the goals of BPR, we must take a hard look at how we produce, serve, manufacture, create, inform, educate, market, and sell health services (Canton, 1994). The structure, values, and norms of an organization may change along with the skills, job roles, and responsibilities (Stoddard and Jarvenpaa, 1994).

At a 1994 conference on restructuring, Judy Ryan, PhD, RN, FAAN concluded that nurses have no choice but to redefine and redesign the way they do their work (Ketter, 1994). From a global/policy viewpoint, nursing leaders are challenged to take the lead and not assume that cuts in full-time equivalents are the only tactics in reengineering.

As with all management strategies, BPR is not without a life cycle. We have seen management by objectives (MBO), transformational leadership, total quality improvement (TQI), and continuous quality improvement (CQI) come and go. King (1994) feels that BPR is a business idea in the debunk part of its life cycle. This is because BPR means different things to different people and the term "BPR" has been misused. However, BPR, or whatever it will be called in years to come, will have a valuable and enduring impact when applied to health care. We will soon get over the herd instinct surrounding BPR whereby everybody is doing it so it must be a good idea (Canton, 1994). In the future, we will see the results of BPR in health care (i.e., improved organizational performance measured by quality and financial indicators).

Hallmark Cards, Taco Bell, Xerox, and Ford are organizations that have successfully employed the principles of BPR. They are cited as companies that made radical changes to reengineer their business (Hammer and Champy, 1993). Integrated delivery systems (IDSs), community health information networks (CHINs), patient-focused care (PFC), and community-based nurse case management are examples of radical redesign for improved performance of healthcare delivery.

There are few reported completed BPR projects in health care, and evaluation has been limited. The measurement of the success of these healthcare reengineering programs is yet to be established. Lakeland Regional Medical Center in Florida is spending $10 million on PFC and expects to save $20 million per year, while the Medical Center of Beaver County, Pennsylvania, is spending $30 million on PFC improvements including bedside information systems and cellular communications (Bergman, 1994). Because of the relative newness of BPR, very little has been published concerning the results of BPR in health care. In the next section, the elements for success and failure of BPR projects will be reviewed.

Critical Success Factors

Reengineering efforts are ongoing in many industries, but the impact of these projects varies greatly. More than half of those responding to a business survey reported that they were reengineering or planning to reengineer their information technology operations. Sixty-five percent of these indicated moderate to significant improvement (Ready for the ReEngineering Challenge, 1994).

In a study of 20 large companies, Hall, Rosenthal, and Wade (1993) found the BPR had little measurable impact on the performance of individual business units. The authors found that for the process to be improved, it must be defined in terms of consumer value (breadth). The process change involves six organizational elements (depth levers): roles and responsibilities, measurements and incentives, organizational structure, information technology, shared values, and skills. Bashein, Markus, and Riley (1994) conducted a study to investigate the conditions that predispose BPR efforts to success and contribute to BPR failure. They found that successful companies' goals for BPR projects were company growth and expansion rather than downsizing and cost cutting. In addition, reengineering that is not driven by customer satisfaction seems to be less successful.

Carr, Dougherty, Johansson, King, and Moran (1992) describe BPR as a growth strategy and found that organizations that had a desire to dominate the competition rather than match it were more successful. Additionally, Carr and colleagues suggest that viewpoints from outside the organization are very important to the foundations of improvement. Successful organizations employing BPR have a culture that values customers, shareholders, suppliers, and employees and recognizes change as a business need. These organizations also understand their own capacity for change and believe that the most valuable core competency is the ability to create change.

Barrett (1994) describes process visualization as the single most important activity for successful BPR programs. Visualization is having a mental picture of a future reengineered business process in advance of its realization. BPR teams visualize the future processes, their function, and the performance improvements that the changed processes will bring. Both a narrative and a graphical depiction is encouraged.

Using a case study research approach, Stoddard, Jarvenpaa, and Littlejohn (1994) found that many of the common assumptions about BPR need to be challenged. They studied a successful reengineering project of a large communications company. In this empirical study, they found that while project design was radical, implementation was incremental and limited by constraints over which management had no control. The focus of implementation was on the "broken pieces," whereby managers would get the most benefits with the least effort. There was a close alliance between the problem and the solutions instead of an attempt to change everything. These authors found that although the design for change was top-down, it must be owned from the bottom up. Ownership and commitment were visible throughout the organization for the success of the project. Finally, the project was designed with information technology as a critical element, but in reality implementation could be initiated without information technology capabilities in place.

In another study, Caron, Jarvenpaa, and Stoddard (1994) described 10 principles that a large insurance and financial services company learned from 5 years of experience in over 20 reengineering projects. The company was very successful in reengineering and not only saved over $100 million but also increased customer satisfaction by 50% and improved quality by 75%. Many of these principles can be applied to reengineering in health care:

1. Diffuse and leverage learning from each project.
2. Learn from failure.
3. Foster commitment and ownership at all levels.
4. Exploit "clean slate" opportunities.
5. Tailor reengineering to the characteristics of the environment.
6. Ascend to higher forms of reengineering.
7. Move with lightning speed.
8. Communicate truthfully, broadly, and via multiple forums.
9. Select the right people.
10. Focus most of all on a mindset change.

In light of these findings, there are several questions nurses should be asking when approaching a reengineering project. The strategic vision of the organization should be clear and easily communicated. Nursing leaders should be able to articulate the needs of the organization and the overall plan for change. Upper management and providers must all be involved in planning and implementing the changes. Readiness of the organization should be assessed and direction planned and communicated. Resources (financing, staffing, support) should be available. Process change should be based on solving problems that impact the nurse and patient care. Use of a formal methodology and an enterprise-wide focus on strategy, operations, and information technology will positively impact the outcomes of the BPR initiative. Finally, the lack of information technology should not hinder implementation of a BPR project. A plan to optimize the systems in place and add additional supporting applications may be enough to get the project underway and completed successfully.

Total Quality Management/Continuous Quality Improvement and Business Process Reengineering

The differences between total quality management/continuous quality improvement (TQM/CQI) and BPR have to do with the approach and focus of the projects (Bergman, 1994). While BPR centers on a top-down management strategy and radical change, TQM/CQI looks at the problems from the bottom up and is based on incremental changes. There is a strategic focus to BPR projects and generally a tactical approach to a problem with TQM/CQI. Finally, the role of information systems is considered with TQM/CQI, but information systems are an enabler to the success of BPR projects. TQM and CQI have laid the foundation for process improvements and reengineering in health care. Once BPR is implemented, CQI must be in place to sustain the benefits of the radical changes in an organization.

What Are The Benefits of BPR?

There are a variety of reasons for healthcare organizations to turn to reengineering. First and foremost is the need to become competitive or to maintain market share. Small incremental change will not bring the cost reductions and efficiencies necessary to compete for and win managed care contracts. Mergers, acquisitions, and the closing of facilities have put great pressure on administrators to change the way care is delivered and improve the quality of the care. Additionally, administrators are questioning the value of traditional models of care and reviewing the elements of integrated delivery systems as patient and staff satisfaction has become an important indicator of quality. Consultants are being engaged by large and small healthcare organizations to assess the present processes and improve profitability and quality through reengineering techniques.

Ideally, BPR is adapted before there is a crisis, but in reality dramatic change may be mandated when there is no other alternative. Reorganizations and downsizing may have been tried, but true BPR methodology is necessary to turn the organization around. A headline in a recent publication said, "The economy is changing. Jobs are changing. The workforce is changing. Is America ready? Rethinking work" (*BusinessWeek*, 1994). This is just what BPR is: changing the way we work.

BPR and Information Management

The selection and implementation of a new computer system is often the impetus for an organization to review business processes. This is because performance improvements are not being delivered through information systems alone. Hammer (1990) says that it is time to stop paving cow paths. Computers are no longer being used to mechanize existing processes.

By first evaluating functions and processes across departments, the need for reengineering before automation becomes evident. Computer systems that make the wrong things happen faster will not assist with organizational goals. For example, Happ (1994) found that the quality of patient care did not improve when bedside information technology was implemented. In this study of point-of-care technology in three hospitals, the technology was examined using patient satisfaction and nursing documentation as quality indicators. Patients on units that had bedside computers were less satisfied with nursing care, and documentation was better on units without computers at the bedside. The recommendations from this study included assessing nursing care delivery for possible streamlining before adoption of automation. In this way, automating the paper process could be avoided. Therefore, BPR may assist with optimizing present and new information technologies.

Information technology may be the transformer for many organizations. In a project at a major academic medical center, modeling the enterprise was the first step in preparation for BPR initiatives. Modeling includes identifying and documenting all the essential processes to baseline the operations of the health care organization. Using a computer aided systems engineering (CASE) tool, each clinical, financial, and administrative process was documented in a diagram and database. This provided process visualization for decision makers because you can only change what you can identify. Modeling provided the benchmark to expose inefficient, overlapping processes. Ideally, modeling brings consensus on opportunity for cross-functional process changes. Concurrent with the modeling, a technical architecture study was performed. Subsequently, when the technical architecture information was added to the model, it exposed the lack of clinical information system support as part of the infrastucture.

Barriers to and Enablers of BPR

There are several major constraints in implementing BPR. Middle management resistance is found to be the greatest barrier to dramatic change in the organization due to fear of job loss and complacency after previous efforts. Various levels in an organization may ask these questions: (Top Level) "Why can't we just get on with it?"; (Middle Level) "I'm not sure where we are going"; (Professional and Support) "What are they doing to us now?" (Caluori, 1994).

Enablers to the success of BPR include sound strategic planning (vision), top leadership support, understanding change management, and economic and/or quality pressures associated with healthcare operations. Aligning people and culture with changes brought about by BPR is the major role of change managers. Change management involves describing change, identifying the focus, determining the actions needed to support change by the individual and group, assessing the readiness for change, defining the new behaviors, and removing the barriers to change.

There are many theories about why BPR works and why it does not. Stoddard and Jarvenpaa (1994) studied the capacity to change and the leadership to guide the radical change in three organizations implementing BPR. The objective of BPR was to build a new business model aimed at increasing both customer satisfaction and company profits. The changes in skills, job roles, and responsibilities along with organizational structure, values, and norms were found to be the major parts of the transformation brought on by BPR. The authors found that revolutionary change (versus evolutionary) presumes technical and social system change at the same time. In contrast to Hammer and Champy (1993), Stoddard and Jarvenpaa found that reengineering may start with a clean slate, but in reality the organizational history, politics, behaviors, structures, and practices impact the implementation negatively. This means that radical change may be planned, but expectations should be tailored because only incremental improvements were sustainable for these three companies.

More than anything else, BPR facilitates organizational flexibility through identifying and implementing value-added processes across functional areas in the healthcare organization. Consensus on planning, organizational mission, and vision is also an outcome of BPR. Successful implementation involves rethinking of business from the board on down with ownership from the bottom up. Information management technology, as an essential enabler and key driver of change, supports the redesigned processes for improved organizational performance.

Getting Started

Most consulting firms have a methodology for planning and implementing a BPR project. For example, Martin (1994) offers a four-step recipe for implementing BPR in a physician group practice: process identification, creative thinking, technology enabling, and risk taking. Generally, a four- to six-step framework may be used in planning and implementing BPR. As with most methodologies, the process is based on the scientific method/nursing process and includes assessment, planning, implementation, and evaluation. The following describes the formal actions critical to reengineer a business process (these high-level steps assume that a strategic plan and team are in place and the mission statement and objectives are written):

1. Assess, identify, and document current processes by overviewing operations through interviews and document examination. Computer assisted software engineering (CASE) tools can be used to complete this effectively. This starts at the top of the organization for consensus building.
2. Analyze the documented processes and prioritize for value impact to the stated goals of the organization. Activity-based costing (assigning costs to processes) may be used to assess which processes have the greatest financial impact and thus need changing. Focus should be on strategic processes.
3. Select the processes to be reengineered and prioritize once again. Benchmarking is often used at this point to examine process performance against other like organizations.
4. Plan the new processes through brainstorming. In the best of all situations, how would the process owners like the whole process to look? Design the new process. Process simulation may assist this activity. Outcomes and expected benefits should be written.

5. Plan and implement the migration to the new reengineered process with evaluation phases. This includes skills and training assessment, cross training, team and consensus building, and implementation of change management techniques.
6. Plan for continuous monitoring and ongoing process improvements and fine-tuning.

Action Plan For Nursing

Professional nurses are integral to the provision of care to patients. It is time to change how care is delivered and managed: the venue has changed, the acuity has changed, the technologies have changed. Business process reengineering is radical change for improvements in organizational performance and quality. With an understanding of this management strategy, nurses have the opportunity to change every phase of nursing care delivery and improve patient care outcomes. Here are seven questions to assist nurses in developing and managing BPR projects (answering each question will facilitate development of an individual action plan for the BPR project):

1. If changes are communicated in the organization, decide if the change is TQM/CQI, downsizing, reorganizing, or actually reengineering. Will consultants facilitate the process? If so, what is the role of administration?
2. If it is a BPR project, who is the owner of the project and who are the stakeholders? How large is the project, and does it involve information systems planning, selection, or implementation?
3. Who is on the BPR team and how can you become part of the team? What tools will be used? What is the methodology?
4. What are the expected outcomes of the project? Are there both economic and quality goals? What is the time frame?
5. How will the results be measured?
6. How will the changes be maintained?
7. Why is the organization undertaking this BPR project now?

Conclusion

This chapter has been presented as a BPR primer for nurses. The opportunities that reengineering presents are challenging, but the rewards are promising. Although the pure definition is evolving, BPR methodology has the potential to improve dramatically the quality of patient care through changes in the delivery process. Tinkering with the present system brings small changes over time; BPR can bring dramatic improvements in the cost and quality of patient care. Reengineering is preliminary to adoption of information systems. To harvest the full benefits that information systems can bring to health care, BPR must be implemented. In the journey to fully integrated healthcare delivery systems, nurses will lead with revolutionary changes to enhance not only the quality of patient care but also their own job satisfaction.

Questions

1. Define and describe BPR in your own words.
2. What are some potential situations in which BPR is indicated in health care?
3. Delineate some of the critical success factors of BPR.
4. What are some of the benefits of implementing BPR?

References

Barrett JL: Process visualization. *Information Systems Management* 1994; 11: 14–20.

Bashein BJ, Markus ML, Riley P: Preconditions for BPR success and how to prevent failures. *Information Systems Management* 1994; 11(2): 7–13.

Bergman R: Reengineering health care. *Hospitals & Health Networks* 1994; February 5: 28–36.

Business Week: Cover. October 17, 1994.

Caluori A: 10 Restructuring don'ts. *Beyond Computing* 1994; September/October: 52–53.

Canton AN: BPR: The arguments every CIO hears. *Information Systems Management* 1994; 11: 87–96.

Caron JR, Jarvenpaa, SL, Stoddard DB: *Business Reengineering at CIGNA Corporation: Experiences and Lessons Learned from the First Five Years.* Boston, MA: Harvard Business School, 1994.

Carr DK, Dougherty KS, Johansson HJ, King RA, Moran DE: *Break Point Business Process Redesign.* Arlington, VA: Coopers & Lybrand, 1992.

Curtis B, Kellner MI, Over J: Process modeling. *Communications of the ACM* 1992; 35(9): 75–90.

Guterl F: The doctor will see you now—just not in person. *Business Week* 1994; October 3: 117.

Hall G, Rosenthal J, Wade J: How to make reengineering really work. *Harvard Business Review* 1993; November/December: 119–131.

Hammer M: Reengineering work: Don't automate, obliterate. *Harvard Business Review* 1990; July/August: 104-112.

Hammer M, Champy JA: *Reengineering the Corporation.* New York: HarperCollins, 1993.

Happ BA: The effect of point of care technology on the quality of patient care. In: Safran C, ed. *Seventeenth Annual Symposium on Computer Applications in Medical Care.* New York: McGraw-Hill, 1994; 183–187.

Ketter J: ANA has strong presence at restructuring conference. *The American Nurse* 1994; September: 5, 9.

King WR: Process reengineering. *Information Systems Management* 1994; 11: 71-73.

Klein MM: Reengineering methodologies and tools. *Information Systems Management* 1994; 11: 30–35.

Martin K: Reengineering a telecommunications system: Lessons learned. *Healthcare Information Management* 1994; (3) 8: 45–47.

Pierson DA, Williams, JB: Compensation via integration. *Hospitals & Health Networks* 1994; September 5: 28–38.

Ready for the re-engineering challenge. *Beyond Computing* 1994; September/October: 10.

Ryan HW: Reinventing the business. *Information Systems Management* 1994; 11: 77–79.

Stoddard DB, Jarvenpaa, SL: *Managing Change in Business Process Reengineering: Three Case Studies.* Harvard Business School Working Paper 9-4080, April 1994.

Stoddard DB, Jarvenpaa SL, Littlejohn M: *Business Reengineering in Reality: Pacific Bell's Centrex Provisioning Process.* Harvard Business School Working Paper 94-079, June 1994.

Unit 5
Research and Nursing Informatics

Unit Introduction

This unit explores the role of research in nursing informatics and its implications for clinical practice. Brennan and Casper offer an update on a chapter in the first edition of this volume. They suggest the modeling of decisions to support the nurse in selecting alternate courses of action or when encountering a problem of great uncertainty with various pathways to resolution. Meyer, Abbott, and Williams offer insight into the integration of research in clinical practice using examples in two veterans' hospitals and a U.S. military hospital. Curran and Hales explore virtual reality and the potential applications for nursing and the broader healthcare arena. Turley expands on the virtual reality concept and discusses the differences between that and augmented reality. He explores the idea of "computing everywhere," also known as ubiquitous computing.

24
Modeling for Decision Support

PATRICIA FLATLEY BRENNAN AND GAIL R. CASPER

Computerized decision-support systems link computer technology with decision-making algorithms to augment, extend, or replace the judgment of the nurse. Decision modeling is one approach to computerized decision support with significant implications for clinical nursing practice. Nurses use decision-modeling systems when further analysis, rather than additional data, is needed to solve a decision problem. Implemented primarily on microcomputers, these systems, which incorporate the probability of events occurring, descriptions of outcomes, and values associated with the predicted outcomes, use decision analytic or multiple criteria models as the structure for analyzing decision problems. More recently, decision modeling has been conceptualized as a means to incorporate patient views or preferences in the decision-making process.

Modeling of decisions is achieved by one of two major approaches to decision support: analysis and advice. Analyzing systems, also called decision-modeling systems, are computer programs specifically designed to help nurses structure problems and explicitly consider values, risk, and uncertainty and, on the basis of these considerations, make selections consistent with a set of defined objectives. Advising systems, on the other hand, recommend solutions to nursing problems—solutions that reflect the judgment of nurse experts regarding the most expedient and effective response to nursing situations. Both modeling and analytic techniques incorporate individual values or preferences for outcomes into the decision-making strategy. These values or preferences may reflect those of the nurse or the patient, dependent on the requisites of the decision problem.

Utilization of decision-analytic techniques also provides nurses the opportunity to incorporate patient preferences for outcomes in the resolution of the decision problem. Incorporation of patient preferences has been promoted from the perspectives of improving the quality of health care and promoting patient autonomy and self-responsibility (Kaplan, 1991). It has been demonstrated that incorporation of patient preferences, rather than healthcare provider preferences, in decision analyses often results in the choice of more conservative treatment approaches (Kasper, Mulley, and Wennberg, 1992).

Modeling Concepts

Models and selected software packages to build models provide clinical practitioners with decision-support capabilities. Many nurses are already familiar with the concept of models. A nurse relies on a model of the renal system each time he or she interprets a patient's fluid balance for a specified period. Nurses employ Bowlby's (1980) model of loss as they attempt to understand why the 4-year-old patient cries when her parents leave her in the hospital. A model of political change guides actions in initiating a new way of assigning nurses to be responsible for the care of patients. The ability to build such models is inherent in the utilization of decision-support software.

In these examples, the models employed serve

- To represent a complex process (kidney function)
- As a template for categorizing and interpreting behavior (separation and loss)
- As a prescriptive pathway for action (change process).

Thus, a model is an observable structure that represents the essential components of the entity of concern. Maps, formulas, and stick figures are all models. In modeling a nursing decision, the nurse uses familiar words and phrases to flesh out the skeleton of the model to produce a small replica of the problem he or she faces. This process of structuring the decision problem results in explicit consideration of alternative options and of the values attached to predicted outcomes of the alternatives.

Following normative decision theory, mathematical functions are the skeletons on which the nurse builds the representation of a decision problem and form the basis on which the optimal action is identified (von Winterfeldt and Edwards, 1986). Two mathematical representations form the core of computerized decision-modeling systems: decision-analytic models (decision trees) and multiple criteria models.

Decision-Analytic Models

Decision-analysis trees provide structure to a decision problem in which the choice of a present course of action depends on the outcome of some future event. Decision trees have a series of components: actions, events, values (utilities), outcome states, and probabilities. For example, in a pain management decision, the nurse may consider two alternative courses of action (chemical analgesic or relaxation coaching) (Corcoran, 1986). The events include the occurrence of side effects of the alternative actions and the relief of pain. The various levels of patient function, such as somnolence or relief of pain, comprise the representative outcome states for this problem. The nurse uses the tree to represent visually the likelihood, or probability, that a particular action leads to certain outcome events. By attaching a numerical assessment of the probability of an outcome to the patient-identified utility or value of each outcome and following the laws of subjective probability, the nurse can compute the expected value of each action under consideration for each individual patient. Normative decision theory dictates that the most desirable action for the individual is the one with the highest expected value for the individual patient.

Decision analysis allows for the explicit incorporation of the value associated with the probable outcomes. These values or utilities may reflect the views of the patient or the nurse involved in the decision situation depending on whose values are more appropriate in resolving the decision problem. Therefore, the desirability of the event occurring as well as the probability of the event occurring are integral to the identification of the optimal solution for the decision problem.

Multiple Criteria Models

Many patient care decisions require that choices simultaneously satisfy numerous values and objectives. Consider, for example, the problem of determining how to prevent patient falls. The nurse could use cloth restraints, have a staff member seated with a patient at all times, or keep the lights on in the patient's room. An effective course of action must be legally appropriate, feasible within the nurse's budget, and respectful of the desires of the patient. No single alternative meets all of these criteria. Multiple criteria models reduce complex decisions such as these into their elemental parts and help the nurse select the alternative that performs best on the summation of all criteria. Weighted sums are computed after determining how well a particular alternative meets each individual criterion and the relative importance of the criteria. Again, decision theory dictates that the best action will be that alternative with the highest cumulative score.

Capabilities

Decision analysis and multiple criteria are two types of mathematical models that can represent the decisions faced by nurses in caring for patients. By collaboratively constructing these models, the nurse and patient both gain greater understanding and insight into the problem at hand. This modeling process, based on a problem description presented in the nurse's and frequently the patient's own words, results in a recommendation for action that may be accepted or rejected by the user. Mathematical modeling of decisions is a specialized skill that previously required the participation of a decision analyst. Substantive developments in computer software now permit many of the analyst's functions to be taken over by an English language interactive query, and healthcare providers can conduct an analysis independently. Three features distinguish these decision-modeling systems from other types of decision support (i.e., advising systems):

- Domain independence (expert knowledge is provided by the user, not embedded in the software program)
- Focus on analysis rather than expert advice
- Intent to augment rather than replace the judgment of the nurse.

Software

Decision-modeling systems may serve as stand-alone decision-support tools or may form the basis for the advising (domain-dependent) decision-support systems. In this section, we describe only the stand-alone systems. Stand-alone decision-modeling systems are domain-independent, content-free decision aids (Brennan, 1986). These models, which act as templates, can serve as general-purpose structures for analyzing a wide variety of problems. For example, a medical/surgical nurse may use a multiple criteria modeling package such as Lightyear to determine what type of aftercare is best for a 45-year-old patient with cancer based on the probability of events occurring and the patient's preference for that event to occur. Because it is domain independent, a pediatric nursing team may use the very same software package to select an exercise routine for a hospitalized adolescent utilizing the same considerations.

Computerized decision-modeling systems are designed to reflect and structure the nurse's knowledge base and the nurse's or patient's preference structure. These systems are process oriented, with the emphasis on detailed understanding of the problem rather than on the recommendation of a solution. Decision-modeling systems show nurses the implications of their values, the patient's values, and associated assumptions. Final recommendations result as a reflection of, rather than a replacement of, the nurse's or patient's judgments.

Types of Computerized Decision-Modeling Systems

Most decision-modeling software packages run on microcomputers. In this section, we describe software designed to support the two major categories of mathematical models: decision analysis and multiple criteria. Advising systems (or expert systems) will not be addressed.

Decision Analysis

Decision-tree programs provide a visual display on the computer screen of the acts/events sequence encountered in a decision problem. The decision problem is graphically represented by a choice node on the left, with sequential branches to the right representing alternative actions and predicted outcomes of these actions. By combining the probability and value information assigned by the user to each outcome, the program computes the desirability or expected utility of each action. SMLTREE, a decision-analysis program developed by Jim Hollenberg in 1985, enables the nurse to construct and evaluate a decision tree. Running on an IBM-compatible personal computer, SMLTREE helps the decision maker model the series of values, actions, and events relevant to the decision problem and to determine the sensitivity of the expected value to variations in probability or utility assignment. SMLTREE can handle the generic class of decision problems in which the uncertain future consequences and values assigned to those consequences must be considered in tandem when selecting a course of action. Analysis in SMLTREE enables the evaluation of solutions on the basis of maximal expected value.

Decision Maker 7.04, created by Stephen Pauker and running on the Apple Macintosh computer, specifically models diagnostic and treatment problems faced by clinical practitioners (Sonnenberg and Pauker, 1986). Decision Maker 7.04 helps the nurse construct decision trees useful in selecting a course of treatment in which the outcome of the treatment and the state of the disease process are uncertain. Using Bayesian models and utility theory (Keeney and Raiffa, 1976; von Neumann and Morganstern, 1947), Decision Maker 7.04 helps the nurse determine the intervention most likely to bring a patient to a particular desired state of health.

Two analytical functions make Decision Maker 7.04 particularly useful for clinical judgment. One is the ability to determine how sensitive the recommended action is to imprecision in the nurse's estimates of disease status and efficacy of treatment. The second is that the preference for anticipated future outcomes (in this case, patient health or functional status) can be specified in terms of quality-adjusted life-years (QALYs). QALYs, which reflect outcomes and desirability of outcomes, represent a more familiar, understandable concept to both nurses and patients.

Multiple Criteria Models

Multiple criteria decision modeling helps nurses choose alternatives when the choice of action depends on satisfying many competing criteria simultaneously. Multiple criteria decision-modeling programs break down complex problems into smaller components that include the options under consideration, the criteria used to determine the best option, and the relative importance of or the assigned values of each option. At the end of the modeling session, these programs provide a printed and/or screen display of the results, including a designation of the most desirable option based on values and probabilities of each option.

Nurses have successfully used MAUD, a multiple criteria decision-modeling program, for clinical management decisions (Brennan, 1986). For example, a nurse may consider several approaches for ongoing treatment of a patient with chronic schizophrenia: hospitalization, day hospitalization, or individual outpatient treatment. Factors critical to this selection include the cost of the program, the patient's need for transportation to and from the site, the patient's preference for site of treatment, and the likelihood of obtaining the needed treatment. MAUD asks the nurse to type in first the alternative sites and then the name of each factor. Once the nurse evaluates each site individually on each factor based on his or her knowledge and patient preference, MAUD elicits the importance of each factor relative to the other factors. Finally, a list including all alternative treatment sites listed in rank order is printed. Other multiple criteria programs and their vendors include Expert Choice (Expert Choice, Inc.), Policy (Exec-Live Software), and Lightyear (Thoughtware). While the underlying models differ, each package is designed to help the decision maker select the best option in light of the complex factors to be considered (Table 24-1).

Use of Decision-Modeling Systems

Selection of a course of action is only one reason for using decision-modeling software. Modeling systems can also help nurses aggregate signs and symptoms to produce diagnostic statements. Some modeling software (such as Confidence Factor, produced by Kepner-Tregoe) specifically focuses on helping the nurse identify new options for creative problem solving. A nurse can consult a decision-modeling package when faced with a novel, important, and difficult decision. The software guides the nurse through the analysis of the decision problem to arrive at a recommendation. Additionally, decision-modeling software helps with post hoc analysis of a decision to verify the nurse's judgment. Use of decision-modeling software requires sessions from 10 to 60 minutes (Brennan, 1986).

TABLE 24-1. What Decision Model Should Be Used?

Decision Problem	Model Type	Software
If the problem involves . . .	Then the decision model is a . . .	And appropriate software is . . .
Selecting one alternative from several	Multiple criteria model	Policy (Decision Techtronics) Lightyear (Thoughtware) Expert Choice (Expert Choice)
Choosing an action now and the best choice depends on uncertain events in the future	Decision-tree analysis	SMLTREE (Hollenberg) Decision Maker 7.04 (Pauker) Data 2.6 (Tree Age)

Group Decision-Support Systems

Many of the decisions faced by nurses must be made in group settings. These groups may include other nurses or members of many disciplines. Computerized group decision-support systems (GDSSs) facilitate group conferencing and communication. In addition to providing the benefits afforded individuals in decision making, GDSSs help members with some group process tasks. For example, in a multiple criteria analysis, the voting power can be divided proportionally to the extent of the influence held by the various members. A discharge planning group may elect to use a GDSS to help a family resolve the issues surrounding aftercare placement of an ill family member.

Most decision-modeling packages are designed to replace the decision analyst and therefore can be used by a nurse without extensive understanding of computers, mathematics, and decision analysis. English language directions guide the nurse through these modeling programs. Printouts and graphical display screens show the results of the decision modeling.

To obtain the greatest benefit from decision-modeling software, the nurse should have a cursory knowledge of the software's underlying models. Familiarity with the assumptions of utility theory and decision analysis will enable the nurse to select the correct decision aid and interpret the results accurately. Several texts (von Winterfeldt and Edwards's *Decision Analysis and Behavioral Research* or Weinstein and Fineberg's *Clinical Decision Analysis*) provide basic introduction to some of the concepts underlying the packages described (von Winterfeldt and Edwards, 1986; Weinstein and Fineberg, 1980). For full appreciation of the power of decision modeling, these texts should be consulted.

Conclusion

When the nurse faces a problem of selecting alternative courses of action, multiple criteria models will serve best. When the nurse encounters a problem of great uncertainty with various pathways to resolution and varying values for potential outcomes exist, the decision-tree models provide the greatest assistance.

Questions

1. What benefits can nurses expect when using decision-support systems?
2. Compare and contrast multiple criteria modeling with decision-tree analysis in terms of problem types and solutions provided.
3. For what types of decision problems and in what circumstances are decision-modeling tools preferable to expert systems?

4. How can the nurse ensure that the analysis produced from a decision-modeling system is correct?
5. How could the nurse obtain the probability estimates required for using a decision-tree analysis package?

References

Bowlby J: *Attachment & Loss—Volume III: Loss.* New York: Basic Books, 1980.
Brennan PF: *The Effects of a Computerized Decision Aid on the Decision Making of Nurse Managers.* Unpublished doctoral dissertation. University of Wisconsin, Madison, 1986.
Corcoran S: Decision analysis: A step by step guide for making clinical decisions. *Nursing and Health Care* 1986; 7: 149–154.
Data 2.6 [computer software]: Boston, MA: Tree Age Software Co., 1995.
Expert Choice 9.0 [computer software]: Pittsburgh, PA: Expert Choice, Inc., 1994.
Hollenberg J: *SMLTREE* [computer software]. New York: Author, 1987.
Humphreys P, Phillips L: *MAUD.* [computer software]. London: Decision Analysis Unit, London School of Economics, 1980.
Kaplan RM: Health-related quality of life in patient decision making. *Journal of Social Issues* 1991; 47: 69–90.
Kasper JF, Mulley AG, Wennberg JE: Developing shared decision-making programs to improve the quality of health care. *Quality Review Bulletin* 1992; June: 183–190.
Keeney R, Raiffa H: *Decisions with Multiple Objectives: Preferences and Value Tradeoffs.* New York: Wiley, 1976.
Lightyear 1.5 [computer software]: Coconut Grove, FL: Thoughtware, Inc., 1987.
Pauker SG: *Decision Maker 7.04* [computer software]. Boston: Pratt Medical Group, 1993.
Sonnenberg FA, Pauker SG: Decision Maker 6.0. In: Salamon R, Blum B, Jorgensen M, eds. *MedInfo 86—Proceedings of the Fifth Conference on Medical Informatics, Vol. 5.* Amsterdam: North-Holland, 1986; 1152.
von Neumann J, Morganstern O: *Theory of Games and Economic Behavior.* 2nd ed. Princeton, NJ: Princeton University Press, 1947.
von Winterfeldt D, Edwards W: *Decision Analysis and Behavioral Research.* Cambridge, UK: Cambridge University Press, 1986.
Weinstein M, Fineberg H: *Clinical Decision Analysis.* Philadelphia: W.B. Saunders, 1980.

25
Integrating Research Data into Clinical Practice

Kerry E. Meyer, Patricia A. Abbott, and David Williams

Healthcare information systems (HISs) are a tremendous resource for professional nurses conducting scientific inquiries in their clinical practice. To take advantage of the capabilities of an HIS, research activity requirements must be defined during the early stages of HIS development or when the commercial HIS is customized.

Informatics nurse specialists (INSs) must participate actively in the development, evaluation, and selection process of a robust HIS to ensure that research requirements are implemented. In this chapter, we discuss issues of integrating research requirements into the HIS. A case presentation illustrates how key issues of integrating research were managed by an INS.

Research Process

Research is the application of the scientific method to problem solving and the expansion of knowledge (Polit and Hungler, 1987). Nursing research involves the scientific investigation of actual or potential health problems. The focus of these investigations includes promoting health and preventing disease, understanding and mitigating the effects of acute and chronic illnesses and disabilities, and delivering nursing services. Nursing research examines the biological, biomedical, and behavioral processes that underlie health care and the environment in which it is delivered (American Nurses Association, 1980). The research process is defined here to include problem definition (phenomenon or clinical problem observed), review of the literature, methodological development (hypotheses formulated, sample sizes determined, and instruments developed and validated), data management (collection, organization, and analysis of data), and dissemination of findings (publication, review, and critique). The goal of nursing research is improvement of nursing practice and patient health (Grant, Fleming, and Calvanico, 1991).

Given this broad definition of research, information processed in an HIS as a result of quality assurance programs; monitoring systems; and financial, administrative, and care planning programs integrates well with information specifically collected for research. The challenge is to address people, data, hardware, software, and procedural issues occurring as a result of this integration.

Nursing Process and Nursing Research

Clinical care is changing rapidly in response to the demands of healthcare reform. During these turbulent times, the nursing process continues to be a stabilizing concept, providing continuity across providers and patients. The content within nursing assessments, planning processes, interventions, and evaluations has changed. However, the structure (or data models) of the nursing process has not changed significantly. When integrating research, these data models can be viewed as a starting point. There are many logical, functional, and conceptual information design parallels between the nursing process models and the process of nursing research (Glass, 1991). With relatively small changes in the data models (e.g., the entities and their relationships) for the nursing process, many broad nursing research requirements can be met. Helping information system managers understand the similarities between the two processes of nursing and research is an important role for the INS.

Issues to Consider When Integrating Research Requirements into the HIS

Problem Statement

Suppose you are the informatics nurse specialist. Further suppose that you have been asked by a team of investigators to address their research information needs with the HIS department. These investigators include staff nurses, providers, administrators, academicians, and clinical specialists. Depending on the scope of the project, existing resources, and the setting, these issues will vary from simple to complex. These issues may impact one or more of the data processing components of the current HIS, including people, data, software programs, hardware, and procedures.

People

Several groups of people need to engage in the software life cycle if research requirements are to be included as part of the HIS. In this instance, the clientele is the nurse investigators. The users may include healthcare providers representing several disciplines, administrators, or research personnel (e.g., biostatisticians) external to the healthcare environment. Operations personnel run the computer and associated equipment. Depending on the requirements, their involvement may be minimal (e.g., changes only to the existing database) or extensive (e.g., installing local area networks). Systems development personnel design and implement the database and its application. This group may involve persons external to the HIS department such as contracted programmers/analysts and consultants as well as internal personnel such as clinicians, clinical information specialists, researchers, and administrators. In addition, the support of the chief executive officer (CEO) may be desirable. A survey conducted by *Modern Healthcare* indicates that there is a new breed of hospital CEOs that will have a major impact on the requirements for an HIS and provide more inroads to building repositories of data for research (Lutz, 1994).

The use of computers in patient interviewing has been studied since the 1960s. Research requirements may include the incorporation of patient end users as part of the HIS strategic plan. It is now well known that patients react favorably, even with enjoyment, to computer-based interviews that are carefully written (Locke et al., 1994).

Managing issues associated with each of the various groups of people involved with the nursing research project is a major task for the INS. Common goals and a common language between and among group participants are required for a successful implementation. Building a common language between the expert researchers, clinicians, administrators, and HIS managers will help reduce problems later. Traditional structured analysis sessions can facilitate a portion of these discussions. Facilitators should be present at all group meetings. Documentation of each session is essential and should be validated with group members. Knowledge engineering techniques have been shown to be effective in research information systems projects (Petrucci, Canfield, and Petrucci, 1992). McGraw and Harbison-Briggs (1989) present a variety of knowledge engineering techniques in their book entitled *Knowledge Acquisition: Principles and Guidelines,* which is an excellent guide for the INS.

Data-Level Issues

Issues surrounding data can be considered at three levels: the data level, the system level, and the process level (Canfield and Petrucci, 1994). Patient care, clinical research, and administrative events are represented at the data level. For example, information contained in the patient's medical record or research record is found at the data level. A key issue to address with nurse researchers and HIS managers is the large problem of standardizing healthcare terminology. Without standards, comprehensive queries performed to support research efforts are difficult. For example, dementia, cognitive dysfunction, or loss of cognition may be documented inconsistently by the same provider over different encounters or across different providers during the same visit.

Input, throughput, and output comprise a simplified representation of the information pathway. As we speak of input in defining data requirements, it is critical to examine the relationship of input to output. In conjunction with determining the data needs of investigators and evaluating the querying process, formal representation of data must occur. Simply put, users need to specify the pieces and format of data to be represented, in what order they need to appear, and the relationships between elements far in advance of designing the input mechanism. This method of backing in to the problem-solving process is frequently used by system developers to stimulate critical thinking on the part of the end users. Discussions of this type not only help clarify the data requirements but often help educate the HIS managers.

System-Level Issues

The system level of the data model includes interfaces to external information systems and, most importantly, to the people that the information system is designed to support. Database managers, system developers, and end users work with graphical user interfaces (GUIs), which are designed to facilitate integration with disparate systems and appeal to users. An interface was designed by the informatics core at the Baltimore VA Medical Center to bridge the gap between a customized clinical database called GERI (discussed later in this chapter) and the VA-wide HIS known as DHCP. This interface provides a seamless display of patient-related data that is generated by two markedly disparate information systems. This interface effort supports the natural work flow of clinicians and researchers and has increased end user acceptance in the Geriatrics Service. An additional example follows, in which a commercial system was customized to address system interface issues.

The INS at the Madigan Army Medical Center in Tacoma, Washington has worked to customize and implement a clinical information system (CIS) that is widely accepted by clinicians and researchers. The CIS captures data from myriad patient monitoring devices and is the lifetime data repository for order transcription, laboratory results, multidisciplinary clinical notes, and selected waveforms. Currently at Madigan, over 400 CIS terminals have been placed to cover every patient care area, and this has resulted in an extremely powerful and user-friendly point-of-care system. The CIS offers a user-friendly process for data entry, viewing, storing, and communicating electronically a gestalt view of relevant patient data to all healthcare providers and ancillary staff.

Interfacing to the Department of Defense legacy HIS (Composite Health Care System [CHCS]), the CIS provides the ability to document patient care at a resolution many times finer than CHCS. A key feature of this project was the attention to system-level requirements while working with an external CIS vendor, including on-site customization, rapid response time (zero wait state), a graphical user interface, and at least 99.95% uptime (measured against scheduled and unscheduled downtime). These CIS characteristics, coupled with the vendor's participation, have produced a system that supports documentation practices with the capability of handling a large number of research requirements across all disciplines. Research requirements are facilitated through the capability of performing queries at the lowest possible resolution, across time and patients.

End User Interface

A user interface for clinicians and researchers supports these queries. Two screen types that enable querying data at such low resolution include flowsheets and notes. Flowsheets are used for quantitative data and limited strings of ASCII text data. The data are selected and placed on the x-axis by clinicians and researchers; the x-axis is stored against the y-axis, time. Examples of data that can be stored in the flowsheets are physiological readings, intake/output, medication administration records, treatment administration records, and neurologic monitoring scales. Notes are the second screen type. Each note is comprised of a template that supports free text entry and choice lists from which to select. Templates are a series of fields that are structured to facilitate the healthcare provider's documentation of the care provided, observations, and rationale of care. The combination of free text and choice lists is the only currently available method to meet all end users' documentation needs. The choice list, if cleverly constructed, may meet up to 90% (but possibly not all) of the conditions that researchers and providers plan to store.

The user interface can also be configured to prompt end users visually to perform a task. The task could be a certain method of documentation or information pertaining to a research protocol. Empirically at Madigan, this prompting in and of itself has not only increased profoundly the quantity and quality of day-to-day documentation but has also significantly increased the end users' probability of documenting in a manner that is being prompted.

System Developer Interface

The clinical information system at Madigan furnishes the system manager with two powerful options: on-site rapid prototyping of templates and the ability to cross-populate data throughout a patient's record. Rapid prototyping produces the best results when the system manager constructs the templates in the physical location of the live environment. Creating templates within the presence of end users, in a matter of minutes, ensures a rapid turnaround, pertinent prompts, and logical document flow and facilitates maximum end user participation and acceptance. Once a research question has been formulated, if the data are not found currently in the

CIS, they can be added easily to a template and queried later. Cross-population data are used when the same data are found in multiple locations in the CIS. Items such as patient demographics, laboratory results, problem lists, and a host of other information can be configured to cross-populate predefined fields automatically when the note is opened or upon demand by the end user. However, experience at Madigan warns the INS that rapid prototyping only works when the process being automated is understood fully. It is also important to allow researchers and clinicians to test the prototype during a working period of about 4 weeks. Implement, evaluate, adjust, and then reevaluate is a continuing process used through the entire CIS and HIS life cycles to meet researcher and clinician needs.

Minimally, the INS will need to negotiate user-friendly, no-frill interfaces from the information systems (IS) managers (or vendors) and obtain satisfactory evaluations from the researchers. In some circumstances, even this task will be difficult to complete. Cost, corporate culture, and constrained resources will impact system-level issues and how such issues can be resolved.

Process-Level Issues

The third level is the process level. These issues relate to the integration of existing HIS processes with necessary research processes (Curtis, Kellner, and Over, 1992). Fortunately, processing issues have been addressed in the literature. Boone, Duisterhour, and Ginneken (1992) discuss a project in which research processes were implemented successfully in a computerized patient record using a distributed, collaborative computing environment. Zielstorff, Jette, and Barnett (1990) have also reported on the experiences of one group in designing a system that serves as both a clinical record system and a database that can assess directly the impact of a coordinated care program for postacute care of the elderly. While large information system vendors are consolidating and increasing their data-collecting capacity, a parallel consolidation is going on among a group of vendors putting the data to good use with intelligent processing (Morrissey, 1994). Hospitals and healthcare systems are still busy building the computer systems that can process data from all sites and departments and make the data universally accessible. Once done, integrating research requirements into the existing process will be simplified greatly.

Software Programs

Research agendas can be software intensive. These may include operating systems, database management systems, application software, communication programs, library systems, and statistical programs. At a minimum, the operating system and the database management system are required. Researchers can interface to the data through forms, reports, and menus automatically provided by the database management system. However, for more complicated research agendas, an application program is usually required. If the research requirements include multiuser systems, the program is required to facilitate concurrent processing. For example, if the research requirements are well suited for local area network (LAN) technology, LAN operating systems and communication control programs must be included in the budget.

A major component of the research process is reviewing the literature. Traditional literature reviews have been accomplished at the library or by telecommunicating with the library system. Existing information and computerized library programs make it possible to bring information stored within the library to nurses in the clinical setting. Graves (1990) points out the difficulties associated with obtaining a relevant set of articles related to the nursing issue in question in a timely fashion.

Statistical programs can range from simple spreadsheet applications to neural networks. Queries to support the statistical analysis must be identified. If researchers want to be able to extract and analyze the finest detail from a particular test using statistical programs, then that finest detail becomes a data requirement. As stated previously, biostatisticians outside the HIS personnel may be required to maximize the use of the statistical programs. The INS should plan to facilitate discussions between any biostatistician and HIS managers. Identifying solutions to issues of security, data access, storage, and control before statistical programs are purchased is important.

Finally, research budgets for software programs warrant a few simple guidelines. The INS can be instrumental in facilitating the purchase of all programs required for research. If these programs are not coordinated with the HIS managers, a good deal of money can be wasted. All programs require support from the vendors directly, a biostatistician, or from HIS personnel.

Hardware

Integrating research requirements into an HIS does require the use of computer hardware. At the very least, the power of an 80286 processor is required. If the research requires workgroups, a local area network and a minicomputer or mainframe may be required. Extracting at least good estimates of the data storage requirements from the researchers early in the definition phase is a key. Many researchers are unfamiliar with data storage requirements. Data storage requirements for the research agenda include source data, metadata, overhead data, and possibly application metadata. Source data are the facts stored in the database. Metadata are the data contained in the data dictionary that make program/data independence possible. Overhead data consist of linked lists, indexes, and other data structures that represent record relationships and serve other roles. Application metadata are the structure of menus, screens, reports, and other application constructs (Kroenke, 1992). HIS managers will appreciate the efforts of the INS who prevents hardware issues from becoming problematic with a thorough evaluation of data storage requirements. Many HISs are being converted to client-server systems. These hardware systems consist of local area networks with a database server and a number of microcomputers. The database server and microcomputers share the processing requirements. This hardware configuration, with the support of the CEO and HIS managers, allows researchers the opportunity to design and implement research applications on their local systems within a distributed computerized environment. In some cases, nursing research requirements may include the monitoring of patient data using specialized hardware. As the size of computers has decreased, the power of hardware monitoring equipment has increased. For example, home cardiac monitors (Ayala and Hermida, 1991) are available for use without the presence of a health provider while the patient performs independent monitoring activities. Having hardware available, such as micromonitors or wireless systems, increases the amount of information available over time and decreases the intervals of data collection from visit to visit to minute to minute outside the confines of a traditional intensive care unit setting. The cost and resources associated with maintaining specialized hardware needs for research efforts may be viewed as outside the scope of the traditional IS department. In special situations, biomedical support personnel will become part of the development team and work closely with IS managers and nurse investigators.

Procedures

To integrate research into the HIS, the INS will be faced with the issue of establishing and documenting procedures. Both users and operations staff need documented procedures describing how the new research system works within the HIS policies and procedures. Ideally, procedures can be programmed into the application. Research budgets often fail to include the costs of developing procedures, educating end users, and enforcing those procedures within the HIS environment. Research staff operating research systems have higher turnover rates than personnel within HIS departments. Rotating graduate students often perform backups and recovery operations that, if not documented, can lead to disastrous situations. Once the student leaves, the knowledge of the research system should not go with him or her. If the research application is actually an extension of the HIS, the database manager must also have procedures to follow. For example, changes to the database may require a community-wide view when multiusers are involved. A change made to benefit one researcher could affect another researcher's agenda. Issues regarding how changes are made to the system, actions to take when the system fails, and responsibilities for new transactions require communication to be resolved effectively.

Case Study: Geriatric Education Research Information

Work was begun in the spring of 1992 to build an adjunct information infrastructure named GERI (Geriatric Education Research Information) within the Baltimore Veterans Affairs (VA) Medical Center specifically to support a new geriatric research education clinical center (GRECC).

People

Strong support for GERI was provided by the director of the GRECC program, who contracted an external consulting team to initiate the project. One of the first recommendations of the consultants was to develop a strong internal information systems management team (hereafter referred to as the GRECC HIS team). Responding to this recommendation, an informatics nurse specialist (INS) and two systems programmer/analysts were hired. The systems development personnel consisted of the consultants, the GRECC HIS team, and key clinical researchers from the GRECC program. The operations personnel for GERI would eventually include the GRECC HIS team and the current systems programmer/analysts working with the VA hospital information system, known as the decentralized hospital computer program (DHCP). Over time, the INS was designated as the project manager for GERI. The end users were clinicians, researchers, and administrators in the GRECC program. Finally, the client of the GERI program was considered to be the director of the GRECC because there were no patients in the GRECC at the time. During the first 6 months, the consultants essentially managed the project while the GRECC HIS team was being developed. Within 9 months, the GRECC HIS team was stable and ready to take full responsibility. All operations and management requirements for the project were brought under the leadership of the INS.

Data

Establishing requirements at the data, system, and process level required a flexible approach that could accommodate a rather ill-defined set of requirements across all levels. A structured methodology was combined with rapid prototyping and several information acquisition techniques. In addition, the team made a commitment to client-server technology early in the definition phase.

The methodology selected to establish data requirements included a combination of structured analysis techniques known as knowledge acquisition development systems (KADS) (Hickman et al., 1989). Expert clinicians and researchers were key end users of the proposed GERI program. Focusing on knowledge using the KADS method helped to identify data at the data, system, and process levels.

Rapid prototyping helped the team work with end users to establish essential processes, such as an automated telephone interview. Lessons learned from early prototyping efforts led to sophisticated design decisions along the way.

Several types of information acquisition methods were implemented by the development team throughout the program. Brainstorming sessions with "expert" teams, face-to-face interviews with individuals and workgroups, structured educational sessions, and formal surveys were the primary acquisition modes. In this environment, it was very difficult for the users to determine the needs under prospective and abstract circumstances. Definitions of queries and reports were being created by researchers in parallel with the development of GERI. The GRECC was 9 months away from seeing its first patient. The diversity within the division was tremendous, the only computing capabilities were within the current hospital information system (DHCP) and with a single VAX terminal left over from a previous study, and many of the new pieces of testing equipment had not been installed. To compound the situation further, the Baltimore VA Medical Center was moving into an entirely new hospital in the downtown area in January of 1993.

The INS worked directly with the end users to define information requirements and gather input, which would eventually lead to the existing application. Mock-ups, printouts, and rapid prototypes were used by the GRECC HIS team to assist users in visualizing and manipulating structures. Under the direction of the GRECC HIS team, the methodology gradually shifted from the process-oriented approach of KADS to defining queries and outputs—now ready for discussion with the research team. Characteristically, users would present a data recording sheet that was currently in use and request that the system mimic the layout. Users were assisted in specifying the pieces and format of data to be structured, the order in which they needed to appear, and the relationships between elements. This change in approach was somewhat difficult for the users initially, but the eventual outcome was a cohesive, concise, and goal-oriented method of data representation.

The GRECC HIS team understood the constant tension between benefit and effort in relation to the recording of data by busy researchers and clinicians. While trying to structure the data for extraction, one walks a fine line between efficiency and exhaustion. Whereas the goal of the system was to capture and code explicit data for research and clinical purposes, the ability to keep an exhaustively descriptive record was beyond the scope or goal of the project. It became a balancing act for users to define which pieces of data contributed to the output and which might be superfluous and noncontributory.

Consensus building among the group was difficult not only due to the previously mentioned elements of no patients, no system, and tremendous diversity but also due to having users involved in the design phase. Many of the clinicians were accustomed to dictated functionality. Being asked to specify what, how, and when was challenging.

Software Programs

A number of communication packages, office automation systems, statistical programs, and graphics packages were purchased. The discussion here is limited to the software purchased to support GERI and the user requirements implemented in GERI.

SQLServer and SQLBase by the Gupta Corporation were selected to develop the GERI application. Data requirements operationalized in GERI are discussed as (1) a linking of knowledge sources (i.e., networks), (2) data acquisition at point of service, (3) situation-specific views of information, and (4) a method for rapid, focused data retrieval.

The team began to formulate software solutions in GERI to these four user requirements. For example, in support of the research goals of the GRECC, a method by which dispersed researchers, clinicians, and associated staff could access the system was mandated, necessitating a LAN. In addition, the ability to access other knowledge sources via the Internet was highly desirable as well as a method to access DHCP data. Metabolic, cardiac, and exercise laboratories needed to be connected to collect and store research data in the repository. Clinic rooms, offices, and classrooms all needed to access the network. It is obvious that data that are all part of the patient research record are not collected in one place, yet it is the GRECC goal to have all such data stored in one place with a formalized and secure data structure.

The idea of a separate LAN dealing with patient data external to DHCP was met with some resistance and cynicism. However, thanks to a progressive information resource management (IRM) department at the Baltimore VA and a good deal of team building by our network administrator, most issues were resolved. In addition to the research database server and application server for the division, the Baltimore VA now links to the University of Maryland at Baltimore (UMAB) system through the geriatrics LAN, giving authorized users access to the Internet and other services available through UMAB. The geriatrics network will link into DHCP by the summer of 1995, once again the work of a team of progressives working together to advance the use of information technology. The success of in-house development hinges on the commitment and "buy-in" of all of those affected by the project.

Requirement 2, data acquisition at point of service, is a true buzzword in healthcare informatics, so it was not surprising to the team that this was one of the four primary user requirements. To support the principal research focus of the GRECC, the system was designed to ready data automatically for extraction while being entered. Therefore, during the normal documentation of the patient visit, or as a laboratory specimen is being analyzed, or as compliance with a dietary regime is being recorded, the data are coded and stored in a state of constant readiness for extraction. The coding is virtually invisible to the user yet is a critical component of using clinical data for research. As we support point-of-service computing and attempt to replace the paper chart (while keeping the demands of recording to a reasonable level), we are looking toward new technologies, such as pen-based or voice-activated devices.

One of the goals of the system is to maintain a comprehensive record of patient-centered data for research management. A strong effort was made to support point-of-care data entry by making the technology and the interface palatable to users, especially the clinicians. As discussed earlier, this requires a constant balance between benefit and effort. In this environment, for example, users decided to adopt a "charting by exception" concept—meaning that normal findings are not recorded. It was deemed unnecessary by clinicians to record 350 "normals" in the standard review of systems. If a finding is deemed abnormal or worthy of comment, only then is the clinician required to document. Structuring the interface in this way was helpful in influencing clinicians to enter data. Moreover, the data collected and recorded in the GRECC are truly geared toward research testing, protocol, and patient management. Therefore, users are collecting data that support direct needs, not as an administrative mandate. This focused approach, which gives users immediate feedback to support work activity, has contributed to the utility of the system. Data for administrative use are (and should be) a byproduct of clinical and research computing. The feedback to users leads us into the next requirement, a method by which to extract specific data for review and analysis (situation-specific views and rapid data extraction).

The requirement for a specific mechanism for examining and extracting the data highlighted the diversity common in the healthcare arena. In our clinical research environment, a marked divergence between clinical researchers and basic science researchers was noted. Clinicians focus on the patient as a whole, in keeping with the traditional healthcare model, whereas the basic scientists focus on very specific data points. For example, the clinician may want to view 10 variables from an exercise treadmill test at two different time periods to examine the patient progress over time. Each of the 10 variables is important to the clinician. An example is the need to examine a change in blood pressure related to a weaning of antihypertensives or to review the progress being made by the patient over time. The basic scientist, however, is only interested in, for example, the VO_2 Max value at baseline and postintervention. This dichotomy required that the system support situation-specific views of information as well as the ability to extract very specific and independent variables.

The clinicians chose a GUI or view resembling a patient record in that it was encounter-based and included progress notes, order sets, results reporting, problem lists, and the like. Basic science researchers, in focusing on specific research protocols, did not want to use a patient-centered record system. The question became how we could meet the specific computing needs of diverse users within the division, especially in the mix of clinical and nonclinical personnel.

Ultimately, GERI was built to support the fine granularity and comprehensive needs of the clinicians, of which the basic researchers' requirements were subsets. However, when the basic scientists were ready to record, review, and extract, they did not want to see the additional layers of data required by clinicians. This mandated the creation of specialized tools and applications to create situation-specific views of data to meet the users' needs. These tools focused on two main areas: input and extraction. Additional months were added to the development process, but the investment was well worth the wait.

A tool for extraction and customized data set assembly was formulated, supporting user-specified searching of all data in the system external to the GERI interface. The tool supports views both across and within patients, thereby providing utility for researchers and clinicians alike. Users can choose a patient or patients within the database, specify the intervention or data of interest, narrow that search by choosing entire tests or subcomponents, and further restrict by specifying research codes, such as baseline or postintervention. The user has thereby created the query for a customized data set, containing only the variables of interest. The touch of a button executes the query, and the user is returned a spreadsheet of data for review, manipulation, or analysis. This method of extraction is popular, widely used, and supports the diversity of users within our division.

Modules were created that allow basic science researchers to maintain independent spreadsheets, which are instantly imported to the central data repository. Basically, the team created additional "front ends" for those averse to the computerized patient record. It has been interesting to note, however, that after the construction and programming of the spreadsheet modules, the only contingent using this method is the blood laboratory located in another section of the hospital. The data from laboratory analysis are entered in spreadsheets and directly imported over the network to GERI. It is generally believed that the user input in the design of the system and the resulting ease of use has shifted the preferred method of documentation to GERI.

Hardware

The GRECC HIS team made an enormous effort to coordinate design decisions regarding communication protocols and hardware needs within the new hospital. This was key in establishing the software, hardware, and processing requirements for the proposed architecture. The Baltimore VAMC is now in the new facility in downtown Baltimore. The LAN is up and fully functional, and the connections to UMAB are in place and operational. Twenty-one networked workstations are connected to the LAN, and the GERI system is now handling over 20 separate research protocols and clinics. Data on 467 research subjects reside on the database server, and the system is growing in quantum leaps.

Procedures

The GRECC HIS team has developed a set of in-house procedures available to end users. Further documentation is planned.

Conclusion

Incorporating research requirements into the HIS is still a complex task. Issues involving the people, data, software programs, hardware, and procedures must be considered carefully by the researchers in conjunction with the INS and HIS team. A great deal of experience has been gained by INSs who have developed and implemented robust systems, such as those at Madigan Army Medical Center and GERI at the Baltimore VAMC.

Research requirements can easily be built on nursing processes that do exist in most healthcare information systems. With the right support, incorporating research agendas is possible. As healthcare information systems move toward client-server environments using intelligent graphical interfaces and the information highway grows, incorporating research agendas will be a common event within the corporate information system strategy.

Questions

1. One data level issue involves the standardization of healthcare terminology. Discuss why this is an important issue.
2. What kinds of software might be utilized in a research environment to help collect and manipulate data?
3. Using the GERI case study as a model, discuss some of the aspects that made this project successful.

References

American Nurses Association: *Nursing: A Social Policy Statement.* Kansas City, MO: Author, 1980.
Ayala DE, Hermida RC: Predictable blood pressure variability in clinically healthy human pregnancy. In: Bank I, Tsitlik J, eds. *Proceedings of the Fourth Annual IEEE Symposium.* Los Alamitos, CA: IEEE Computer Society Press, 1991; 54–61.

Boone W, Duisterhour J, Ginneken A: New functional requirements for electronic medical records. In: Degoulet P, Piemme T, Rienhoff O, eds. *MedInfo '92, Proceedings of the Seventh Congress on Medical Informatics: Vol. 1.* Amsterdam: North-Holland, 1992; 697–702.

Canfield K, Petrucci KE: Issues in Enterprise Data Modeling for Open CIS. In: *1994 HIMSS Proceedings, Vol. 1.* Chicago, 1994; 403–412.

Curtis B, Kellner M, Over J: Process modeling. *Communications of the ACM* 1992; 35: 5–90.

Glass EC: Importance of Research to Practice. In: Mateo MA, Kirchhoff KT, eds. *Conducting and Using Nursing Research in the Clinical Setting.* Baltimore: Williams & Wilkins, 1991; 1–8.

Grant M, Fleming I, Calvanico A: Importance of research to practice. In: Mateo MA, Kirchhoff KT, eds. *Conducting and Using Nursing Research in the Clinical Setting.* Baltimore: Williams & Wilkins, 1991; 8–21.

Graves JR: A research-knowledge system (ARKS) for storing, managing, and modeling knowledge from the scientific literature. *Advances in Nursing Science* 1990; 13(2): 34–45.

Hickman FR, Killin JL, Land L, Mulhall T, Porter D, Taylor RM: *Analysis for Knowledge-Based Systems.* New York: Wiley, 1989.

Kroenke DM: *Database Processing: Fundamentals, Design, Implementation.* New York: Macmillan, 1992.

Locke SE, Kowaloff HB, Hoff, RG, Safran C, Popovski MA, Cotton DJ, Finkelstein DM, Page P, Slack WV: Computer interview for screening blood donors for risk of HIV transmission. *M.D. Computing* 1994; 11(1): 26–32.

Lutz S: The new CEOs. *Modern Healthcare* 1994; 10: 37–46.

McGraw KL, Harbison-Briggs K: *Knowledge Acquisition: Principles and Guidelines.* Englewood Cliffs, NJ: Prentice Hall, 1989.

Morrissey J: Firms interpreting data for integration. *Modern Healthcare* 1994; 24(38): 13, 19.

Petrucci KE, Canfield K, Petrucci P: A knowledge acquisition framework for planning problems in health care: A qualitative study. In: Degoulet P, Piemme T, Rienhoff O, eds. *MedInfo '92, Proceedings of the Seventh Congress on Medical Informatics: Vol. 1.* Amsterdam: North-Holland, 1992; 440–446.

Polit DF, Hungler BP: *Nursing Research: Principles and Methods.* 3rd ed. Philadelphia: Lippincott, 1987.

SQLBase, Gupta Corporation. 1600 Marsh Road, Menlo Park, CA 94025.

SQLServer, Gupta Corporation. 1600 Marsh Road, Menlo Park, CA 94025.

Zielstorff RD, Jette AM, Barnett GO: Issues in designing an automated record system for clinical care and research. *Advances in Nursing Science* 1990; 13: 75–88.

26
Virtual Reality

CHRISTINE R. CURRAN AND GARY D. HALES

What Is Virtual Reality?

Virtual reality has been described as the ultimate human-computer interface (Arthur, 1992). It attempts to eliminate the boundary between the user and the computer and to provide a means for interacting and processing information naturally and intuitively. It is a way for humans to visualize, manipulate, and interact with extremely complex data via a computer-generated environment (Aukstakalnis and Blatner, 1992). Virtual reality was pioneered about 30 years ago when Ivan Sutherland, a computer scientist, built his own head-mounted display (Antonoff, 1993). The term "virtual reality" was coined in the mid-1980s by Jaron Lanier, founder of VPL Research, Inc., in Foster City, California (the first company dedicated to virtual reality environments) (Hamilton, Smith, McWilliams, Schwartz, and Carey, 1992). While "virtual reality" is the popular term, some authors and researchers prefer terms such as "immersive simulation," "artificial reality," "telepresence," "virtual world," "cyberspace," or "virtual environment" to label the concept (Peterson, 1992a).

Scientists working on virtual reality applications believe that intelligence amplification (or augmentation) is more powerful than the use of computers for artificial intelligence. Dr. Frederick Brooks of the University of North Carolina, Chapel Hill, describes three areas in which he believes human minds are superior to any algorithms designed for artificial intelligence: pattern recognition, evaluations, and context (Rheingold, 1991).

Virtual reality gets its power from the fact that people comprehend images quicker than they can grasp numbers and text. A key assumption of virtual reality work is that the brain can process information better when it is presented data in a multiplicity of senses (Hamilton et al., 1992). Visual cues and eye-hand coordination are particularly important. In humans, one's eyes play the dominant role in interpreting the environment (Arthur, 1992). Almost half of the neurons in one's brain are dedicated to processing and evaluating visual information (Aukstakalnis and Blatner, 1992, p. 50).

Characteristics of Virtual Reality Systems

Three predominant characteristics of virtual reality systems are (1) a computer-generated environment (generally calculated moment by moment from basic physical principles depending on where one looks and goes), (2) a three-dimensional (3-D) presentation of information (e.g., visual and auditory), and (3) conveyance of information by multiple senses (Peterson, 1992a). The senses most developed in virtual reality systems are vision, hearing, and touch.

Aukstakalnis and Blatner (1992) describe three levels of virtual reality systems: the passive, exploratory, and interactive stages. In the passive stage, the virtual world moves around the viewer as in a "fly-by." During the exploratory stage, the individual gets to explore the virtual world by crawling or walking around but cannot manipulate objects. The most powerful stage is the interactive stage. In this stage, one actually experiences the virtual world. Objects can be moved, resistance can be felt, and sounds are 3-D.

The ability of the individual to become immersed in the virtual world is integral to the experience. In the virtual world, simulated beings do not have to be exceptionally smart or even complex (human-like in form) for a user to be immersed in the virtual environment. A simulated character that keeps quiet most of the time can appear quite knowing (Peterson, 1992b). What is important is that the user be engrossed in the interaction.

To that end, Joseph Bates and his team of researchers at Carnegie Mellon University have created animated characters (bouncing blobs with eyes who can change color or speed) that display emotion. They were programmed based on theories of behavior. Because of this, the blobs appear to take on "personalities" and people identify with them. The researchers' goal is to build creatures that are believable enough that people have to choose whether to treat them as objects or as living things (Peterson, 1992b).

The key to success in displaying computer-generated animated images is to have a low latency and a high frame-refresh rate concurrently. Latency is the measure of time between when an individual moves and when the computer registers the movement. There are presently five basic position-sensing methods in use: mechanical, ultrasonic, magnetic, optical, and image extraction. The frame-refresh rate is the number of frames that a computer can generate in a given amount of time. This rate is usually measured in number of frames per second (Aukstakalnis and Blatner, 1992, pp. 31, 265).

Technology

The concept of virtual reality is a quantum leap in human-computer interfaces. The major reason that virtual reality is still predominantly done only in research labs is the current limitations of technology, especially hardware. In many ways, the current technology for virtual reality is still considered primitive (Grimes, 1991; Pausch, 1993). The technology is intrusive, computer tracking systems are sluggish, and programming is difficult.

The technology involved includes input devices (e.g., data gloves; rigid exoskeletons or body suits, to sense movements; 3-D mice; and voice recognition), databases that can create essentially any virtual world, display devices (e.g., two head-mounted displays), and high-powered interactive computer systems. Data gloves and bodysuits tend to stretch out of shape and lose their sensing ability. They also respond poorly to subtle gestures but are good at sweeping motions (Grimes, 1991; Peterson, 1992a). Rigid exoskeletons are an attempt to correct some of these problems.

The head gear is cumbersome. Individuals who wear glasses often have difficulty with fogging of their lenses. Head-mounted displays are slow to respond to eye movements. There is a problem with motion sickness if the display lag time hits a critical window of response time (Antonoff, 1993). Motion sickness also occurs due to the sensation of self-motion without the corresponding physical cues (Aukstakalnis and Blatner, 1992).

Systems are getting better but are still very expensive. Good systems can cost between a quarter to three quarters of a million dollars. Often multiple computing systems are needed to gain sufficient power to have response time approximate real time. Unlike other graphics programs, virtual reality images are generated "as you go" (i.e., depending on where you look and move). Thus, model construction frequently takes 6 months or more (Grimes, 1991). Recently, several organizations have joined forces to develop a modular virtual-environment operating system (VEOS), the only one of its kind known to be planned or under development to date (Dutton, 1992).

Virtual Reality Applications

Uses for virtual reality are diverse. Science, health care, education, architecture, and entertainment have all found potential applications for virtual reality. Imagine a novice surgeon learning how to operate by placing his or her hand over that of an expert surgeon in a virtual world. A nurse who is physically remote from the patient could perform an assessment and intervene as necessary. One could even tour a virtual work environment before taking a position with the organization. These will be common events in a world with virtual reality capabilities.

However, implemented applications of virtual reality in actual practice are few. Perhaps one of the most widely known and earlier applications is flight simulation. Used by the military to train airplane pilots, this system is credited with improving safety for pilots. Virtual reality systems also allow correction of potential design flaws in new aircraft as well as other equipment. The military use of virtual reality systems exceeds that available for the general public.

The first general public virtual reality display, Battle Tech Center, located in Chicago, Illinois, opened in June 1990. It is a super arcade with 16 machines. This entertainment center has been extremely popular and profitable from opening day (Grimes, 1991). Japan produced the first marketplace application of virtual reality. The "virtual kitchen" opened in April 1991. A customer can try out a specified kitchen before purchasing it and make any necessary modifications to the plans (Bylinsky, 1991).

A few medical applications are emerging. Surgeons can now practice on a virtual leg (Bains, 1991). Henry Fuchs and colleagues at the University of North Carolina at Chapel Hill are using real-world ultrasonic images of a fetus superimposed over the mother's abdomen to visualize the position of a fetus in utero. This technique is called augmented reality (Stix, 1992). Radiologic applications are getting a lot of attention (e.g., 3-D imaging for radiation therapy), and psychiatrists are beginning to use virtual reality systems to treat patients with phobias (Aukstakalnis and Blatner, 1992).

Virtual Reality and Nursing

At present, nursing applications of virtual reality systems are nonexistent. In fact, fewer than five articles on the topic appear in nursing literature at present. Most of the other literature does not even mention nursing as a potential market but rather focuses on business, industry, space, or medical applications. There is, however, a nursing conceptual framework that has promise for the study of this topic.

Conceptual Framework

Staggers and Parks (1993a) have developed a framework for studying elements important to the nurse-computer interaction process. Since virtual reality is a human-computer interaction, this framework is appropriate to study virtual reality systems in nursing.

The Staggers and Parks Nurse-Computer Interaction Framework is a synthesis of concepts from the disciplines of human-computer interaction, nursing informatics, and developmental psychology (Staggers and Parks, 1993b). Framework elements include nursing context, nursing characteristics, nurse behaviors, a task, computer interface actions, computer characteristics, and a nursing informatics development trajectory (see Fig. 26-1).

Nurse behaviors and computer interface actions

Nurse behaviors are defined as "observable motor movements, influenced by nurse characteristics as well as other framework elements" (Staggers and Parks, 1993b, p. 284). They are classified as initiatory or responsive actions. Initiatory behaviors relate to the nurse using an interface device

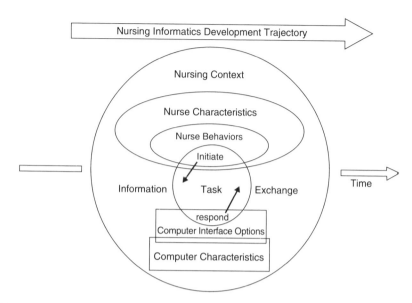

FIGURE 26-1. The Staggers and Parks Nurse-Computer Interaction Framework. Reprinted with permission from Amer. Med. Inform. Assoc., *Proceedings of the Sixteenth Annual Symposium on Computer Applications in Medical Care* (p. 663). New York: McGraw-Hill, 1993. Copyright 1993 by McGraw-Hill.

(e.g., using a mouse, typing in data or a command), while responsive actions occur as a result of information displayed on the computer interface.

Computer interface actions are computer-initiated or computer-responsive displays or sounds. For example, a computer-initiated display may be a query for more information. A computer response may be a beep as an error message (Staggers and Parks, 1993b).

In this framework, the nurse is depicted larger than the computer to reflect his or her difference in importance to the process. The nurse drives the interaction process (Staggers and Parks, 1993b). This would also be true when using a virtual reality system. The nurse would decide what virtual world to explore and where to go. He or she could change course in mid-exploration, stay on the current path, or abort the journey at any point in time.

Task information exchange process

In the Staggers and Parks Interaction Framework, some nurse behaviors and characteristics and computer interface actions fall outside the stated task domain because nurses, as well as computers, generally use only a portion of their available actions during a given nurse-computer interchange. The task component of the framework depicts information flowing from the nurse to the computer and back again in a potentially perpetual feedback loop (Staggers and Parks, 1993b).

In virtual reality systems, this feedback loop is integral to the interactive component but is also a cyclical process. The movements of the nurse would be "sensed" via the body suit, a data glove, or other direct manipulation device, and the computer would then display a response (e.g., via the head-mounted display). The process then repeats.

Nurse and computer characteristics

According to Staggers and Parks (1993b), nurse characteristics are personal attributes that are measurable but not necessarily observable (e.g., computer knowledge). Computer characteristics are attributes related to specific hardware and software.

Nursing informatics developmental trajectory

The idea of nurse-computer interactions (or even human-computer interactions) occurring as a developmental process is a unique concept to this framework (Staggers and Parks, 1993b). No other human-computer interaction frameworks have an element of time as part of their model (see Fig. 26-1).

Like other computer systems, virtual reality continues to have an evolutionary development. There are new hybrid virtual reality systems that contain knowledge-based systems (Hedberg, 1993). These systems have the ability to create "intelligent agents" that can direct you to shortcuts or answer your questions. Virtual reality will revolutionize computer-based training and teaching more than any technology thus far conceived. This technology is to computer assisted instruction (CAI) as CAI was to early attempts at programmed learning with paper and pencil.

Nursing context

In the Staggers and Parks Framework (1993b), the computer system is separate from the environment. The nurse-computer dyad is embedded in a nursing context. In virtual reality, the system and the environment become one (see Fig. 26-2). This is the only portion of the Staggers and Parks Nurse-Computer Interaction Framework that does not represent the virtual reality system correctly. However, other models or frameworks that include context have the same problem.

Virtual Reality, Nursing, and the Staggers and Parks Interaction Framework

In thinking ahead about virtual reality systems for nurse-users, the design of information systems for nursing, communication patterns of nurses as affected by virtual reality systems, and the impact of virtual reality on nurses' work flow, the following applications might be considered. We have placed our thoughts within each particular concept of the framework to give examples of possible topics for investigation.

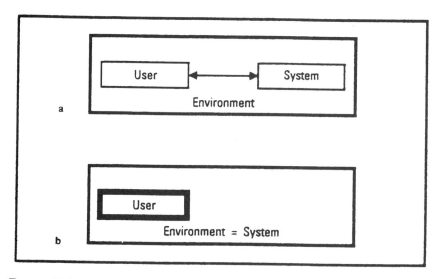

FIGURE 26-2. Conventional user/computer interface (a) and virtual reality interface (b). Reprinted with permission from J. Grimes, "Virtual Reality 91 Anticipates Future Reality," *IEEE Computer Graphics & Applications, Vol. 11,* 1991, p. 81. © 1991 IEEE.

Task information exchange process

Experimental prototyping is the single most talked about use for virtual reality (Antonoff, 1993). Nurses could create virtual nursing units and new delivery systems to try them out before they would actually be implemented. The ability not only to see these units but to work in these units would allow the nurse to understand the strengths and limitations of the design. What is the impact of a specific geographical layout on nurses' work flow? Possible modifications could then be made in the system, the system could be reexplored, and so forth, until a viable working model was achieved.

Similar experiments could be done in planning patient care or with patient interventions. Nurses could try out a plan or an intervention on a virtual patient before needing to do it for an actual patient. Virtual reality would allow debugging before use.

Nurses could learn skills such as intravenous catheter insertion with the help of augmented systems. The actual path of the vein could be portrayed over the patient's arm to guide catheter insertion. The same would be true for other catheters as well, such as indwelling urinary catheters and nasogastric tubes.

Nurses could make more accurate judgments about when to turn patients if the effect of positioning on circulation and ventilation were evident. Data about both systems could be superimposed over the patient and monitored.

When a significant compromise to either system was detected, the system would alert the nurse to reposition the patient.

Discharge instructions for patients could include what would actually occur at home since virtual reality could simulate the patient's actual home environment. A patient who was to receive an amputation could anticipate his or her change in mobility by trying out an artificial limb even before surgery.

Virtual reality removes the limits of language to express a concept or interpret an idea or data. Think about a nurse researcher "flying" around data to get a different perspective on patterns that are present. Would one need to do the same or any statistical tests on these data? One could manipulate the data right there by picking up the data and moving it to see what consequences emerge (just like a "what-if" scenario).

Nurse behaviors

What if we designed a virtual reality system for an entire group (e.g., a unit) of nurses and not just the individual nurse? Interactions between individuals could be studied as system changes were made. Communication patterns and work flow would become evident. Even the impact on other services could be evaluated.

Nursing students would be able to train on virtual patients in virtual settings. Students could learn from unique cases in remote areas. Students would have access to a leading expert regardless of his or her place of residence. How to function in high-risk events, such as code situations, could be taught to the nurses in a virtual environment.

Nursing recruitment would also be different in a world with virtual reality. Candidates would not have to come to the potential employment site. Managers could have the applicant take care of virtual patients to assess their skills before they were hired. Patients could do the same. In fact, it is likely that patients would choose their own nurse in this type of environment.

Computer interface actions

Quadriplegics and patients with other disabilities would be able to regain their full functionality in a virtual world through an interactive interface device designed to meet their unique needs. This would empower the disabled and allow them to gain independence and broaden opportunities of employment. For example, they could learn how to construct virtual reality prototype systems for customers.

Nurses could directly manipulate objects for patients who are receiving hazardous treatments (e.g., radiation implant treatments) or who are in isolation for some reason (e.g., tuberculosis or a virulent viral strain). Because visualization and manipulation are present in virtual reality, the patient would be able to interact with the nurse, both visually and tactually, and not have a sense of isolation, as often occurs now.

Nurse characteristics

Nurses could put themselves in the patient's shoes in a virtual world. Empathy would be generated as the nurse could experience the patient's situation and not just cognitively understand what it is like.

A nurse who may be uncomfortable about seeing an autopsy could experience a virtual one first. Likewise, nurses who are shy about presenting in front of a group could practice the speech in a virtual conference. If the system has a knowledge-based component, the nurse could even get a critique of his or her presentation by the computer.

Computer characteristics and nursing context

Because the system and the context become one in virtual reality, this chapter addresses them together. Currently the computer system for virtual reality requires intrusive equipment to use the system. What are the health effects on nurses who use this equipment? What is the stress level of virtual reality users? What types of environments do nurses use most frequently in virtual reality systems? What is the most effective design of a virtual reality system for practical use on a nursing unit?

Nursing informatics developmental trajectory

It will be important to study the longitudinal impact of nurses' use of virtual reality systems. Studies of frequent users of computerized arcade games have found that users display addictive-type behaviors (e.g., distortions in thinking) (Arthur, 1992). Can similar behaviors be found in frequent virtual reality users? Will nurses (and others) begin to confuse virtual worlds and the real world as systems get so sophisticated that they exactly replicate the real world? As virtual reality systems use less intrusive interaction devices, what will the effect be on use, satisfaction, and attitude about the system?

Conclusion

Virtual reality has significant promise as an enabling technology. For nursing, virtual reality is an unexplored technology. No systems exist in actual nursing practice today, and no nursing studies of virtual reality were found. Having a nursing conceptual framework from which to generate research questions places nursing in a better position to evaluate the impact of this exciting technology when it emerges in the field of nursing.

Questions

1. What are potential applications for virtual reality in health care?
2. What are some barriers to the implementation of virtual reality for nursing?

3. Do you agree that the Staggers and Parks Framework is appropriate to use in the study of virtual reality and nursing? Why or why not?

References

Antonoff M: Living in a virtual world. *Popular Science* 1993; 242: 83–86, 124–125.
Arthur C: Did reality move for you? *New Scientist* 1992; 134: 22–27.
Aukstakalnis S, Blatner D: *Silicon Mirage: The Art and Science of Virtual Reality.* Berkeley, CA: Peachpit Press, 1992.
Bains S: Surgeons slice virtual leg. *New Scientist* 1991; 131: 28.
Bylinsky G: The marvels of virtual reality. *Fortune* 1991; 123(11): 138–139, 142, 146, 150.
Dutton G: A virtual operating system to handle virtually anything. *IEEE Software* 1992; 9: 100–101.
Grimes J: Virtual reality 91 anticipates future reality. *IEEE Computer Graphics & Applications* 1991; 11: 81–83.
Hamilton JO, Smith ET, McWilliams G, Schwartz EI, Carey J: Virtual reality: How a computer-generated world could change the real world. *Business Week* 1992; October 5: 97–105.
Hedberg S: See, hear, learn. *Byte* 1993; 18: 119, 121, 123, 125, 127–128.
Pausch R: Three views of virtual reality. *Computer* 1993; 26(2): 79–83.
Peterson I: Looking-glass worlds. *Science News* 1992a; 141: 8–15.
Peterson I: Wizard of Oz: Bringing drama to virtual reality. *Science News* 1992b; 142: 440–441.
Rheingold H: *Virtual Reality.* New York: Simon & Schuster, 1991.
Staggers N, Parks PA: Collaboration between unlikely disciplines in the creation of a conceptual framework for nurse-computer interactions. In: Frisse, ME, ed. *Proceedings of the Sixteenth Annual Symposium on Computer Applications in Medical Care.* New York: McGraw-Hill, 1993a; 661–665.
Staggers N, Parks PA: Description and initial application of the Staggers & Parks Nurse-Computer Interaction Framework. *Computers in Nursing* 1993b; 11(6): 282–290.
Stix G: See-through view. *Scientific American* 1992; 267: 166.

27
Nursing's Future: Ubiquitous Computing, Virtual Reality, and Augmented Reality

JAMES P. TURLEY

Ubiquitous computing, virtual reality, and augmented reality indicate new directions for computer use in nursing practice. Nursing has not been on the front line of computer implementation in health care; that may change in the future. Computers are integrated into some healthcare areas more than others. Laboratory systems would not be possible without computer-based automation. Large numbers of samples are tested; the results are promptly and efficiently reported. Billing and finance are completely dependent on computer-based information for insurance expensing, record checking, and, in many cases, the scheduling of patients, equipment, and staff.

Computers have entered into a number of clinical arenas. Computers are embedded in a number of bedside products. Intravenous (IV) pumps, ventilators, and monitors are managed by computer. Until recently, these machines ran independently of each other; lately these products have begun to communicate with each other, sharing information related to patient treatment and recordkeeping. Information services have been among the last areas in health care to receive assistance from computing technology. As the future looms, new generations of computing will become commonplace throughout the healthcare arena.

This chapter will review some of the possibilities for computerized nursing in the future, examine some of the problems, and explore some of the features. It is clear that computers will become ubiquitous in the healthcare and nursing environments. Computerization in health care will progress in some unexpected ways: First is the notion of ubiquitous computing discussed by Mark Weiser of Xerox Corporation; second is the notion of virtual reality (projects are under way in industrial and defense areas, and examples exist in medical education); and third is the notion of augmented reality, which combines some of the aspects of ubiquitous computing and virtual reality to provide what may be the critical elements for nursing. All of these are computer-intensive environments, and all will impact the delivery of nursing and health care in the future.

Ubiquitous Computing

Weiser (1991, 1993) developed the concept of ubiquitous computing. The main tenets are conceptually simple but technologically difficult to implement. In ubiquitous computing, common everyday devices can and will be augmented by computer technology. Once these devices have embedded computers, the devices will be brought into a mode whereby they can communicate with each other. The result will be a work area similar to what we already know and understand; however, the work area will be enriched because the devices will be able to communicate with each other and provide data in the most appropriate format for the user.

This process has begun and can be seen in everyday areas. Many people carry electronic appointment organizers. These organizers are microcomputers with the ability to store names, addresses, telephone numbers, messages, and a variety of other personal information. These personal organizers can be linked to desktop computers. The linking allows the sharing of information between the two computers. Currently the linking is accomplished by running a cable between the two computers, loading special software on each, and instructing them to pass information to each other. This linking may allow the two machines to rationalize different data between the two machines and organize the most current data. With coming advances, the communication between the computers will become wireless and occur on a regular, less disruptive basis. The data will always be current, and no separate steps will need to be taken to ensure that there is consistency between the machines.

Addresses and telephone numbers are located in my pocket organizer and are also located in my desktop computer. If a new office phone number is entered into the pocket organizer, when the pocket organizer is linked to the desktop computer, the desktop database will be updated by the pocket organizer because the pocket organizer has the most current information on the phone number. Similarly, the desktop machine can update the pocket organizer when it contains the most current information. These updates can occur automatically or they can ask for input of the owner. Likewise, pocket organizers such as the Newton®, Envoy®, and others can be linked to remote fax machines and other computer-driven devices. Communication between devices will be independent of location, operating system, and manufacturer.

Ubiquitous computing allows for the development of a number of independent computing devices that are then brought together. These devices will communicate with each other to present information in a way useful to the user. Multiple devices will be developed to allow different approaches to the manipulation of information; one device may appear as a Post-it™ note while another device may display the same information as a record in a database. The result is that computers will be embedded in a series of everyday devices. Some of these devices can and will mimic devices that we currently use; others will appear as new products. New devices can be developed that more completely reflect the way we are working and the way we want to work.

How will these devices function in nursing arenas? Computerized devices are not currently in common use in nursing areas; therefore, the future leads to speculation. A common device used on many nursing units is a clipboard. The clipboard is used frequently during the day to collect vital signs or to list reminders to be done by the person using the clipboard, rather like a set of portable Post-it™ notes. The clipboard is an example of a device that can be computerized. The screen on the clipboard may contain a list of patients who need to have their morning vital signs taken. The vital signs can be entered on the electronic clipboard screen by using a pen device. The data entered on the clipboard would be stored not only on the screen but immediately uploaded to the patient's electronic record. At other times during the day, the clipboard could be used to record and calculate intake and output (I&O) information. Typically this information is recorded throughout the day as the I&O is recorded. At the end of shift or end of day, the nurse sits down with a calculator to total the I&O and bring the balance forward. The sheet is placed into the permanent record. With an electronic clipboard, the items can be entered and the clipboard itself would calculate an automatic running total. This total could also maintain a running I&O summary from the time the order for I&O was initiated to the current time. Likewise, if the I&O balance exceeded preset limits, the appropriate people could be notified immediately rather than waiting for the end-of-shift or end-of-day totals. The electronic clipboard could send messages to the pagers of the appropriate people.

The medication kardex could also be computerized. The medication kardex is often separate from the patient's record. To examine the current state of medication administration, it is necessary to locate the medication kardex, often on the medication cart—it is never near the patient record. Using an electronic kardex, the patient could be identified automatically using a smart card or a bar code on the wrist identification bracelet. Likewise, the medication nurse could be identified using a bar code on the institution's ID badge or using a smart card. The medication itself could be similarly labeled. By simply scanning the device for the medication nurse, the patient, and the medication, the time, date, and dosage of the medication could be recorded. Further, the electronic kardex could update the patient record immediately. Searching for the kardex could become a thing of the past. With all of the medications marked and all of the patients coded, it could be possible for the electronic kardex to check each medication against the patient's profile, check for interaction among the medications, check the appropriateness of the doses, and record the time the medication is given and by whom. Eventually the electronic kardex could notify physicians when automatic renewals are needed for medications (e.g., antibiotics). The electronic kardex could also prenotify the medication nurse 10 minutes before the time a critical medication was scheduled to be given.

Devices like electronic clipboards and electronic kardexes will communicate with beepers or personal information devices worn by staff. When a critical event occurs, people could be notified immediately to prevent risk to the patient. Automated scheduling of these events could reduce the time and effort needed to renew medication orders and prevent missed or improper medication and other traumatic situations.

In other areas of the nursing environment, computers are currently embedded in existing systems. Bedside patient monitors, IV pumps, ventilators, and other devices are already computerized. These devices typically have a limited ability to communicate with other devices. Each of the devices is designed to be a stand-alone device reporting information with a series of beeps, whistles, flashing lights, or a liquid crystal display (LCD) of information. While efficient, these devices are not intended for easy or intuitive communication. Future designs of these products will allow them to communicate with other devices. Eventually, they will communicate directly with the electronic patient record, storing appropriate data, and with the nursing caregivers, providing status reports, warnings, and alerts. Appropriate and timely data will be displayed in appropriate ways and locations useful for the delivery of nursing care.

Patient monitoring systems in the future will be designed to communicate with other devices either through the patient record or directly with each other. A bedside patient monitor might note that a patient's blood pressure was dropping below a predetermined limit. The bedside monitor would then note that an IV pump was also connected. Looking through the patient record, the bedside system would note that a vasopressor was included in the IV solution and would direct the IV pump to increase the medication dosage. At the same time, the bedside monitor would send a message to the nurse caring for the patient about the status of the situation and what had been done about it. A note would be entered into the patient record that the bedside monitor had noted the drop in blood pressure, and the monitor would identify what rule or algorithm had directed it to change the IV flow rate, note that the IV flow rate had been altered, and record the time, date, and name of the nurse who had been notified. Such systems would include more complex decision making than is currently available. However, prototype systems that include artificial consciousness are being developed. Artificial consciousness will give the computer-based decision systems a greater ability to self-regulate.

Similarly, the bedside monitors could communicate with ventilators; if pulmonary pressures started to rise, the bedside monitoring system could communicate with the ventilator to modify settings. What is important in the discussion of all of these devices is the ability to communicate. Communication includes the need for standards in the communication process, the need for a level of embedded intelligence that can direct the communication, and finally the ability to document all that has occurred in the patient record as part of the communication process.

The technology that will allow this to occur is already being introduced into the nursing environment. Standards such as HL7, MEDIX, and the Hospital Information Bus are creating the communication standards that all of these devices will use. The Computer-Based Patient Record Institute (CPRI) concept model committee is developing a model for a computer-based record that will allow for the recording of patient information in real time. In addition, the CPRI concept model will direct the electronic record to attach to external databases and knowledge bases, which can be used inside the electronic record to assist with logical controls and communications such as those described earlier.

Slowly, the healthcare arena will see the development of a patient-based local area network. The patient network will allow for the free flow of data and information around the patient. This will include information from the monitors and devices that are attached to the patient and hence are part of the interventions. Another nurse-based network will surround the nurse and support the planning, decision making, and intervention strategies that the nurse performs to deliver patient-centered care. There will be a clear interconnection between the patient-based network and the nurse-based network. Similar networks will be developed for physicians, pharmacists, and any of the other healthcare providers who are responsible for care for a given patient. The result will be a complex set of interconnecting networks, each connected to several embedded devices. These networks will make possible patient-centered care using information on demand as the critical focus for the delivery of care. The delivery of patient-centered care is knowledge and data intensive. New devices with their strong communication orientations will finally act to support clinicians in their practice, improving patient outcomes.

Virtual Reality

Virtual reality (VR) has long been a topic for science fiction. Whether it was the holodeck on "Star Trek: The Next Generation" or some other world, VR seems to have been defined, developed, and refined in science fiction. Most of the references to VR have truly belonged to fiction. The major exceptions have been the use of VR in flight training simulators and games. However, recent developments in VR have generated possibilities for use in health care.

VR can be defined as the generation of a complete environment. Larijani (1994) describes the six basic subsystems necessary for the development of a VR system. Each of the subsystems can vary in their complexity depending on the implementation. The six subsystems are (1) audio (earphones, acoutestrons, microphones, synthesizers), (2) visual (glasses, goggles, projectors, screens), (3) tactile (smells, pins, gloves, bodysuits), (4) hardware (host computers, peripherals), (5) electronics (power supply, signal conversion, accessories), and (6) software (operating system, simulation software).

In a VR system, a person receives multiple sensory inputs that are either computer generated or mediated. At a basic level, VR systems include binaural video screens that display pictures of a world designed using a computer graphics program. Stereo audio in the headphones may include synthesized voice, music, or other sounds that are purported to belong to the designed world. Typically, these audio/visual worlds are displayed using a headset that includes the binaural video displays and the stereo headphones. In turn, the headset is linked to external sensors. Thus, when the person physically turns or looks to the right, the video display adapts and shifts in a similar direction. The same occurs looking up or down. The sounds likewise adjust to when they appear to be forward or behind the person. The sounds likewise shift as the head is turned.

Newer technology will allow the display of more complex data forms in VR. Transducers embedded in gloves and bodysuits can give the sensations of temperature and pressure. Newer display technology can add peripheral vision. VR can be interpreted as the opposite of ubiquitous computing. In ubiquitous computing, computers are embedded in all of the devices that are part of everyday experience. In VR, the person has become embedded in a computer-generated world. Even when elements of the visual world are from videotapes of a real situation, the person's interaction and experience of the generated world is moderated through the computer.

Holusha (1993) described the use of VR for the training of surgeons. Using VR techniques, a surgeon could practice an operation a number of times before approaching the first patient. VR would allow a surgeon to practice the same surgery using a number of different approaches. The system would even allow a recording of how the practice had been done, so that the surgeon could observe the procedure that had just been performed. Certainly this decreases the risk to the patient and increases the ability to "play" with alternatives and explore variations on a procedure to produce the best surgical solution. The National Library of Medicine (NLM) established standards for the development of organs and organ systems for use in VR (Merril, Raju, and Roy, 1994). Derived from computed tomography (CT) and magnetic resonance imaging (MRI) scans, this set of standards for electronic organs is referred to as the Visible Human Project. As these standards evolve, it will be possible for companies and organizations to assemble organs from different companies, to establish a virtual patient.

With the development of more sophisticated feedback instruments, it will be possible for student nurses to feel the sensations as venous catheters are inserted into virtual patients; similarly, students will feel the insertion of nasogastric (NG) tubes. The tactile information has always been the most difficult for instructors to impart to students. VR can allow all students to have the same patient so that they can discuss how things feel. When using the same technique with different patients, individual variation could limit the amount of generalization when describing a procedure or situation. Conversely, the use of VR can allow the instructor to change the experience structurally for each student with a known amount of variation. This can assess the student's ability to discriminate changes to a situation that may be known only to the instructor.

VR may have some novel implications for nursing. Much of the data and information that nurses use is very complex. Physician data tends to be abstract and independent of the patient. The results of lab tests (e.g., complete blood counts [CBCs], blood gases, and the like) can be interpreted independently of the patient. Many physicians can do their diagnostic work using only the data gathered by other sources and do not need to see the patient directly. By contrast, nursing data are not as abstract. Nursing data are often embedded in the way the patient responds to a given situation or illness. Different patients do have different responses to the same stimulus. Patients who are one or two days postoperative after abdominal surgery can have widely varied responses to abdominal pain. Some will cough and breathe deeply with little complaint, others will attempt short walks, and others will be reluctant to move at all. Unlike the data used by physicians, wherein the relationships between the laboratory tests and the disease are patient independent, nursing data are often patient specific.

Nursing often works with cues that are less well defined than, for example, the "postabdominal surgery patient." Nurses talk about patients as "looking good," "sounding poorly," etc. This type of data is completely embedded in the patient response to a situation. Nurses are often not able to decompose the elements of this gestalt. Even with the components, the complete response is often a more complex interaction among the components than an identification of the components alone. VR techniques may allow the capture of such patient-specific responses. VR may allow nurses to use more complex data for identification of the patterns of a patient response to situations than what is available currently. The use of paper records restricts the data types that can be used for the recording and identification of patient problems. VR techniques can be linked to electronic patient records, expanding the data types that are available for the identification and recording of patient-specific responses. As nursing continues to explore ways to understand, codify, and display embedded information, VR techniques will become increasingly important to the profession. Nursing understanding of patient responses to situations can be modeled using VR. This will give researchers and practitioners new avenues to describe, investigate, and report on complex patient responses.

VR may also become an important tool in patient education. In complex situations such as patients preparing for surgery or MRI, no amount of verbal explanation or paper drawings seems to prepare patients for the experiences that they are likely to encounter. VR techniques can immerse the patients in the sound, feel, look, and sensation of the environments that they will be encountering. With that as a basis, nurses will be able to discuss patients' response to the situation before the actual situation has occurred. Creating a safe experience with which patients can experience a situation may allow for a better understanding of what is occurring and why and increase patient compliance. Such approaches may be important to children who have a limited ability to conceptualize something they have not experienced. Using VR, parents and children could both experience a procedure before it occurs, giving them a common basis to address the child's fears and concerns.

VR will not be the solution to all problems. It is simply the application of an existing technology to the areas of health and nursing. In and of itself, VR is neither a solution nor an obstacle. As with any other technology, VR will be more useful when it is seen merely as a technology. Any technology must be applied for a specific purpose. When the purpose is clear (e.g., the teaching of the tactile sense of IV insertion), then and only then can the appropriate technology be selected and evaluated regarding how well it meets that purpose. VR as a technology can assist nursing with the process of describing and understanding a complex phenomenon. While useful for describing and presenting the phenomenon, VR will not solve nursing's need to formalize its concepts and language. As a technology, it may prove useful in this process, but the work needs to be done by nurse investigators.

Augmented Reality

Augmented reality is a computing approach that has received little discussion. Augmented reality can be thought of as a combination of the aspects of ubiquitous computing and virtual reality. With ubiquitous computing, the computers were embedded into a variety of products and the computers tended to disappear as unique products. Ubiquitous computing works because of the focus on communication among the computing devices. Communication allows the data or information to be presented in a variety of display-appropriate formats. With VR, external reality tends to disappear as everything presented to the observer is mediated by the computer. Complex data and information can be presented in VR. By being immersed in VR, a person can sense, feel, and be immersed in a situation, not just look at the data. Augmented reality combines elements of both ubiquitous computing and VR.

In augmented reality (AR), the user has a headset or viewer that allows the user to view both a computer-generated image as well as what is going on in front of him or her. External reality is not blocked out, as it is when using an enclosed VR headset. In AR, the user tends to wear a single earpiece, and there is a single-image video screen mounted to a visor. This is similar to rearview mirrors that bicyclists attach to their glasses or helmets. The cyclist learns to focus on the rearview mirror when necessary and ignore it while focusing forward the remainder of the time. Systems using augmented reality have been developed for use in industry and the military. Boeing Aircraft uses augmented reality to assist people who are involved with aircraft repair. The "manual"—which has the complete set of instructions necessary for a repair as well as the associated diagrams and flowcharts that contain the logic for troubleshooting—is contained on a CD-ROM subsystem that the person wears. The CD-ROM is displayed on a view monitor over the right eye. The repair person is free to focus either on the part of the airplane that is being repaired or on the monitor which displays the repair manual. Audio sounds can be played using an earphone in one ear. The repair person is free to commute between the VR world generated by the computer system and the actual airplane engine that is in the process of being repaired. The result is that the manual is available at the same time that the work is being performed. It is not necessary to interrupt the work being done to consult the manual. It is possible for the worker to compare the diagrams in the manual with the work that is in the process of being completed. The real world is augmented with computer-generated assistance (hence augmented reality).

With AR, the user can decide on the spot how much time and attention should be given to the computer-generated view and how much attention should be given to the work being performed. As the worker becomes more proficient in performing the task, it is likely that he or she will alter the allocation of time given to the electronic manual versus the time spent actively working on the engine repair. Many of the advantages of the VR system are available with augmented reality: (1) Complex data can be displayed, (2) audio and video data can be combined, and (3) using sensors, the system can alter the display when the worker changes position or location.

The flexibility of AR, which allows the user to migrate between the computer-generated world and the real world, is one of its major strengths. Typically the users of augmented reality systems wear complete computer systems. Often the display is a small monitor so that the monitor appears to float in front of the user. A CD-ROM is used to store large amounts of information, which is rapidly searchable. The size is no larger than a portable audio CD player. The central processing unit (CPU) for the computer can likewise be shrunk to a package no larger than the CD-ROM. Companies such as NEC have shown entry keypads that are worn like a wide bracelet on the wrist. With the combination of package shrinking and redefining the traditional keyboards, a wearable computer becomes a reality. In 1992, NEC hosted a fashion show of wearable computers. While at first this seems humorous, the use of a computer fashion show indicates the need to see the computer as part of the personal environment and not simply as an external device that one uses in the office. Further, exploring computing as a fashion issue will allow for innovative ways to design input devices. In the future, these wearable computers will be connected by wireless communication to other computers in the work environment. The AR worker will receive the most current information and data from other computers embedded elsewhere in the work environment. This aspect of AR combines many of the strong communications features of ubiquitous computing.

AR may be the technology with the greatest application in nursing environments. As AR systems are integrated into the notion of personal networks and patient networks, AR technology can supply nurses with data and information while they are in the process of delivering patient care. Using AR, the nurse can have available the instructions for performing a complex task at the same time that the task is being performed. The instructions can be available in a hands-free form, which allows the nurse to focus on the patient while care is provided. For example, if the nurse was involved in a complex assessment of newborns, the augmented reality system could display pictures of what the nurse might be observing. Thus even if the nurse could not precisely describe what was being observed in the newborn, the nurse could compare the newborn with photos of other newborns and use visual comparison techniques to access more information from resources or to compare the newborn's presentation with what had been observed 24 hours ago or a shift previous. Since nursing phenomena are complex and embedded in the patient situation, photos, videos, and sound may be necessary for comparisons and developing contrasts. On a paper record, normals of lab tests can be printed as numbers per milligram percent; however, nurses may need more complex data formats to display patient responses as normal. AR can do that. Admittedly, however, some social and cultural modifications may be necessary before patients easily accept nurses wearing AR systems.

AR will open a variety of new possibilities for nurses in clinical practice. Many of the applications for AR technology have not yet been considered. AR techniques will allow the nurse to have access to previous data, pictures, and sounds and to be able to compare previous data with the current state of the patient. An electronic patient record would then provide for the recording of the current state, the previous state, and the changes that have occurred.

Summary

Ubiquitous computing, virtual reality, and augmented reality are technologies that have great potential to assist in the delivery of future nursing care. These technologies will have importance for the teaching of nursing, delivery of nursing care, and research into nursing practice with concomitant impact on the outcomes of nursing interventions. However, it must first be remembered that these are technologies. As technologies, they are neither solutions nor obstacles. They are of importance only to the degree that we understand nursing practice and what nursing practice is attempting to achieve. Within the goal of assisting patients to return to a life of health-seeking behaviors, these technologies can have impact on some specific areas. The technologies will not be solutions to all problems.

Nursing has a long cultural history of being technophobic (Turley and Connelly, 1993). For these technologies to have an impact on nursing, nursing must be willing to look outward and embrace technologies that can improve nursing practice. Nursing has had a history of reticence when considering the adoption of computer technology. In many cases, this has been because the existing computer technology has not addressed the needs identified by nurses. However, nurses cannot stand by and wait for others to adapt technology to nursing practice. Nurses must seek out the technology that will improve the quality and efficiency of nursing practice. When the use of the technology can also improve patient outcomes, an ideal match will be found. The technology included in ubiquitous systems, virtual reality, and augmented reality may be that technology.

Questions

1. Create an example of the use of ubiquitous computing in any setting.
2. How does virtual reality differ from ubiquitous computing?
3. What is the potential for augmented reality in the field of nursing?

References

Holusha J: Carving out real-life uses for virtual reality. *New York Times* 1993; October 31:11.
Larijani C: Homo faber or homo sapiens? *Virtual Reality Systems* 1994; 1:7–10.
Merril J, Raju R, Roy R: VR applications in medical education. *Virtual Reality Systems* 1994; 1:61–64.
Turley J, Connelly D: The relationship between nursing and medical culture: Implications for the design and implementation of a clinician's workstation. In Safran C, ed. *Proceedings of the 17th Annual Symposium on Computer Applications in Medical Care.* New York: McGraw-Hill, 1993; 233–237.
Weiser M: The computer for the twenty-first century. *Scientific American* 1991; September: 94–104.
Weiser M: Some computer science problems in ubiquitous computing. *Communication of the ACM* 1993; July: 137–143.

Unit 6
Education and Nursing Informatics

Unit Introduction

Gassert begins the section with a viewpoint on academic preparation in nursing informatics. She lists the activities that describe nursing informatics practice and details the curricula from two U.S. universities. Next, Edwards discusses the many educational uses of computers for basic nursing education, continuing education, and patient education. She includes criteria for the evaluation of educational software.

28
Academic Preparation in Nursing Informatics

CAROLE A. GASSERT

The dream of many professional nurses is to become involved in an initiative with tremendous potential for impacting the outcomes of healthcare delivery. Nursing informatics (NI) is such an initiative. Its activities are positioned to facilitate nursing's entry, along with other healthcare providers, onto the information highway. Informatics practitioners, including nurses, are being sought to help employers manage information competitively. Increased interest in information technology and informatics specialists will allow even more nurses to contribute to the development and implementation of information structures and tools needed to deliver effective and efficient care in a constantly changing healthcare environment. What an exciting initiative informatics is for nurses!

Within the last 10 years, nursing informatics has been named, recognized as a specialty, and defined by the nursing profession. Academic programs to prepare nurses within the field have also been developed. In addition, standards for the practice of nursing informatics have been written. Finally, the American Nurses Credentialing Center (ANCC) has developed a certification examination to credential as informatics nurses those individuals who demonstrate beginning levels of competency in nursing informatics.

The purpose of this chapter is to discuss educational preparation of nurses in nursing informatics. While the focus is on describing academic programs, it is necessary to examine nursing informatics as a specialty, discussing its definition, specialty attributes, scope of practice, and standards as they influence academic program development.

Evolving Definition of Nursing Informatics

Since the 1970s, nurses have been helping to install and use information systems in hospitals, contributing to the design of information systems, and consulting with healthcare agencies about selecting and using information technology. In 1992, their roles were professionally acknowledged when the American Nurses Association (ANA) recognized nursing informatics as an area of specialty practice in nursing (Milholland, 1992). While many nurses practice in the rapidly growing specialty, others ask, "What is nursing informatics?"

The delineation of nursing informatics has been dynamic, changing to reflect growth within the field. As initially identified in the literature by Ball and Hannah (1984), NI was defined as the discipline of applying computer science to nursing processes. A year later, nursing informatics was described as a focus that uses information technology to perform functions within nursing (Hannah, 1985). This later definition was easily understood and therefore widely dispersed in nursing to explain the new practice area. Although useful, the definition failed to acknowledge NI activities beyond the use of computer applications.

Subsequent definitions presented a more widely delineated practice, including reference to a theoretical basis for practice. In 1988, Grobe described nursing informatics as "the application of the principles of information science and theory to the study, scientific analysis, and management of nursing information for purposes of establishing a body of nursing knowledge" (Grobe, 1988b, p. 29). A more widely disseminated and accepted definition appeared in a classic article that describes the study of nursing informatics. In their article, the authors define nursing informatics as "the combination of nursing science, information science and computer science to manage and process nursing data, information and knowledge to facilitate the delivery of health care" (Graves and Corcoran, 1989, p. 227). Computers are acknowledged as tools used in the NI field.

Both the Grobe and Graves and Corcoran definitions are important for three reasons. First, they more accurately describe the field, allowing information processing, language development, application of the systems life cycle, and human-computer interface issues to be identified as part of NI. Second, these definitions have implications for content to be included in curricula used to prepare informatics nurses. Finally, these definitions serve as a foundation for ANA's definition, which states that nursing informatics "is the specialty that integrates nursing science, computer science, and information science in identifying, collecting, processing, and managing data and information to support nursing practice, administration, education, research and the expansion of nursing knowledge" (ANA, 1994, p. 3).

Specialty Attributes of Nursing Informatics

Designation of an interest area of nursing as a specialty is a multifaceted process (Panniers and Gassert, 1995). A specialty must demonstrate the following attributes: a differentiated practice; a research program; representation of the specialty by at least one organized body; a mechanism for credentialing nurses in the specialty; and educational programs for preparing nurses to practice in the specialty (Styles, 1989).

As stated earlier, nurses have worked in informatics roles for the past two decades (Hersher, 1985; Romano, 1984). Their work experiences have been focused primarily in acute care agencies, but job opportunities are increasingly more varied as the skills of informatics nurses are discovered and appreciated by potential employers in more diverse areas of health care (Anderson, 1992; Gassert, 1991a; Meintz, 1993; Taira, 1992). Even with today's shrinking job market, there is continued demand for nurses prepared in informatics. Such opportunity reflects the differentiated nature of NI practice.

Nursing informatics has met a second attribute required for recognition as a specialty by establishing a specific research program. When Schwirian proposed a research framework for nursing informatics, there was little reported scientific inquiry in the field (Schwirian, 1986). Since that time, however, an increasing number of NI researchers have reported their work at national and international conferences and in the literature. For example, several authors have reported on the development of nursing language (Grobe, 1990; Henry, Holzemer, Reilly, and Campbell, 1994; McCloskey and Bulechek, 1993; Ozbolt, Fruchtnight, and Hayden, 1994; Saba et al., 1991; and Zielstorff, Cimino, Barnett, Hassan, and Blewett, 1993). Others have studied the impact of systems (Brennan, 1993), examined the design of information systems (Staggers and Parks, 1993), or developed and evaluated a nursing informatics model (Gassert, 1989a, 1990, 1991b, 1994, 1995). As a final example, NI researchers have investigated decision-making processes of nurses (Fonteyn and Grobe, 1994; Panniers and Walker, 1994; Thompson and Ryan, 1994). All of these examples support topics identified as research priorities for NI by the National Institute for Nursing Research at the National Institutes of Health (NCNR, 1993).

A third attribute needed as a specialty is to be represented by at least one organized body. Several formal organizations have established special interest groups targeted for NI membership, including the ANA and the National League for Nursing (NLN), two major nursing organizations (Carty, 1994). Likewise, the Center for Health Information Management (CHIM) and the American Medical Informatics Association (AMIA) have nursing informatics workgroups. At the international level, the International Medical Informatics Association (IMIA) has a nursing informatics workgroup with representation from member countries. Regionally and statewide, less formal interest groups promote information sharing among NI members. The formation and maintenance of NI special interest groups is extremely important in providing educational experiences for informatics nurses. With the support of so many organizations, NI has more than met the attribute of representation.

A mechanism for credentialing members of an interest area is the fourth attribute needed for recognition as a specialty. The certification process for NI is currently being developed through the ANA and its affiliate, the

ANCC. Two separate task forces of nurses representing NI practice, education, and administration were appointed by the ANA to develop the scope of practice document and standards for NI practice. Efforts were coordinated by the ANA's Council for Nursing Systems and Administration (formerly the Council of Computer Applications in Nursing). A certification examination for credentialing nurses as generalists in NI is currently being developed under the direction of ANCC. A specialist certification examination planned for future development will complete the credentialing mechanism (J. Bowers, personal communication, April 1994).

As a final attribute, a specialty must have educational programs to prepare nurses to practice within that field. Nursing informatics education will be discussed later in this chapter.

Nursing Informatics Practice

The scope of practice document outlines in detail what is and is not nursing informatics practice. In terms of educational preparation, it is important to note that although nurses practicing NI are expected to be competent in the use of applications software, the use of software alone is insufficient to define NI practice. The scope of practice further describes the boundaries, core, intersections, and dimensions of NI. In essence, the document states that while the field focuses on the nursing perspective of data, information, and knowledge, NI recognizes that collaboration within the larger umbrella of health informatics is requisite to developing integrated information tools that will benefit both providers and recipients of health care (ANA, 1994). Hence NI education should be interdisciplinary.

Political activities within the past 2 years have prompted discussion of whether nursing informatics practice is clinical or administrative in nature (Simpson, 1993). Some have defined clinical NI and administrative NI as distinct entities. The federal government's decision in 1992 to eliminate funding for informatics educational programs because they were viewed as administrative has caused a general rethinking of how to describe the nature of NI practice. Efforts to distinguish NI as clinical or administrative are understandable, but such a distinction seems artificial. Since NI activities have as a foundation the handling of clinical data and information, it seems best to describe all NI as a clinical practice, one in which the informatics practitioner moves back and forth between a direct or an indirect practice focus depending on the patient/client needs. Handling individual patient data in the clinical setting could be considered direct informatics practice, while handling aggregate-level data for allocating resources could be indirect informatics practice. Educational programs in NI should provide students with knowledge and experience from both the direct and indirect practice focuses.

Nursing informatics is generally practiced in one of five arenas: health-care agencies, consulting firms, vendor corporations, academic settings, and private business practices. As health care shifts its focus to nontraditional environments, such as outpatient and home care, NI practice will need to move into these areas. Specific practice activities may vary from one setting to another, but the following list of activities generally describes NI practice.

Developing applications, tools, processes, and structures that assist nurses to manage data

Evaluating applications, tools, processes, and structures to determine their effectiveness for nursing

Adapting existing information technologies to meet nurses' needs

Managing system selection, implementation, and evaluation

Collaborating with other healthcare informatics professionals in developing solutions to previously identified information needs for nurses

Using informatics theories and principles to develop and test computerized educational systems, such as an interactive videodisk system

Developing and testing informatics models and theories pertaining to handling, communicating, or transforming nursing information

Developing a taxonomy or naming system to describe and order nursing phenomena

Conducting research to advance the knowledge base of nursing informatics

Consulting with patients and clients about nursing informatics

Teaching the theory and practice of nursing informatics.

As the field of NI matures, different activities may be added to the list. As an example, Meintz (1993) has suggested that supercomputers offer nurses an opportunity to focus on the role activities of "nurmetrics." Nurmetrics is defined as a conceptual branch of nursing that "applies statistical techniques to the testing, estimation, and quantification of nursing theories and solutions to nursing problems" (Meintz, 1993, p. 143). In presenting the concept, Meintz indicates that nurmetrics embodies NI. Given the definition and nature of NI, it seems more accurate to consider nurmetrics as a focus area within NI. Other focus areas that could be identified currently are telemetrics, computer-based instruction, and clinical reasoning. Nevertheless, it will be interesting to follow the evolution of nurmetrics and its activities.

Informatics Nurse Specialist Role

According to the scope of practice, nurses who practice in the field of NI are designated either as informatics nurses (INs) or informatics nurse specialists (INS), depending on whether they are prepared at the baccalaureate or graduate levels in nursing (ANA, 1994). This specification is consistent with ANA requirements that specialists have graduate education in nursing. Most INs have graduate preparation outside of nursing but in fields that support nursing informatics, such as business or computer science (Carty, 1994; Gassert, 1994). Regardless of their academic degree, all INs and INSs bring NI practice experience to their roles.

Nurse specialists have traditionally described their roles by identifying different components or parts of their practice. It seems appropriate, therefore, to describe informatics nurse specialists' roles in terms of the components of practice, consultation, research, marketing, education, and management. The practice component covers such activities as design, development, selection, testing, implementation, enhancement, and use of information technology. The consultation component includes advising and assisting others to reach solutions related to information technology. The research component covers investigation of such problems as research methodology, symbolic representation of data, clinical decision making, ergonomics, human-computer interface issues, and information system impact. Marketing activities include selling both products and ideas related to information and information technology. The educational role component includes training, presentation of both informal and formal programs in informatics, and development of learning technologies. Management, the final component, involves overseeing issues of change, quality, redesign, adoption-innovation, project planning, and cost. Just as activities are dependent on the practice setting, the INS's primary role component may change with the setting or priorities of the employer.

Nursing Informatics Competencies

A competency is defined as "having sufficient knowledge, judgment, skill or strength" (Grobe, 1988a, p. 4). Identifying competencies for a specialty and certifying nurses who meet those competencies promotes higher quality in specialty practice (Parker, 1994). IMIA's working group on nursing informatics initially identified levels of informatics competencies (Peterson and Gerdin Jelger, 1988). The statements of competency were intended to describe preparation of the general population of nurses relative to informatics as they accomplished their roles of practicing nurse, nurse administrator, nurse educator, and nurse researcher (Grobe, 1989). The working group's designation of levels of preparation, however, has been used as the basis for organizing specialty programs in nursing informatics at the University of Maryland at Baltimore (UMAB) (Gassert, Mills, and Heller, 1992).

Nurses prepared with level 1 competencies are considered to be information technology users. These individuals know, understand, use, and interact with computer applications and healthcare information systems. These nurses must also be prepared to collect relevant data for patient care, access information needed for providing nursing services, and implement policies to assure the privacy, confidentiality, and security of data. Such preparation should take place in baccalaureate (basic) nursing programs. The scope of practice for NI states that these competencies are required for all nurses (ANA, 1994). In reality, nursing education programs have been slow to incorporate informatics competencies into the curriculum, and many nurses lack user-level competencies upon completing their basic nursing programs.

Nurses with level 2 competencies are recognized as information technology modifiers who analyze, manage, critique, develop, modify, and evaluate information technology for nursing. In addition to information technology skills, modifiers apply theoretical knowledge of nursing science, information science, computer science, and business to their practice. Modifiers' practices are focused in nursing informatics, and they are expected to conduct research to contribute to the body of knowledge. Modifiers are the informatics nurse specialists prepared at the master's level in graduate specialty programs in nursing informatics.

Nurses with level 3 competencies are identified as information technology innovators. These nurses design and develop research-based information technology for nursing, analyze and define the structure of nursing language, and explain the processing of information by nurses as they make both clinical and administrative decisions. Innovators are prepared at the doctoral level in nursing. With highly sophisticated preparation in research, nursing science, and information/computer science, innovators should contribute significantly to the body of NI knowledge and design information technology that truly supports nurses in delivering patient care.

Nursing Informatics Standards of Practice (ANA, 1995) defines the responsibilities for practice and professional performance for which generalist-level (initially competent) informatics nurses (INs) are held accountable. There are six standards that address the practice activities of INs. Eight standards speak to the professional performance of INs, and six additional standards delineate expectations for performance relative to the domain or field of NI. Informatics nurses are expected to meet each of the 20 standards but not every measurement criterion within each of the standards. The scope of practice document, competency lists, and standards should serve as the basis for developing educational programs in nursing informatics.

Nurse educators interested in acquiring nursing informatics programs should consider the use of lists of expected competencies requisite to developing the curriculum. Such lists are available in Peterson and Gerdin Jelger's publication (1988) and in the ANA scope of practice document (1994). The standards are also distributed through the ANA (1995).

Professional Development in Nursing Informatics

Most educational opportunities in NI have been available through professional development (continuing education) workshops and conferences sponsored by professional nursing organizations, healthcare organizations, informatics organizations, private foundations, special interest groups, and the literature. The following are examples of ongoing workshops and conferences available for nurses. The ANA sponsors a software demonstration theater at its biennial conventions and cosponsors the Rutgers University Annual Nursing Computer Conference. In collaboration with other councils in its organization, the NLN Nursing Informatics Council sponsors an annual conference focusing in part on NI. The Healthcare Information Management Systems Society (HIMSS) has conducted an annual informatics conference that includes nursing informatics issues. Through HIMSS, nurses are also invited to learn about clinical information systems issues by joining an interdisciplinary special interest group.

Professional development opportunities are also available through AMIA's fall Symposium on Computer Applications in Medical Care (SCAMC) and their Spring Congress. IMIA holds MedInfo, an interdisciplinary international informatics conference, every 3 years. The nursing informatics working group of IMIA sponsors an excellent international NI conference every 3 years, but not the same years as MedInfo. Finally, New York University conducts an annual NI conference in the spring, the University of Virginia offers an annual fall NI conference, and the National Institutes of Health (NIH) Clinical Center conducts periodic NI conferences.

An increased number of workshop and conference announcements are appearing in journals, in the U.S. mail, and on electronic bulletin boards, augmenting the availability of learning opportunities in NI. Most conferences provide an excellent opportunity to learn about the state-of-the-art technology and informatics issues, but some nurses, particularly those who enter informatics without academic preparation in the field, are looking for programs to help them learn how to perform their role. In addition, few conferences focus on the theories and concepts needed to practice NI as delineated by the standards.

The Summer Institute in Nursing Informatics was established in 1991 at the UMAB School of Nursing to meet the needs of NI practitioners newer to the field or nurses interested in learning about NI (Gassert, 1994). The institute has been offered each July with the help of the Information Services Division, the University of Maryland Medical System, and the Veterans Affairs Medical Center on the UMAB campus. It targets nurse managers, nurse executives, nurses interfacing with information system departments, and managers of information systems for nursing. To allow participants the opportunity to network and exchange information with the experts and among themselves, enrollment in the institute is limited.

The purpose of the six-day summer institute is to prepare nurses for information system selection, implementation, and evaluation. Therefore, the institute focuses on information technology and its effects on administrative and clinical nursing practice, information system selection and evaluation, strategies for system implementation, and informatics trends and issues from the nursing perspective. Experts in nursing and healthcare informatics expose participants to didactic sessions, group discussion, software/hardware demonstrations, field observation of information systems, and workshops focusing on informatics techniques and computerized information management tools. Networking opportunities are provided through various social events. The institute faculty come from academic centers, healthcare agencies, vendor corporations, and consulting firms throughout the United States to provide the learning opportunities. Evaluations from the participants indicate that the institute provides them with new knowledge about NI that will be helpful in their practice.

Specialization in Nursing Informatics

In meeting the need to prepare nurses in informatics, a number of nursing schools have reported adding informatics courses and a graduate focus in NI to their curricula (Carty, 1994). Travis and Youngblut (1994) describe three courses included in the undergraduate curriculum to prepare their students to be sophisticated users of information and information technology. McGonigle and Eggers (1991) describe a certificate program that could be used with practicing nurses and students to prepare them to be users of information technology. Magnus, Co, and Derkach (1994) also outline an informatics course that prepares students to be users of information technology, but this course is targeted for graduate students. Lawless (1993) discusses experiences with two nursing informatics courses included in the graduate nursing administration program. Although the courses help students acquire some of the role activity skills, they do not prepare specialists in NI. Because programs offered vary significantly in the level of informatics preparation, potential students are advised to investigate all curricula carefully to assure that their goals and program offerings are compatible.

Professional development programs have supported informatics nurses and expanded their role performance, but with the growing use of information technology in nursing practice, a need for more formalized educational opportunities within NI was recognized. Therefore, the first graduate specialization program in NI opened at the UMAB School of Nursing in 1988 (Gassert, 1989b; Heller, Romano, Moray, and Gassert, 1989). An additional specialized program opened in 1990 at the University of Utah. To date these are the "only two graduate programs awarding master's degrees in nursing informatics" (Carty, 1994).

The purpose of graduate specialization programs in NI is to prepare informatics nurse specialists, the modifiers of information technology and its supporting structures and processes. Expected role activities and competencies have been discussed previously.

With no existing model programs, it has been extremely interesting to develop and implement the NI specialty programs at UMAB. Continuous formative and summary evaluation of the program and its graduates has resulted in several minor course revisions within the curriculum. It has also helped this author to formulate the following assumptions for master's specialty education in NI. First, one of two focuses of course work must be nursing science. Students must have baccalaureate preparation in nursing to allow them to increase their body of nursing knowledge at the graduate level. Increased theoretical understanding of nursing and nursing research facilitates the INS's ability to represent accurately nursing's view of informatics issues and solutions. Second, the additional focus must be interdisciplinary course work in either information systems management or biomedical computing. The second concentration of course work builds the student's knowledge base of technical and management issues related to information and information systems. Learning with another discipline also prepares the INS to view issues and solutions from more than an isolated nursing perspective. The end result should be more representative and integrated information systems for health care.

A third assumption is that state-of-the-art technology must be available to support students' technological growth. Not only must students have access to the latest technologies in one architecture, but they must be able to use multiple platforms of technology. Information technology and healthcare systems are no longer monolithic; increasingly, information is accessed across many different technical environments. The INS must be flexible and able to move with advances in technology. Implied in the third assumption is that NI programs will have personnel available to support students (and faculty) technologically. It should be obvious that availability of equipment alone will not assure that students can use it. The nursing informatics faculty can help with technological support but should not be viewed as the primary providers of this service. Program expectations of teaching, scholarship, and service for faculty necessitate the hiring of full-time technological support to maximize student (and faculty) technological development.

The fourth assumption is that adequate sites for student practicum experiences must be available to students. This allows students to pursue their specific career interests by practicing different NI activities under guidance and supervision. Experiences with traditional and nontraditional agencies that provide health care, vendor corporations, and consulting firms must be available. Having additional experiences available in organizations setting policies for informatics, academic technology learning laboratories, and entrepreneurial NI practices would be helpful.

The final assumption is that students must be prepared in basic computer competencies before starting NI specialty and interdisciplinary courses. The NI scope of practice document indicates that all graduates of basic nursing programs should be able to use informatics applications that have been designed for the clinical practice of nursing (ANA, 1994). To expand on this thinking, if students decide to specialize in NI, which uses the computer as a tool, they should be expected to know basic microcomputer skills of word processing, spreadsheet and database manipulation, electronic mail, and use of simple graphics. In addition, NI specialty students should not be intimidated by computers but inquisitive and self-directed in learning new computer applications.

Nursing Informatics Master's Curricula

Curricula from both the University of Maryland at Baltimore and the University of Utah will be discussed. First, the specialty program in NI at the University of Maryland at Baltimore will be presented with a discussion of credit allocation, courses, and learning activities. Consistent with other master's curricula at UMAB, the NI program consists of 42 semester credits (Heller et al., 1989). Twelve of those credits are for core courses in nursing theory, research, and policy. The core courses help to expand students' theoretical, professional, and research knowledge bases in nursing. NI students interact with other master's students in the core courses and contribute a unique perspective to projects and discussions.

There are 15 credits allocated to the NI major at UMAB. Six credits are assigned to nursing administration courses in organizational theory and managerial health finance. The courses are considered to be essential to support role component activities of the INS. In addition, nine credits are assigned to three NI courses that are sequentially offered to facilitate logical expansion of students' knowledge in the NI field.

The first course is essentially a computer applications in nursing course. It focuses on analyzing nursing data and information and applications used to process and manage these entities. Social, ethical, and legal issues associated with use of applications are also examined. Learning activities are as follows: Communicate with faculty/peers via electronic mail, word process all written assignments, develop a spreadsheet for an information problem in nursing, critique a computer-based instruction program, conduct a bibliographic search, develop a database, make a formal presentation using computer-generated audiovisuals, investigate available clinical systems, examine nursing management systems, develop data flow diagrams, analyze a system's life cycle, and identify critical nursing data elements for a specific information problem. It is important to note that the first six activities are basic and should have been taught in students' baccalaureate programs. The activities have been included to accommodate students' deficits in computer competency. Only the last five activities are unique to NI practice. Work is currently in progress to raise the level of expected competencies demonstrated by those entering and completing the course.

The second course, called an NI concepts course, examines NI models and conceptual frameworks. It also analyzes in detail NI practice activities, including the following: selection, implementation, and evaluation of systems; management of ongoing systems; impact analysis; cost-benefit analysis, and trend analysis. Professional development of NI as a specialty is also explored. Three major learning activities include preparing a selection document for an information system that supports specific clients' needs, discussing an implementation plan for that component selected, and critiquing a trend in nursing, health care, computer science, or information science in terms of its impact on the design of information systems that support nursing in delivering quality patient care.

A practicum, the third NI course, enables students to practice the INS role in an agency or corporation while assigned to a master's-prepared nurse preceptor who works in the field of nursing informatics. Students spend at least 96 hours in their assigned agency, where they perform a systems analysis, plan the evaluation of a system within the agency, examine research activities related to informatics within the agency, complete an informatics project for the agency, and complete additional objectives as selected from a list of 15 possible targeted goals for the practicum. The practicum is scheduled for the final semester to allow students to develop their knowledge of NI as much as possible before practicing INS roles.

To provide the interdisciplinary focus, NI students take nine semester credits in information systems management (IFSM) from any of three designated campuses within the University of Maryland system. The purpose of IFSM courses is to help the NI students acquire technical and information system management skills to perform their role activities successfully. The courses are taught by the IFSM faculty and have a business focus. Students' projects require application of technologies studied in class. Once the initial course in systems analysis is completed, students are advised to choose from courses in data communications and networks, artificial intelligence/expert systems, data security, project management, database development, and human-computer interface.

The final six credits in the NI program are used for a thesis/nonthesis option. Thesis students receive six credits for their research. Students who elect not to do a thesis receive three credits for an NI paper or project and use the last three credits for an elective, usually in IFSM.

The master's specialization program at the University of Utah consists of 63 quarter credits (equal to 42 semester credits). Eighteen quarter credits are allocated for core courses in theory, research, issues, teaching, management, and advanced nursing. Instead of taking administrative courses, Utah's NI students take nine credits of physiological nursing. There are 27 credits of NI courses that focus on programming, introduction to NI, database design, systems analysis and design, NIS support and clinical decision making, and implementation, management, and evaluation of systems. Finally, Utah's students can do either a thesis or a project for nine credits. There are many similarities between Maryland's and Utah's programs. That is not surprising since both are preparing an INS. A noticeable difference, besides their geographical location, is that Maryland's program has been placed within the administration department and Utah's program has been put within adult health. Both are very successful NI specialization programs in preparing INSs that are highly sought in the job market. Graduates of NI specialization programs also have an opportunity to continue their study at Massachusetts General Hospital in its nursing informatics fellowship program (Zielstorff, personal communication, March 1993).

Doctoral Specialization in Nursing Informatics

The purpose of a doctoral program in NI is to prepare innovators or nursing informatics scientists. The NI scientist will be able to conceptualize nursing information requirements for the future; design effective nursing information systems; create innovative information technology; conduct research regarding integration of technology with nursing practice, administration, education, and research; develop theoretical, practice, and evaluation models for nursing informatics; and augment work to develop taxonomies and lexicons for atomic-level nursing data. Given the expected activities, the NI scientist focuses on the role components of researcher and designer/developer. Employment opportunities could be available as appointments in academic institutions, as directors of research and/or information systems in healthcare facilities, in research and development for software companies, as appointments to government agencies, and as consultants in research for information systems.

This author believes that doctoral programs should be built on the following assumptions. Because of the level of expected informatics activities, the doctoral program should build on a master's degree in nursing informatics. Included in this assumption is a belief that students must have sophisticated computer competencies before entering the doctoral program. Since the number of master's specialization programs is limited, students may need to be admitted without such a degree but must take additional courses to build their foundational knowledge base in NI. A second assumption for a doctoral program is that an interdisciplinary approach must be maintained. Students take doctoral-level courses required for information system management students with an emphasis on improving their capabilities of designing and developing information technology. A third assumption is that adequate state-of-the-art technology and technological support must be available to students, as discussed previously. In addition, the physical environment should allow doctoral students to be assigned to their own computer and work space to facilitate design and development efforts. The final assumption of doctoral study is that adequate informatics researchers must be available in the academic community to support student research activities.

As of this writing, the only doctoral program in NI that has a prescribed curriculum with substantive courses in NI is at UMAB (Gassert et al., 1992). Like the master's program, there was no model to use in developing the doctoral program. Experience in developing, implementing, and coordinating the master's-level program; thoughtful conceptualization of doctoral study in the field; and the advice of colleagues in NI throughout the United States were essential in writing the curriculum. The NI doctoral curriculum consists of 64 semester credits. Thirty-one of those credits are assigned to core courses, 14 credits to nursing theory courses, and 17 credits to nursing research and statistics courses.

Fifteen additional credits are assigned to NI emphasis courses. Six credits are for specific NI courses that have been developed with the help of Drs. Brennan, Chang, Grobe, Holzemer, and Saba, all leaders in nursing informatics. The first course examines judgment and clinical decision making in NI. The focus is on data relative to decision making of individuals. The second course examines quality of care in NI. The focus is on aggregate-level data used for making decisions. The last nine credits in the NI emphasis are IFSM courses in database development, advanced system design, and human-computer interface. Students who enter the doctoral program with a master's degree in nursing informatics have six elective credits to build their knowledge base relative to their chosen research. In addition, there are 12 credits of dissertation research in the doctoral program.

Although only UMAB offers a prescribed NI doctoral program, many other universities offer students an opportunity for doctoral study in NI. Examples are the University of Utah, University of Texas at Austin, University of California San Francisco, Case Western Reserve, State University of New York at Buffalo, and University of Rochester. Since doctoral study varies, potential students are again advised to investigate curricula carefully to assure that their goals and program offerings are compatible.

Summary

In summary, nursing informatics is maturing and has been recognized as a specialty within nursing. The development of a scope of practice document and standards of practice will help build continuity and consistency in describing the NI as a specialty and will facilitate curriculum development. A mechanism for certification will add legitimacy to the specialty. Finally, various educational opportunities for preparing nurses to practice in this exciting initiative have been developed. However, the development of additional specialization programs, particularly at the master's level, is needed to prepare a cadre of INSs to continue to move the nursing informatics specialty to higher levels of achievement.

Questions

1. Define nursing informatics.
2. How has nursing informatics qualified to be designated as a specialty practice by the American Nurses Association (what attributes are present)?
3. Discuss your beliefs regarding whether nursing informatics is a clinical or an administrative practice.
4. List specific activities that may be included in the practice of an informatics nurse specialist.
5. Compare and contrast the master's-level program from the two universities discussed in this chapter.
6. How does preparation of a nursing informatics specialist differ at the doctoral level from the master's level?

References

American Nurses Association: *Scope of Practice for Nursing Informatics.* Washington, DC: American Nurses Publishing, 1994.

American Nurses Association: *Nursing Informatics Standards of Practice.* Washington, DC: American Nurses Publishing, 1995.

Anderson BL: Nursing informatics: Career opportunities inside and out. *Computers in Nursing* 1992; 10: 165–170.

Ball MJ, Hannah KJ: *Using Computers in Nursing.* Reston, VA: Reston Publishers, 1984.

Brennan PF: Computer networks promote caregiving collaboration: The Computer-Link project. In: Frisse ME, ed. *Proceedings of the Sixteenth Annual Symposium on Computer Applications in Medical Care.* New York: McGraw-Hill, 1993; 392–396.

Carty B: The protean nature of the nurse informaticist. *Nursing & Health Care* 1994; 15(4): 174–177.

Fonteyn ME, Grobe SJ: Expert system development in nursing: Implications for critical care nursing practices. *Heart & Lung* 1994; 23(7): 80–87.

Gassert CA: Defining nursing information system requirements: A linked model. In: Kingsland LC, ed. *Proceedings of the Thirteenth Annual Symposium on Computer Applications in Medical Care.* Washington, DC: IEEE Computer Society Press, 1989a; 779–783.

Gassert CA: Opportunities to study nursing informatics. *Input/Output* 1989b; 5(2): 1–2.

Gassert CA: Structured analysis: A methodology for developing a model for defining nursing information system requirements. *Advances in Nursing Science* 1990; 13(2): 53–62.

Gassert CA: Preparing for a career in nursing informatics. In: Marr PB, Axford RL, Newbold SK, eds. *Nursing Informatics '91: Proceedings of the Post Conference on Health Care Information Technology: Implications for Change.* New York: Springer-Verlag, 1991a; 163–166.

Gassert CA: Validating a model for defining nursing information system requirements. In: Hovenga EJS, McCormick KA, Hannah KJ, Ronald JS, eds. *Proceedings of Nursing Informatics '91.* New York: Springer-Verlag, 1991b; 215–219.

Gassert CA, Mills ME, Heller BR: Doctoral specialization in nursing informatics. In: Clayton PD, ed. *Proceedings of the Fifteenth Annual Symposium on Computer Applications in Medical Care.* New York: McGraw-Hill, 1992; 263–267.

Gassert CA: Summer Institute: Providing continued learning in nursing informatics. In: Grobe SJ, Pluyter-Wenting ESP, eds. *Nursing Informatics '94: An International Overview for Nursing in a Technological Era.* Amsterdam: Elsevier, 1994; 536–539.

Gassert CA: A model for defining information requirements. In: Heller BR, Mills ME, Romano CA, eds. *Information Management in Nursing and Health Care.* Springhouse, PA: Springhouse Corporation, 1995.

Graves JR, Corcoran S: The study of nursing informatics. *Image: Journal of Nursing Scholarship* 1989; 21(4): 227–231.

Grobe SJ: Introduction. In: Peterson HE, Gerdin Jelger U, eds. *Preparing Nurses for Using Information Systems: Recommended Informatics Competencies.* New York: National League for Nursing, 1988a; 4.

Grobe SJ: Nursing informatics competencies for nurse educators and researchers. In: Peterson HE, Gerdin Jelger U, eds. *Preparing Nurses for Using Information Systems: Recommended Informatics Competencies.* New York: National League for Nursing, 1988b; 25–33.

Grobe SJ: Nursing informatics competencies. *Methods of Information in Medicine* 1989; 28(4): 267–269.

Grobe SJ: Nursing intervention lexicon and taxonomy study: Language and classification methods. *Advances in Nursing Science* 1990; 13(2): 22–33.

Hannah KJ: Current trends in nursing informatics: Implications for curriculum planning. In: Hannah KJ, Guillemin EJ, Conklin DN, eds. *Nursing Uses of Computer and Information Science.* Amsterdam: Elsevier, 1985; 181–187.

Heller BR, Romano CA, Moray LR, Gassert CA: Special follow-up report: The implementation of the first graduate program in nursing informatics. *Computers in Nursing* 1989; 7(5): 209–213.

Henry SB, Holzemer WL, Reilly CA, Campbell KE: Terms used by nurses to describe patient problems. *Journal of the American Medical Informatics Association* 1994; 1(1): 61–74.

Hersher BS: The job search and information systems opportunities for nurses. *Nursing Clinics of North America* 1985; 20(3): 585–594.

Lawless KA: Nursing informatics as a needed emphasis in graduate nursing administration education: The student perspective. *Computers in Nursing* 1993; 11(6): 263–268.

Magnus MM, Co MC, Derkach C: A first-level graduate studies experience in nursing informatics. *Computers in Nursing* 1994; 12(4): 189–192.

McCloskey J, Bulechek G: The NIC taxonomy structure: Iowa intervention project. *Image* 1993; 25(3): 187–192.

McGonigle D, Eggers R: Establishing a nursing informatics program. *Computers in Nursing* 1991; 9(5): 184–189.

Meintz SL: Super computers open window of opportunity for nursing. *Computers in Nursing* 1993; 11(3): 140–144.

Milholland DK: Congress says informatics is nursing specialty. *American Nurse* 1992; July/August: 1.

NCNR Priority Expert Panel for Nursing Informatics: *Nursing Informatics: Enhancing Patient Care.* Bethesda, MD: NIH, 1993.

Ozbolt JG, Fruchtnight JN, Hayden JR: Toward data standards for clinical nursing information. *Journal of the American Medical Informatics Association* 1994; 1(2), 175–185.

Panniers TL, Walker EK: A decision-analytic approach to clinical nursing. *Nursing Research* 1994; 43(4), 245–249.

Panniers TL, Gassert CA: Standards of practice and preparation for certification. In: Heller BR, Mills ME, Romano CA, eds. *Information Management in Nursing and Health Care.* Springhouse, PA: Springhouse Corporation, 1995.

Parker J: Development of the American Board of Nursing Specialties (1991–1993). *Nursing Management* 1994; 25(1): 33–35.

Peterson HE, Gerdin Jelger U: *Preparing Nursing for Using Information Systems: Recommended Informatics Competencies.* New York: National League for Nursing, 1988.

Romano CA: Computer technology and emerging roles. *Computers in Nursing* 1984; 2(3): 80–84.

Saba VK, O'Hara PA, Zuckerman AE, Boondas J, Levine E, Oatway DM: A nursing intervention taxonomy for home health care. *Nursing & Health Care* 1991; 12(6): 296–299.

Schwirian PM: The NI pyramid—a model for research in nursing informatics. *Computers in Nursing* 1986; 4(3): 134–136.

Simpson RL: Shifting perceptions: Defining nursing informatics as clinical specialty. *Nursing Management* 1993; 24(12): 20–21.

Staggers N, Parks P: Description and initial applications of the Staggers & Parks nurse-computer interaction framework. *Computers in Nursing* 1993; 11(6): 282–290.

Styles MM: *On Specialization in Nursing: Toward a New Empowerment.* Kansas City, MO: American Nurses Foundation, Inc., 1989.

Taira F: Consider becoming a computer lab coordinator. *Computers in Nursing* 1992; 10(6): 235–236.

Thompson CB, Ryan SA: Knowledge solicitation from expert nurse clinicians. In: Grobe SJ, Pluyter-Wenting ESP, eds. *Nursing Informatics '94: An International Overview for Nursing in a Technological Era.* Amsterdam: Elsevier, 1994; 326–330.

Travis LL, Youngblut J: Supporting patient centered computing through an undergraduate nursing informatics curriculum. In: Safran C, ed. *Proceedings of the Seventeenth Annual Symposium on Computer Applications in Medical Care.* New York: McGraw-Hill, 1994; 757–761.

Zielstorff RD, Cimino C, Barnett GO, Hassan L, Blewett DR: Representation of the nursing terminology in the UMLS metathesaurus: A pilot study. In: Frisse ME, ed. *Proceedings of the Sixteenth Annual Symposium on Computer Applications in Medical Care.* New York: McGraw-Hill, 1993; 392–396.

29
Using Computers in Basic Nursing Education, Continuing Education, and Patient Education

Margaret J.A. Edwards

Introduction

As the use of computers and information science in nursing practice, education, and administration increases, the need also increases for nurses who possess the skill and knowledge to use and manage information technology in nursing environments. Our task as nursing educators is changing. Our new responsibility is to teach our students and colleagues to become discriminating users of information. Nurses need to have expertise in the use of computer-based information systems in the healthcare organizations and agencies in which they are employed. They must also come to use the technology as a tool to practice their chosen profession rather than practicing their profession to suit the needs of technology. In the delivery of health care, nurses have traditionally provided the interface between the client and the healthcare system. They will fulfill this function in new ways in a technologically advanced environment.

This chapter will provide an overview of the opportunities and issues related to the use of computers in formal nursing education, both undergraduate and graduate, continuing nursing education, and patient education. One issue that crosses all these areas—evaluation of educational software—begins the chapter.

Evaluating Educational Software

As nurse educators and continuing education coordinators have gained experience with educational software, they have become more sophisticated and selective in evaluating software before purchase. On the basis of previous experience, these nurses have often established personal criteria for evaluating software for their particular needs. There remains, however, a large number of nurses responsible for purchasing educational software who have no prior knowledge or experience in this area. The next section is designed as a resource for those nurses without a personal framework for evaluating educational software. The principles apply to formal nursing education, continuing education for nurses, and patient education. Educational criteria, quality assessment, and cost analysis will be discussed.

Educational Criteria

Nursing educators must make a conscious effort to acquire the skills necessary for evaluating software. In choosing among alternative computer assisted learning (CAL) software or between CAL and other teaching/learning strategies, nurse educators must compare alternatives on the basis of effectiveness, quality, and cost. Each of these variables must be included in the evaluation of each alternative and the comparison among different alternatives. This will result in increasing pressure on the marketplace to improve the quality of software products.

The evaluation process must address a number of key considerations. To begin, the evaluation team must take into account the fact that not all content is equally well taught by different teaching methodologies. For example, group process terminology or concepts can be taught using instructional computing, but group process interaction skills cannot. At present, there are few criteria for discriminating among teaching strategies to identify those most appropriate for learning specific content.

The evaluation team must also make a concerted effort to determine the congruence between instructional objectives and the objectives of a particular CAL program. Although to some this may appear obvious, experience suggests that decisions to purchase instructional computing software are sometimes made without examining the objectives of that software and comparing them to the program, course, or learning unit objectives.

Quality/Utility Assessment

Numerous guides, checklists, and evaluation tools are available to assist the nurse in judging the worth of a particular CAL package for a specific instructional purpose (Ball, Hannah, Gerdin Jelger, and Peterson, 1988; Bork, 1984; Caissy, 1984; Hannafin and Peck, 1988; Hudgings and Meehan, 1984; Komoski, 1984; Posel, 1993; Sawyer, 1984). Table 29-1 summarizes the most frequently used criteria in evaluating the quality and utility of instructional computing software.

Cost Analysis

When comparing commercial CAL software, usually only the purchase price is considered because all other costs are considered to be equal. In comparing commercially available CAL to locally developed CAL, usually only direct rather than full costs are considered. Direct costs are those costs

TABLE 29-1. Criteria Frequently Used for Evaluating Instructional Computing Software for Nursing Education

Content	Documentation Style
Accurate	Scholarship
Relevant	Parsimony
Current	Use of humor
Format	Personalization
Frames	Strategies
Graphics	Predominant type
Ergonomics	Variety
Psychosocial	Remediation
Physical	

related specifically to the alternative under consideration. Full costs are all costs associated with an alternative including direct costs as well as indirect overhead costs, such as a proportion of utilities or administration. However, direct costs of locally developed CAL materials must include design, development, and operation of the CAL software program.

Comparison between CAL and other alternative teaching/learning strategies involves more elaborate and sophisticated calculations than when making comparisons between different CAL software programs. When comparing CAL with other teaching/learning strategies, the following categories of costs should be included:

- Personnel salaries and benefits
- Administrative fees or salaries and benefits
- Services such as printing, postage, telephone, and equipment rental
- Hardware
- Software
- Facilities.

The most useful method of comparison would permit comparison among alternatives using all of the aforementioned variables (i.e., effectiveness, quality, and cost).

Cost-Benefit Analysis

Cost-benefit analysis involves the calculation of the monetary costs and benefits of alternatives. The relative attractiveness of each alternative is then assessed by determining which alternative has the lowest dollar cost and highest dollar benefit (Fig. 29-1), where B represents the benefits in

$$B_1 - C_1 \geq B_2 - C_2$$

FIGURE 29-1. Cost-benefit analysis model.

dollars and C represents the costs in dollars. Cost-benefit analysis provides for the use of quantitative objective data to compare two alternatives. Unfortunately, many benefits and costs in nursing education are not quantitative: rather; they are qualitative. This model does not allow consideration of measures of either the effectiveness or quality variables. Therefore, in the author's opinion this model is usually not useful for evaluating instructional computing software for nursing education.

Cost-Utility Analysis

Cost-utility analysis provides comparison of ratios between alternatives. The costs of an alternative are calculated. The decision makers determine the utility or usefulness of the alternative. These two factors are then compared to the same factors for other alternatives under consideration (Fig. 29-2) where C represents costs in dollars and U represents subjective judgment by decision makers of the perceived utility of the software. The cost-utility analysis method relies on a combination of quantitative and qualitative data, but unfortunately only the quantitative data are objective. The utility (qualitative) data are based on the subjective judgment by the decision maker of the alternative's utility.

Cost-Effectiveness Analysis

Cost-effectiveness analysis also establishes a ratio. In this case, the ratio is between the measure of the extent to which an alternative is effective in achieving a predetermined goal and the cost of the alternative in dollars. Ratios for different alternatives are then compared (Fig. 29-3) where GE represents measures of goal effectiveness, and C represents costs in dollars. In this method, both quantitative (costs) and qualitative (goal effectiveness) data are considered and objective measures are gathered for both types of data. This method of comparison permits both the effectiveness and quality variables identified to be considered as goals. Thus cost-effectiveness analysis is the superior method for choosing among instructional alternatives.

$$\frac{C_1}{U_1} \geq \frac{C_2}{U_2}$$

FIGURE 29-2. Cost-utility analysis model.

$$\frac{GE_1}{C_1} \geq \frac{GE_2}{C_2}$$

FIGURE 29-3. Cost-effectiveness analysis model.

Formal Nursing Education

Today, student learning needs in informatics are changing. With computer literacy almost a universal requirement for graduation from high school, an increasing number of students enter the nursing curriculum with advanced keyboarding skills and an understanding of computer terms, concepts, and history as well as computer applications in nursing. Often, they have out-distanced their nursing instructors in understanding and applying computer technology to their educational process.

The past decade has seen enormous changes in the quality and availability of instructional software for nurses. The increasing use of computer assisted video instruction (CAVI) and the advent of personal computer (PC)-based CD-ROM technology has changed the face of educational computing. Nurse educators, many of whom were educated before computers became a mainstay of instructional strategies, have struggled in the past to even keep up with this rapidly evolving technology. Faculty computer courses and the increased use of personal computers have helped increase the confidence with which nurse educators now approach the solutions that computer technology can offer.

The amount of literature documenting nursing educational uses of computers is growing exponentially. The studies cited in this section are meant only to be illustrative but not exhaustive of the available literature. Nurse educators are using the computer in a number of ways to manage the educational environment of both undergraduate and graduate nursing students:

- To instruct (Cohen and Dacanay, 1994; Froman, Hence, and Neafsey, 1993; Koch and McGovern, 1993; Strength and Keen-Payne, 1991; Weiner, Gordon, and Gilman, 1993; Wood, 1992).
- To evaluate (Abraham et al., 1991; Donabedian and Donabedian, 1993; Gilbert and Kolacz, 1993; Henry and Holzhemer, 1993: Wong, Wong, and Richard, 1992).
- To identify individual students' learning problems (Abbott, 1993; Lawless, 1993; McGonigle and Eggers, 1991; Wilson, 1991).
- To gather data on how learning takes place (Gonce-Winder, Kidd, and Lenz, 1993; Hanson, Foster, Nasseh, Hodson, and Dillard, 1994; Sawyer, 1984; Scarpa, Smeltzer, and Jasion, 1992; Thomas, White, Delaney, and Weiler, 1992).
- To manipulate data for research purposes (Napholz and McCanse, 1994).
- To direct continuing education (Carter and Axford, 1993; Tiano and White, 1990; Whiteside, McCulloch, and Whiteside, 1990; Williams and Benedict, 1990.

In the first edition of this book (Ball, Hannah, Gerdin Jelger, and Peterson, 1988), a major concern was the lack of quality software. Nurse educators had often been sold hardware to solve their instructional problems but then were unable to find either software to run on their particular configuration or the time and expertise to design their own software. The listing of software in the previous edition of this book (Bolwell, 1988) cited over 600 nursing educational software packages and over 70 vendors, while the current listing (Bolwell, 1995) cites over 300 packages from only 22 vendors. The expertise in software development is now concentrated within a small number of vendors producing high-quality software. The problem no longer is the availability of quality software but the vision, understanding, and expertise of nurse educators in knowing how to use this technology to full advantage.

Nursing educators must accept the responsibility of becoming knowledgeable about the use of computers in nursing practice and nursing education to make rational curriculum decisions about the integration of nursing informatics content into nursing curricula. In the meantime, they can make use of the model curricula described in the literature. They should also expect guidance and advice from professional organizations, such as the International Medical Informatics Association, the Alberta Association of Registered Nurses, the National League for Nursing, the American Nurses Association, the British Computer Society, and the Computer Applications in Nursing Special Interest Group of the Royal Australian Nursing Federation, all of which have active groups addressing the need for nursing informatics content in nursing education curricula. In addition, curriculum planners must locate instructional materials, evaluate their utility, and use them to support the teaching of nursing informatics. Finally they must accept the responsibility of being proactive in anticipation of the need to prepare graduates who are discriminating users of information and not hampered by the technology.

Continuing Nursing Education

Information is being generated at explosive rates. Between 6000 and 7000 scientific papers are written each day, and knowledge is expected to double every 20 months in the decade ahead. Therefore, 5 years after a nursing student graduates from school, more than 50% of the knowledge acquired will be obsolete (McCormick, 1984).

Staff development and continuous learning are a major responsibility of nursing management. Staff development can be viewed as synonymous with continuing nursing education. Continuing nursing education can be defined as all those learning activities that registered nurses undertake following basic nursing education that enhance their nursing competence. The main goal of this ongoing professional educational process is to maintain and improve the quality of health care by providing educational opportunities directed toward the personal and professional growth of the individual nurse.

Staff development includes, but is not limited to, those activities directed at orienting new staff to a facility, updating technical competency, progressing toward professional and career goals (including development of leadership potential and of decision-making and problem-solving skills), and enhancing professional roles and accountability.

Although the use of computerized instruction in nursing education has focused on basic nursing education in the past, many of the indications for using CAI in formal nursing education also apply to continuing education for nurses. In many areas, the focus in hospitals and community agencies has been on using computer technology to address administrative tasks, including bedside documentation. This focus has allowed many nurses to become familiar with specific uses of computers. Education departments of hospitals and community agencies have not been the focus of computerization efforts. Often the only relationship between continuing education for nurses and computers occurs when the nurse is oriented to new applications on the agency computer system. The use of computers in continuing education for nurses varies widely across the continent. The amount of literature related to computerized continuing education for nurses is growing. However, many articles are similar to those published 10 years ago about the use of computer assisted instruction for nursing students. Site-specific programs that have been developed for local use are reported.

The American Heart Association CPR Learning System is the most frequently documented wide-reaching use of computers in continuing nursing education. The literature reports efficient, cost-effective, and time-saving results (Edwards and Hannah, 1985; Hekelman, Phillips, and Bierer, 1990; Shehee, 1989; Umlauf, 1990). However, after the first rush of enthusiasm, unless careful attention was paid to administrative systems, the use of the CPR learning system tailed off, in many institutions to the point of nonuse.

The temptation to produce or purchase a learning system that will solve all related educational concerns must be resisted. However, sophisticated, computer supported learning cannot stand alone. The administrative processes and systems must be available to support the technology if computerized continuing education for nurses is to have an impact on nurses and their practices.

Nurse managers must familiarize themselves with the concepts of computer assisted learning as a means of maximizing the resources available for staff development. These are important factors considering that "training and education departments are frequently viewed as the most expendable units in an agency when budget cutbacks are necessary" (Porter, 1978, p. 161). Nurse managers must acquire sufficient understanding of the technology to make rational decisions about selection and implementation of such a learning system for use in staff development. In a period of economic constraints, relatively modest expenditures have the potential to create significant benefits. With CAL, these benefits range from the availability of learning materials, to productivity increases and savings resulting from reduced learning time and hence less time away from assigned duties, to improved staff morale associated with maintaining the commitment to staff development.

Patient Education

Computer assisted instruction has been identified as a unique ally for the nurse in delivering patient education (Bell, 1986; Sinclair, 1985; Tibbles, Lewis, Reisine, Rippey, and Donald, 1992). The benefits of patient education are now universally accepted. However, lack of time, lack of adequate resources, varying degrees of subject knowledge, and a perception among nurses that time spent in patient teaching is not valued by management have led to inconsistent and sporadic delivery of health education to patients. Computer assisted instruction is an ideal technology for addressing many of these concerns.

Advantages and Limitations of Using Computers in Patient Education

Advantages of using computers in patient education documented by Sinclair (1985) and Tibbles et al. (1992) include the following:

- Standardized content and delivery of educational material
- Ability to individualize both instruction and evaluation
- Decreased anxiety and embarrassment in learning new material, due to privacy
- Time and cost efficiency, once developed
- Availability outside traditional instruction times.

Although there are many benefits of using computers in patient education, one overriding limitation exists: There is a significant lack of quality commercial courseware, and the cost associated with development is prohibitive to most agencies. The state of patient education software is similar to that of nursing education in the past. Small numbers of individual developers have produced site-specific software; however, the quality of these varies widely.

Categories of Patient Education Courseware

Three categories of patient education courseware have been identified: (1) instruction on acute health problems, (2) teaching aimed at chronic health problems, and (3) wellness education (Sinclair, 1985). The following examples of these categories of patient education courseware are meant to be illustrative and not exhaustive.

1. Instruction on acute health problems. This category includes pre- and postoperative teaching and cardiac rehabilitation topics (Masten and Conover, 1990; Tibbles et al., 1992).

2. Teaching aimed at chronic health problems. Teaching self-management to young people with cystic fibrosis (Cooper, 1992) or nutrition to new diabetics (McKiel, 1991) are examples of this category.
3. Wellness education. The literature notes very few current examples of the use of computers in wellness education (Kahn, 1993; Vargo, 1991). However, while the professional community has not made significant progress in providing courseware for wellness education, commercial vendors have. While the reliability of some programs could be questioned, there is an abundance of courseware related to topics such as healthful eating, nutrition, and stress management that healthcare consumers can use on their personal computers at home.

Influencing Factors

Societal trends have accelerated the need for timely health education delivered in a manner that is both time- and cost-efficient. The increase in life expectancy has also included an increase in the number of people with long-term illnesses and disabilities. Because no cure exists for many of these conditions, such as diabetes or arthritis, patients need ongoing education to enable them to make decisions related to the personal and medical management of their illnesses. Increasing healthcare costs are compelling all healthcare providers to examine alternative ways of delivering their services. Often, in such an economic climate, concerted efforts at developing patient education materials or programs are abandoned in favor of the individual nurse fitting in patient teaching as time permits. With the increasing use of minimally trained auxiliary staff in healthcare institutions supervised by a nurse, the time available for that nurse to provide individualized patient teaching has decreased dramatically. Finally, healthcare consumers are not only more knowledgable about their health, but they expect to continue to gain knowledge especially as it applies to themselves when they are ill.

Conclusion

Patient education using computers is currently where nursing education and continuing nursing education were a decade ago. There is a need for concerted development of quality, commercially available courseware if this technology is to make inroads into the delivery of patient education.

In both formal nursing education and continuing education, quality courseware is available. Only the vision of educators now limits the use of computers to facilitate the learning of students.

Questions

1. What are ways in which nurse educators are using the computer to manage the educational environment of both undergraduate and graduate nursing students?
2. Discuss advantages and limitations of using computers in patient education.
3. List sample criteria that can be used for the evaluation of educational software. Consider educational criteria, quality assessment, and cost analysis.

References

Abbott K: Student nurses' conceptions of computer use in hospitals. *Computers in Nursing* 1993; 11(2): 78–87.

Abraham I, Evers G, Hasman A, Tanghe H, Silkens R, Hein F: A summer institute on computer applications for nursing management: background, curriculum, and evaluation. *Journal of Continuing Education in Nursing* 1991; 22(4): 136–142.

Ball MJ, Hannah KJ, Gerdin Jelger U, Peterson H. *Nursing Informatics: Where Caring and Technology Meet.* New York: Springer-Verlag, 1988.

Bell J: The role of microcomputers in patient education. *Computers in Nursing* 1986; 4(6): 255–258.

Bolwell C: Index to computer-assisted instructional (CAI) software for nursing education. In: Ball MJ, Hannah KJ, Gerdin Jelger U, Peterson H, eds. *Nursing Informatics: Where Caring and Technology Meet.* New York: Springer-Verlag, 1988; 371–391.

Bolwell C: Index to computer-assisted instruction for nursing education. In: Ball MJ, Hannah KJ, Newbold S, Douglas J, eds. *Nursing Informatics: Where Caring and Technology Meet.* 2nd ed. New York: Springer-Verlag, 1995.

Bork A: Computers in education today—and some possible futures. *Phi Delta Kappan* 1984; 65–66: 239–243.

Caissy G: Evaluating educational software: A practitioner's guide. *Phi Delta Kappan* 1984; 65–66: 249–250.

Carter BE, Axford RL: Assessment of computer learning needs and priorities of registered nurses practicing in hospitals. *Computers in Nursing* 1993; 11: 122–126.

Cohen PA, Dacanay LS: A meta-analysis of computer-based instruction in nursing education. *Computers in Nursing* 1994; 12(2): 89–97.

Cooper M: Playing the game . . . computer games . . . to teach young people selfcare in cystic fibrosis. *Nursing Standard* 1992; 6(21): 22–23.

Donabedian D, Donabedian A: Effectiveness of computer-aided learning in community health nursing. *Computers in Nursing* 1993; 11(3): 101–112.

Edwards MJ, Hannah KJ: An examination of the use of interactive videodisc cardiopulmonary resuscitation instruction for the lay community. *Computers in Nursing* 1985; 3(6): 250–252.

Froman RD, Hence C, Neafsey PJ: A comparative assessment of interactive videodisc instruction. *Computers in Nursing* 1993; 11(5): 236–241.

Gilbert DA, Kolacz NG: Effectiveness of computer assisted instruction and small-group review in teaching clinical calculation. *Computers in Nursing* 1993; 11(2): 72–77.

Gonce-Winder C, Kidd RO, Lenz ER: Optimizing computer-based system use in health professions' education programs. *Computers in Nursing* 1993; 11(4): 197–202.

Hannafin MJ, Peck KL: *The Design, Development, and Evaluation of Instructional Software.* New York: Macmillan, 1988.

Hannah KJ: Using computers to educate nurses. In: Ball MJ, Hannah KJ, Gerdin Jelger U, Peterson H, eds. *Nursing Informatics: Where Caring and Technology Meet.* New York: Springer-Verlag, 1988; 289–300.

Hanson AC, Foster SM, Nasseh B, Hodson KE, Dillard N: Design and development of an expert system for student use in a school of nursing. *Computers in Nursing* 1994; 12: 29–34.

Hekelman FP, Phillips JA, Bierer LA: An interactive videodisk training program in basic cardiac life support: Implications for staff development. *Journal of Continuing Education in Nursing* 1990; 21(6): 245–247.

Henry SB, Holzemer WL: The relationship between performance on computer-based clinical simulations and two written methods of evaluation: Cognitive examination and self-evaluation of expertise. *Computers in Nursing* 1993; 11(1): 29–34.

Hudgings C, Meehan N: Software evaluation for nursing educators. *Computers in Nursing* 1984; 2: 35–37.

Kahn G: Computer-based patient education: A progress report. *MD Computing* 1993; 10(2): 93–99.

Koch B, McGovern J: EXTEND: A prototype expert system for teaching nursing diagnosis. *Computers in Nursing* 1993; 11(1): 35–41.

Komoski K: Educational computing: The burden of ensuring quality. *Phi Delta Kappan* 1984; 65–66: 244–248.

Lawless KA: Nursing informatics as a needed emphasis in graduate nursing administration education: The student perspective. *Computers in Nursing* 1993; 11(6): 263–268.

Masten Y, Conover KP: Automated continuing education and patient education. *Computers in Nursing* 1990; 8(4): 144–150.

McCormick KA: Nursing in the computer revolution. *Computers in Nursing* 1984; 2: 4, 30.

McGonigle D, Eggers R: Establishing a nursing informatics program. *Computers in Nursing* 1991; 9(5): 184–189.

McKiel E: Computer-assisted instruction: Its efficacy for diabetes education. *Beta Release* 1991; 15(3): 85–87.

Napholz L, McCanse R: Interactive video instruction increases efficiency in cognitive learning in a baccalaureate nursing education program. *Computers in Nursing* 1994; 12(3): 149–153.

Porter S: Application of computer-assisted instruction to continuing education in nursing: Review of the literature. In: Zielstorff RD, ed. *Computers in Nursing.* Rockville, MD: Aspen, 1978; 161–169.

Posel N: Guidelines for the evaluation of instructional software by hospital nursing departments. *Computers in Nursing* 1993; 11(6): 273–276.

Sawyer T: Human factors considerations in computer-assisted instruction. *Journal of Computer-Based Instruction* 1984; 12: 17–20.

Scarpa R, Smeltzer SC, Jasion B: Attitudes of nurses toward computerization: A replication. *Computers in Nursing* 1992; 10(2): 72–80.

Shehee A: Computer-certified CPR. *Journal of Nursing* 1989; 89(4): 548.

Sinclair V: The computer as partner in health care instruction. *Computers in Nursing* 1985; 3(5): 212–216.

Strength DE, Keen-Payne R: Computerized patient care documentation: Educational applications in the baccalaureate curriculum. *Computers in Nursing* 1991; 9(1): 22–26.

Thomas BS, White Delaney C, Weiler K: The affective outcomes of course work on computer technology in nursing. *Journal of Nursing Education* 1992; 31(4): 165–170.

Tiano JJ, White AH: Effective training of nursing staff enhances hospital information system efficiency. *Journal of Continuing Education in Nursing* 1990; 21(6): 257–259.

Tibbles L, Lewis C, Reisine S, Rippey R, Donald M: Computer assisted instruction for preoperative and postoperative patient education in joint replacement surgery. *Computers in Nursing* 1992; 10(5): 208–212.

Umlauf MG: How to provide around-the-clock CPR certification without losing any sleep. *Journal of Continuing Education in Nursing* 1990; 21(6): 248–251.

Vargo GS: Computer assisted patient education in the ambulatory care setting. *Computers in Nursing* 1991; 9(5): 168–169.

Weiner EE, Gordon JS, Gilman BR: Evaluation of a labor and delivery videodisc simulation. *Computers in Nursing* 1993; 11(4): 191–196.

Whiteside MF, McCulloch J, Whiteside JA: Helping hospital educators and clinical nurse specialists learn to use and develop computer-assisted instruction. *Journal of Continuing Education in Nursing* 1990; 21(3): 113–117.

Williams RD, Benedict S: RN education flexibility utilizing laptop computers. *Computers in Nursing* 1990; 8(5): 201–203.

Wilson BA: Computer anxiety in nursing students. *Journal of Nursing Education* 1991; 30(2): 52–56.

Wong J, Wong S, Richard J: Implementing computer simulations as a strategy for evaluating decision-making skills of nursing students. *Computers in Nursing* 1992; 10(6): 264–269.

Wood CL: A computer-based AIDS education program for nursing students. *Computers in Nursing* 1992; 10(1): 25–35.

Appendices

Appendix A
Order Communications/ Nursing System Requirements Questionnaire

MARY ETTA MILLS

Order Communications/Nursing

M/D*	Enter Orders	Available	Not Available
M	1. Ability to enter all patient care orders via high-level user-oriented data entry methodology and validate		
M	2. Ability to restrict the entry of patient care orders to specific personnel based on user identification		
M	3. Ability to flash back the order for review before completion of the order entry process and price per test		
M	4. Ability to invoke order verification procedures based on the user's authority		
M	5. Ability to automatically generate protocol orders and hospital policy orders based on the patient's physician, age, sex, etc.		
M	6. Ability to enter multiple department orders and start/stop times for continuing orders following the selection of a single patient on a single screen		
M	7. Ability to enter and modify protocol orders		
M	8. Ability to enter physician words or other special comments		

*M = Mandatory; D = Desirable

365

M/D*	Enter Orders (*continued*)	Available	Not Available
M	9. Ability to modify procedure preps based on patient's condition, physician orders, etc.		
M	10. Ability to cancel verified orders		
M	11. Ability to receive hard copy of all transactions required to be charted		
M	12. Ability to display each selection on the subsequent screen		
M	13. Ability to validate online some basic orders modifiers (e.g. frequency, duration, form, route, etc.)		

Manage Orders

M	1. Ability to print display orders for professional verification, by patient, nursing station, physician, ancillary department, etc.		
M	2. Ability to hold orders in suspense until the appropriate verification has been completed		
M	3. Ability to require physician verification after the fact for physician representative (i.e., nurse) of verified orders either online or by signing a printed order		
M	4. Ability to automatically direct the order for procedures and preps to the correct locations		
M	5. Ability to generate multiple requisitions from individual orders, which are continuing or have a frequency of greater than once per day		
M	6. Ability to explode orders into various procedures and preps to the correct locations		
M	7. Ability to interface with stand-alone computer(s) on a real-time basis		
M	8. Ability to notify the proper personnel when special handling is required		

*M = Mandatory; D = Desirable

M/D*	Manage Orders (*continued*)	Available	Not Available
M	9. Ability to print requisitions immediately for a. STAT orders b. Orders from specific nursing units		
M	10. Ability to maintain all orders and their status online until purged as part of the medical records reporting applications until discharge		
M	11. Ability to print/display all orders for a patient or ancillary department with its station indicated		
M	12. Ability to print all orders scheduled to expire within the next 24 hours by patient, nursing station, or physician		
M	13. Ability to print/display all incomplete orders for an ancillary department on demand or at a specified time		
M	14. Ability to print/display all incomplete orders entered from a specified date forward for a patient by ancillary department		
M	15. Ability to display, print all orders sequenced by a. Department b. Order type		
M	16. Ability to monitor orders. Inquire as to status		
M	17. Check for duplicate orders		

Update Standard Orders Directory

M	1. Ability to establish standard orders by physician, nursing care plans, service, hospital policy, diagnosis, and patient condition		
M	2. Ability to update a directory of standard order either a. Online or b. Batch		

*M = Mandatory; D = Desirable

M/D*	Produce Billing Transactions	Available	Not Available
M	1. Ability to interface to the patient accounting system for automatic charging of procedures		
M	2. Ability to generate a charge for each procedure/test according to charging criteria contained in the procedure directory (i.e., order entry, order verification, procedure, test complete, result entry, etc.)		
M	3. Ability to issue a credit for a test/procedure that was not performed either a. Manually b. Automatically when test is canceled		
D	4. Ability to support point-of-sale billing		

Update Procedure Directory

M/D*		Available	Not Available
M	1. Ability to update a directory of procedures and associated preps either a. Online or b. Batch		
M	2. Ability to link specific comment screens to each procedure		
M	3. Ability to link procedures that serve as preps to other procedures		
M	4. Ability to include the time relationships between the procedure and associated preps		
M	5. Ability to indicate the following for each procedure a. Frequency of the procedure/prep, if frequency is not selected b. Performance times (either available or required) c. Whether or not a requisition is to be printed d. The standard requisition print location e. Department to perform the procedures prep		

*M = Mandatory; D = Desirable

M/D*	Update Procedure Directory (*continued*)	Available	Not Available
	f. Reports where the procedure is to appear (i.e., nursing care worksheet, care plan, medication plan)		
	g. Alternate requisition-print location dependent on account type		
M	6. Provide option, at time of order entry, to review test preparation information or identify other test requirements specific to each other		
D	7. Ability to maintain procedure standard price, price required, or no charge with the hospital and professional components		
D	8. Ability to maintain STAT and special handling surcharges for each procedure		
M	9. Ability to indicate when no charge for each procedure (i.e., order verification, specimen received, procedure/test complete, result entry, etc.)		
M	10. Ability to indicate if professional verification is required and by which categories and authority level before processing the order		
M	11. Ability to update standard formats for procedure requisitions either		
	a. Online or		
	b. Batch		

Enter Results

M/D*	Enter Results	Available	Not Available
M	1. Ability to enter all results via light pen or other high-tech user-oriented data entry techniques		
M	2. Ability to automatically format the screen to accommodate the results for the ordered procedure		
M	3. Ability to interface with stand-alone computer(s) or automated instruments on a real-time basis		

*M = Mandatory; D = Desirable

M/D*	Enter Results (*continued*)	Available	Not Available

M   4. Ability to automatically update the order status on entering results

D   5. Ability to prevent the entry of results without a price for price-required procedures

Manage Results

M   1. Ability to automatically direct test results to the proper location or multiple locations (i.e., nursing station, operating room, emergency room, ancillary department, etc.)

M   2. Ability to print results immediately for STAT orders and patients located in specific units (i.e., ICU, CCU, emergency room, operating room, etc.)

M   3. Ability to print results immediately from specified ancillary departments

D   4. Ability to hold results from specified ancillary departments or specific tests for review and verification before being released for printing or display outside the ancillary department

M   5. Ability to maintain all results online until purged as part of the medical records reporting application

M   6. Ability to print/display all ancillary results for a specific patient, results from a specified date forward or for a specific order

M   7. Ability to print results suitable for chart

Update Procedure Directory

M   1. Ability to indicate the following additional information on each procedure record
     a. Time allowed to obtain result: flag if exceeds maximum time
     b. Result format

*M = Mandatory; D = Desirable

M/D*	Update Abstract Code Directories	Available	Not Available

M   1. Ability to update a directory of abstracting codes for various ancillary department results reporting

Print/Display Order/Result Directories

M   1. Ability to print/display the order result directories, in part or in total, and various sort sequences

Inventory Control

M   1. Ability to maintain inventory control system in ancillary area

Patient Scheduling

M   1. Ability to print/display all unscheduled procedures for an ancillary department with the pertinent scheduling information on demand or on a scheduled basis

M   2. Ability to schedule a procedure for a specific time period for any active patient (i.e., preadmitted, in house, pre registered, and registered)

M   3. Ability to automatically preregister a nonactive patient by entering the appropriate information when scheduling an ancillary department procedure

M   4. Ability to automatically check for conflicts in the patient's schedule

M   5. Ability to schedule an appointment by
    a. Service
    b. Room/equipment
    c. Personnel
    d. Procedure test

M   6. Ability to indicate where the patient is served (i.e., ancillary department, patient room, etc.) or what procedure is being performed

*M = Mandatory; D = Desirable

M/D*	Patient Scheduling (*continued*)	Available	Not Available
M	7. Ability to reschedule the appointment without canceling and reentering		
M	8. Ability to automatically cancel the appointment when the procedure order is canceled		
M	9. Ability to maintain standard hours of availability for services, room/equipment, and personnel		
M	10. Ability to modify standard hours on an exception basis		
M	11. Ability to maintain an unlimited number of services, room/equipment, and personnel		
M	12. Ability to schedule 3 months in advance		
D	13. Ability to print/display the schedules for a specific date, procedure, test		
D	14. Ability to print/display the room equipment, physician, and personnel schedules for a specific date, procedure, test		
D	15. Ability to print/display future procedures scheduled		
D	16. Ability to print/display all procedures requiring scheduling that have not yet been scheduled		
D	17. Ability to print time patient tests in and time out		

Care Planning

M	1. Ability to enter special activities when standard activities within the care category are inappropriate		
M	2. Ability to update a patient's care plan by entering additional physician and nursing orders or canceling existing orders		
D	3. Ability to update all vital signs for each patient		

*M = Mandatory; D = Desirable

Not

M/D*	Care Planning (*continued*)	Available	Not Available

M 4. Ability to indicate compliance with care activities or the justification or noncompliance

D 5. Ability to print/display care activities not complied with and no justification given

D 6. Ability to print/display the entire care plan for a patient

D 7. Ability to print/display the care activities over a specified time period for a patient

D 8. Ability to print care plans limited to activities for a specified time period for a patient

D 9. Ability to group activities by care categories and include pertinent patient data (i.e., allergies, diagnosis, etc.) when printing or displaying care plans

D 10. Ability to print/display a cumulative all-vital-signs summary over a specified time period for a patient

Infection Control

M 1. Ability to print Infection Control notes

Determine Patient Care Requirements

M 1. Ability to interface to a clinical or communication system to obtain acuity classification of all patients in-house

M 2. Ability of Nurse Staffing system to determine the patient's acuity level using nursing input for each acuity criterion

M 3. Ability to computerize the patient care units for a patient based on
   a. Care activity
   b. Its frequency
   c. Patient's acuity level

*M = Mandatory; D = Desirable

	Determine Patient Care Requirements (*continued*)	Available	Not Available
M/D*			

d. By nursing stations
e. For each shift

M 4. Ability to total the patient care units for continuing patients and patients pending discharge from each nursing station by shift on a real-time basis

Compute Nurse Staffing Requirements

D 1. Ability to compute the number of nursing care units required
a. For each nursing station
b. By shift
c. Based on the number of patient care units required on that shift
d. Scheduled admissions and pending discharges for that shift
e. Number of patients on the nursing station

D 2. Ability to translate the number of nursing personnel by job category required for each nursing station and assigned preadmitted patients based on a predefined staffing mix specified for that nursing station

D 3. Ability to consider skill mix in computing staffing requirements

D 4. Ability to allow interunit floating

D 5. Ability to report on-call requirements by skill level

*M = Mandatory; D = Desirable

Appendix B
Site Visit Checklist

KAREN LAFFERTY ZIMMERMAN

Preliminary Points

- Site visits are more important today than ever due to the increasingly rapid changes in technology and the influx of new vendors scrambling to take advantage of these exciting new technologies.
- The purpose of site visits, therefore, is to validate what the vendor has sold, what has been learned about a product, and what is the level of client satisfaction. Site visits should not be used as a means of obtaining base knowledge about the vendor or the product.
- Do your homework prior to scheduling a site visit. Site visits should follow a request for information/request for proposal (RFI/RFP) evaluation process, detailed system demonstrations by finalist vendors, and thorough telephone reference calls. Additionally, send a list of questions to the host site in advance of your visit, including a list of areas you desire to visit, and set up appointments one on one with key contacts with whom you desire to speak without the vendor being present. Verify that you will have access to speak to end users.
- Ensure that the hosting site has key elements in common with your institution. The importance of similarities in size, specialty, programs, multihospital versus stand-alone, philosophy, size of the data processing shop, budget for the project, degree of administrative support for system installation, size of nursing stations, and type of nursing care delivery system cannot be overestimated. The variables for success are in common. Expending the funds to travel further to visit a site with more commonalities with your own site is a good investment.
- Many times your site visit and presentations will represent a full package, but a "scaled-down" version has been proposed and priced. Be confident of what you are seeing as compared to what has been proposed and priced.
- Do not leave the site until you are satisfied that you have seen what you have been sold. "Kick tires" to feel confident about the product.

General Observations

These are questions and observations that should be made during a site visit regardless of the category of system being evaluated.

_____   1. Go to the specific work area involved. Observe the work flow processes that are automated and those that are manual. Determine the reason for the manual processes.

_____   2. Observe a wide variety of transactions being entered on the system. What percentage of the transactions are being entered via:

        _____   a. Light pen
        _____   b. Keyboard
        _____   c. Mouse
        _____   d. Touch screen
        _____   e. Portable, handheld device
        _____   f. Voice activation

_____   3. Ask the users of the system what they like most about the system and what they like least about it.

_____   4. Ask how long the database, including orders, results, visit specifics, and demographics, is maintained online.

_____   5. Who from the hospital comprised the project team for system selection? For system implementation?

_____   6. Ask for details about implementation strategies and organizational structures that can assist in your own process.

_____   7. Ask about the decision-making process. How did the hospital select the installed vendor?

_____   8. What were the goals for the hospital/department/area in implementing the system? Have the goals been realized?

_____   9. Ask about the knowledge and experience of the vendor's implementation personnel. Were health care professionals on the team?

_____   10. Ask about current and planned projects for computerization in the area being visited. Do plans include interfacing or integrating products?

_____   11. What would the users like the system to do that it currently does not do?

_____ 12. Review all computer-generated reports/documents/forms. How flexible is the design and content? How easy are changes to implement?

_____ 13. Take the time to closely look at screens, content, layout, depth and breadth of available information, and ease of use. This is especially important if you make site visits before seeing a demonstration.

_____ 14. What is the response time (time elapsed between entering data on one screen and being able to enter data on a new screen)?

_____ 15. What is the hardware used to run the system? What is the average downtime—both scheduled and unscheduled?

_____ 16. What is the total number of terminals operational on the system?

_____ 17. Does the system offer a user friendly report writer that end users can easily learn and use?

_____ 18. Does the vendor have an active and productive user group? How would they rate the responsiveness of the vendor to requests for changes?

Hospital Information Systems (HIS)

These are questions and observations to make specifically related to site visits to evaluate an HIS.

On the patient care unit:

_____ 1. Look at the patient's hard copy chart. What is manual and what is computer generated?

_____ 2. Record the time you arrive on the unit. Record the number of phone calls while you are on the unit. Record the time you leave the unit. Record the type and size of the unit. Compare this information to your own environment.

_____ 3. While on the unit, record who is using the system (i.e., pharmacists, ward clerks, physicians, nurses, etc.).

_____ 4. How many terminals are on the unit? What is the ratio of devices to patients? What is the complement of devices between handheld, bedside, wireless, and those mounted at the nursing station?

_____ 5. Observe your guide or a user obtaining the following in a live situation:

_____ a. A medication administration guide
_____ b. A radiology result
_____ c. A laboratory result
_____ d. A pharmacy profile complete with historical medication administrations
_____ e. A current diet list and a historical diet list
_____ f. A clinical history of previous hospitalizations and outpatient visits
_____ g. An online user-defined report
_____ h. A unit management report

_____ 6. Ask about the ratio of direct to indirect hours of patient care.

_____ 7. Ask to see the "explosion of orders" from entering one standard order set. Verify that the explosion resulted in actual active orders, not verification tickets that must be reentered as active orders by nursing and ancillary personnel.

_____ 8. Spend a minimum of 1 hour on the patient care unit. If all your questions are answered in less time, ask to observe.

_____ 9. Go to at least two patient care areas. The second unit visit may be brief, but be confident that the system is fully operational on more than one unit.

_____ 10. Verify that all functionality is available in the outpatient areas for outpatients.

_____ 11. Ask to speak to the Vice President of Nursing to gain an administrative-level perspective of the system. This works best if prearranged.

_____ 12. Ask about the cost per patient day of the system.

In the ancillary areas:

_____ 13. What ancillary areas are supported by the system: Pharmacy, Radiology, Laboratory, Medical Records, Central Supply, Dietary, Cardiology, Physical Therapy, Respiratory, etc.?

_____ 14. What is the level of ancillary support?
_____ a. Order entry
_____ b. Results reporting
_____ c. Worklists
_____ d. Management reports
_____ e. Interface support for demographics to a stand-alone system and acceptance of results back

_____ 15. Can pharmacy review and update a nursing database, including patient allergies, height, weight, etc.?

_____ 16. Does pharmacy have a cart refill list for unit dose dispensing?

_____ 17. Does pharmacy have reports for drug utilization?

_____ 18. Does pharmacy and nursing have IV and hyperalimentation support? What is the support?

_____ 19. Is nursing charting medication administration on the system or charting manually using tools generated by the system, such as a medication administration record?

_____ 20. Does the automated medication procedure shorten the steps and potential error in a manual medication procedure?

_____ 21. Do clinical data automatically pass to the medical records system?

_____ 22. Is all ancillary system support available for outpatients and clinic patients?

_____ 23. Are the patient accounting system and the HIS interfaced or integrated? How are billing problems reconciled?

Nursing Information Systems (NIS)

These are questions and observations to make specifically related to site visits to evaluate a NIS.

_____ 1. Observe your guide or a user obtaining the following in a live situation:
  _____ a. A care plan
  _____ b. A nursing worksheet (kardex replacement)
  _____ c. An assessment document
  _____ d. A discharge planning guide for a specific patient
  _____ e. A quality assurance record
  _____ f. A nurse charting record

_____ 2. Is the charting system flexible enough to support a variety of methodologies (i.e., ABC, SOAP, exception, etc.)?

_____ 3. Is the care planning system flexible enough to support a variety of methodologies (i.e., diagnosis oriented, problem oriented, etc.)?

_____ 4. Ask to see end users charting, updating a care plan, initiating a care plan, entering a nurse treatment order, confirming a nurse treatment order and a physician-ordered treatment, and entering and updating a patient assessment.

_____ 5. Are NIS applications integrated with the HIS applications?

—— 6. Are physician orders automatically loaded into the NIS application and available in the care plan, nursing worksheet, assessment report, and discharge planning record without any redundant entry?

—— 7. Is nursing database information entered on the HIS automatically available in the NIS without redundant entry?

—— 8. Ask to see the research and quality assurance reporting out of the system.

—— 9. Are all the NIS applications available for use for outpatients?

—— 10. Spend a minimum of 1 hour on the patient care unit. If all your questions are answered in less time, ask to observe.

—— 11. Go to at least two patient care areas. The second unit visit may be brief, but be confident that the system is fully operational on more than one unit.

—— 12. Ask to speak to the Vice President of Nursing to gain an administrative-level perspective of the system. This works best if prearranged.

Clinical Information Systems (CIS)

These are questions and observations to make specifically related to site visits to evaluate CIS.

—— 1. Does the system offer abilities to view and control remote application via X-windows? See examples.

—— 2. Can data be imported and exported from the HIS and standalone systems for laboratory and pharmacy? See examples.

—— 3. Can each workstation operate as a
   —— a. Bedside monitor
   —— b. Central terminal
   —— c. Clinical terminal

—— 4. How accessible are the bedside devices? How are they mounted? Do they provide pivot between beds in a semiprivate room? How is data security maintained?

—— 5. Does the system provide decision support? See examples.

—— 6. Does the system support loading billing information directly into the CIS database? Can this billing information be automatically passed directly into the hospital's billing system through an interface?

_____ 7. Is the system installed in ICUs, Med-Surg units, the emergency department (ED), ORs, and ambulatory care settings? Why or why not?

_____ 8. Ask if system implementation has
    _____ a. Improved QI
    _____ b. Improved patient response times
    _____ c. Improved quality and accuracy of documentation
    _____ d. Reduced nursing overtime
    _____ e. Decreased Medicare/Medicaid denials
    _____ f. Decreased physician time reviewing the chart

_____ 9. Are HL7 communication interface protocols used?

_____ 10. What device interfaces are supported? Record the manufacturers for
    _____ a. Ventilators
    _____ b. Infusion pumps
    _____ c. Cardiac monitoring
    _____ d. Urometer
    _____ e. Physiology monitoring
    _____ f. Pulse oximeter
    _____ g. Cardiac output
    _____ h. Blood pressure
    _____ i. Fetal monitoring

_____ 11. Applications to view in a live situation:
    _____ a. Medication charting
    _____ b. Discharge planning
    _____ c. Quality assurance
    _____ d. I&O charting
    _____ e. Treatment charting
    _____ f. Patient assessment
    _____ g. Nursing notes
    _____ h. Neuro checks
    _____ i. Decision support

_____ 12. Do physicians use the system?

Portable, Wireless Point-of-Care Systems

These are questions and observations to make specifically related to site visits to evaluate portable, wireless point-of-care systems.

_____ 1. Are the devices
    _____ a. Pen based

_____ b. Voice activated
_____ c. Touch screen

_____ 2. Where are the devices being used?
    _____ a. ICUs
    _____ b. General med-surg
    _____ c. Specialized care areas
    _____ d. Ambulatory care settings
    _____ e. Emergency Department

_____ 3. Does the system have an integrated graphical user interface? Ask to see examples.

_____ 4. What is the weight of the device? Try to hold it for 4 to 5 minutes. Try to enter transactions using the right and the left hand. Try to enter transactions with the hand holding the device.

_____ 5. What is the average life expectancy of the batteries?

_____ 6. Do capabilities exist for integration with
    _____ a. Voice
    _____ b. Data
    _____ c. Image
    _____ d. Fax
    _____ e. Video
    _____   Note any examples of the host using any of the above capabilities.

_____ 7. What are the connectivity options?
    _____ a. Cable
    _____ b. Cellular

_____ 8. What is the downtime rate for the devices?

_____ 9. Determine the security of the data stored on the devices.

_____ 10. What is the practical signal range?

Automated Patient Classification Systems (PCS)

These are questions and observations to make specifically related to site visits to evaluate the PCS.

_____ 1. Determine if the system is open formatted to support a variety of acuity methodologies:
    _____ a. See your methodology automated by the primary vendor.

_____ b. See your methodology automated by an external vendor.

_____ 2. If the acuity methodology is factor based, what level of integration is developed between the HIS and the NIS and the PCS?
  _____ a. Demographics
  _____ b. Physician orders
  _____ c. Nursing orders
  _____ • Education needs
  _____ • Emotional needs
  _____ • Nursing process (i.e., assessment, care planning)
  _____ d. Medication orders
  _____ e. Activity orders
  _____ f. Treatment orders
  _____ g. Billing system (data to bill for nursing services)

_____ 3. What is the degree of integration between the PCS and the Staffing and Scheduling System? Is it the same or a different vendor?

_____ 4. Can modifications to the critical factors be maintained online or scheduled for future release?

_____ 5. Can methodologies be specific and unique per patient care area?

_____ 6. Is access to other patient care areas' data only available by selected individuals?

_____ 7. Can each patient care area access current and historical data online?

_____ 8. Review computer-generated reports received by the patient care area and by the administrative office.

_____ 9. What is the data entry methodology? Do nurses have to go to a separate/unique device to enter acuity data versus entering data on the same devices that access HIS and NIS applications?

_____ 10. See the data the system provides for quality assurance/quality improvement (QA/QI).

_____ 11. Can the system support patients in the ambulatory, ED, and outpatient settings?

Staffing and Scheduling Systems

These are questions and observations to make specifically related to site visits to evaluate staffing and scheduling systems.

_____ 1. Verify that staff's preferred hours are considered in scheduling.

_____ 2. Does the system consider employee skill levels in generating the schedule?

_____ 3. Does the vendor provide comparison data from other client sites over a regional and national geography?

_____ 4. Verify that the system schedules for a minimum of six weeks into the future.

_____ 5. Observe the process of changing the scheduled staffing for a shift today and for a future shift.

_____ 6. See an interface download using the staffing/scheduling system as the source. Watch as the data are then used in the external program to add to a database to generate graphics, etc.

_____ 7. What options are available for acuity?
   _____ a. Integrated
   _____ b. Interfaced with external vendor
   _____ c. Interfaced with home-grown product

_____ 8. Does an interface exist between the Personnel System and the Staffing and Scheduling System? If so, determine what data automatically pass. If not, determine why.

_____ 9. Does information pass both to and from the Staffing and Scheduling System and the Time and Attendance system?
   _____ a. Do scheduled data (i.e., vacation, holidays, etc.) pass to the Time and Attendance System?
   _____ b. Is time ticket entry eliminated through scheduling verification?
   _____ c. Does Staffing and Scheduling pass detailed work data to the Payroll System?

_____ 10. Are Staffing and Scheduling data available on every terminal at every patient care unit?

Home Health Systems

These are questions and observations to make specifically related to site visits to evaluate home health systems.

_____ 1. Do applications include
        _____ a. Assessment
        _____ b. Care planning
        _____ c. Nursing intervention
        _____ d. Charge capture
        _____ e. Case management
        _____ f. Scheduling
        _____ Ask to see each of these used in a live situation.

_____ 2. Does the system support real-time remote transmission of data to the base station 24 hours a day?

_____ 3. How many remote point-of-care devices can be supported by the base system? At what point (number of remote devices) is additional modem support recommended?

_____ 4. Is data entry via handheld devices that can be operated with one hand?

_____ 5. May historical data be retrieved online, including prior visits, medications, and care plans? For how long?

_____ 6. Does the system provide reminder functions for interventions? Ask to see examples.

_____ 7. Ensure that all data entry, data retrieval, and updating functions are available in the home setting.

_____ 8. Does the system meet all regulatory and reimbursement requirements? Does the system meet all managed care requirements?
        _____ a. HCFA forms 485, 486, 487
        _____ b. UB-92s

_____ 9. Can case assignments be received via the handheld device from remote locations? Do data received include
        _____ a. Demographics
        _____ b. Clinicals
        _____ c. Billing
        _____ d. Directions to the home

_____ 10. Is information transfer from the base to the handheld device via a standard telephone line and modem? Is cellular transmission supported? See examples.

_____ 11. Is rotary or touch tone phone access supported? See examples.

_____ 12. Are interfaces available to and from existing administrative/billing systems? Verify that no redundant entry is required for billing.

_____ 13. Can schedules be based on the orders for services? See examples.

_____ 14. Is time ticket entry eliminated through scheduling verification?

_____ 15. Are perpetual services set up one time, then automatically generated?

_____ 16. Can "help" screens be attached to any field?

_____ 17. Is the system used by other disciplines in addition to nursing (i.e., physical therapy, speech therapy, hospice, etc.)?

Appendix C
Request for Proposal for an Automated Quality Improvement System for a Nurse-Managed Center

Susan K. Newbold

Letter of Transmittal

This is a cover letter that will be sent to the vendors requested to bid on the quality improvement request for proposal (RFP).

Vendor Instructions

This section will include the purpose of the RFP, instructions on communications regarding the proposal, a proposal schedule, number of copies to submit by what date and to whom, how vendor presentations will be conducted, and methodology for contract negotiation. Other items to include are contractual contents, vendor selection, notification of vendor selection, RFP addenda, proposed preparation costs, effective dates of bid, and marketing references. Provide a profile of the vendor to include a brief history of the company, annual revenues for each of the previous 4 years, and the extent of vendor responsibility for monitoring federal and state regulatory proposals and mandates to identify required changes to application code.

Proposal Guidelines

This section will include notes on how the vendor should submit a response to the RFP.

Proposal Introduction

This RFP is for a quality improvement (QI) system for a nurse-managed clinic. QI for the purposes of this RFP is defined as "a structured and comprehensive system to monitor and evaluate the entire ambulatory clinical care program and to resolve deficiencies in that care when discovered."

Profile of the Nurse-Managed Center

(Note: This is a draft sample statement. Pull the profile from the RFP for the administrative/clinical/financial computer system and update it.) This nurse-managed ambulatory care health center is located in the inner city of a major mid-Atlantic community and serves the formerly underserved neighborhoods of _____ and _____.
The center is jointly funded by private foundation money and the University of _____. The Center is currently staffed by three full-time nurse practioners, a full-time director, and one secretarial support staff. The center opened in _____ and is staffed to handle an average of 24 patients per week. It is open _____ hours per week over _____ days per week. The patient load is expected to be _____ over _____ period of time.

Currently, there are no data processing capabilities, but a product called _____ sold by _____ Systems has been purchased. This system is for patient billing, scheduling (limited) medical records, and registration. The system uses RISC technology and runs on IBM-compatible hardware.

Quality Assurance Application Requirements

Instructions for Application Requirements Completion

For each requirement, indicate how this feature will be provided according to the following definitions:

A = available—The described application specification currently exists in the vendor's system and is available to the Center. All the application specifications marked as A are included in the proposed software application price and are currently demonstrable.

E = enhancement—The described application specification does not currently exist; however, the vendor will make this specification available to the Center at no additional cost. Each enhancement will have an outside completion date mutually agreed on by the vendor and the Center.

C = custom—The described application specification does not currently exist; however, the vendor will make this specification available to the Center for an additional cost. Each customization will have an outside completion date and additional charge mutually agreed on by the vendor and the Center.

U = unavailable—The described application specification does not currently exist and will not be made available to the Center at any cost.

Quality Improvement Application Requirements	Vendor Status	Comments

Accessibility—ability to track time from initiation of patient telephone call to receipt of professional advice

Appropriateness of service—ability to input, modify, and delete protocols

Audits—results of audits can be displayed graphically and in report format

Backup of data—describe recommendations for the backup and recovery of data

Can data collection be modified to fit needs of the Center?

Case identification—criteria can be input to search for cases that meet specified parameters

Compare plan of care to established standards and protocols

Completeness and deficiencies. Ability to determine when key information is missing.

Continuity of care—ability to track patient over all episodes of care

Cost of Service—ability to track costs

Describe additional features not defined in remainder of requirements

Documentation—technical. Provide samples of technical documentation.

Documentation—user. Provide samples of user documentation.

Ease-of-use features for experienced and frequent users. Please describe.

Ease-of-use features for new users. Please describe.

Quality Improvement Application Requirements	Vendor Status	Comments
Identify potential problems—patient risk minimization		
Incidents: Ability to collect, track, and report information on incidents, including		
Incidents—lab errors		
Incidents—medication errors		
Incidents—miscellaneous		
Incidents—narcotic count errors		
Incidents—patient/personnel security problem		
Incidents—treatment errors		
Incidents—valuables missing		
Interfaces to medical records systems, particularly _____, and statistical packages		
Number of software updates per year		
Patient compliance—ability to indicate whether patient understands his or her health care plan		
Patient satisfaction—ability to track waiting time		
Patient satisfaction—ability to trend patient surveys related to satisfaction		
Performance of provider staff—ability to maintain employee credentials		
Performance of support staff—ability to maintain information on support staff		
Presentation mechanisms: tables, graphic presentations, bar charts, etc.		
Random selection of criteria for evaluation		
Reports—can be generated on an ad hoc basis.		
Reports—list standard reports		

Quality Improvement Application Requirements	Vendor Status	Comments
Security and Confidentiality—describe measures		
Statistics: ability to perform analysis of variance, pattern analysis, descriptive differential techniques, etc.		
Technical—describe the implementation support provided by the company, including training. Describe in detail your recommended strategy.		
Technical—describe the postimplementation support provided by the company. Include hotline support and hours of service.		
Technical—describe proposed communications architecture		
Technical—hardware platform. Provide a schematic diagram of the proposed hardware. Describe the hardware requirements including the CPU, main memory size, disk size, terminals, printers, other input/output devices, and communication devices.		
Technical—performance. Based on the volume statistics provided in the Center Profile, provide statistics showing expected peak load response times.		
Technical—software platform. Describe the system's software and any support tools (report writers, database managers, graphics, or statistical packages, etc.).		
What are your future plans for development of this system?		

Evaluation Criteria:
 Functionality: 50%
 Cost: 25%
 Technical Considerations: 25%—hardware, software platform, interfaces to other systems (especially UNIX), number of sites using system

Appendix D
Index to Computer Assisted Instructional Software for Nursing Education

CHRISTINE BOLWELL

CAI Software Vendors

AJN (American Journal of Nursing Company)
555 West 57th Street
New York, NY 10019
(800) 582-8820
In New York state call
(212) 582-8820

Applied Microsystems, Inc.
PO Box 832
Roswell, GA 30077
(404) 552-9000

Cardionics, Inc.
1100 Hercules, Suite 210
Houston, TX 77058
(713) 488-5901

C&D Enterprises
PO Box 2278
Glen Ellyn, IL 60138-2278

CES (Computerized Educational Systems)
Florida Hospital Association
Management Corp
PO Box 536905
Orlando, FL 32853-6905
(407) 841-6230, ext. 215

College of DuPage
Office of Instructional Design
22nd Street and Lambert Avenue
Glen Ellyn, IL 60137
(312) 858-2800, ext. 2490

Diamond Custom Training Software
PO Box 6952
Boise, ID 83707-6932
(800) 359-2996

Health Science Consortium (HSC)
201 Silver Cedar Court
Chapel Hill, NC 27514-1517
(919) 942-8731

Jackson & Milne, Associates
12679 14th Avenue
Surrey, BC, Canada V4A 1H3
(604) 540-4630

J.B. Lippincott Co.
Department of Audio Visual Media
227 East Washington Square
Philadelphia, PA 19106-3780
(800) 523-2945
In Pennsylvania call collect
(215) 238-4443

**Medi-Sim/W&W (Medi-Sim/
Williams & Wilkins)**
Electronic Media Division
428 East Preston Street
Baltimore, MD 21202
(800) 527-5597 or (410) 528-4000

Medware
768 Faxon Avenue
San Francisco, CA 94112
(415) 586-8219

National Nursing Review
342 State Street, Suite 6
Los Altos, CA 94022
(800) 950-4095

Open Learning Agency
Marketing Department
4355 Mathissi Place
Burnaby, B.C., Canada V5G 4S8
(604) 431-3210 or (800) 663-1653

P11 Enterprises
PO Box 5185
Bridgeport, CT 06610
(203) 366-0258

**PDS (Professional Development
Software)**
PO Box 2063
Chapel Hill, NC 27515
(919) 932-5013

PixSoft
3A-2020 Portage Avenue
Winnipeg, Manitoba, Canada
R3J OK4
(204) 885-4936

R.A. Williams, PhD, RN, FAAN
University of Michigan
2028 Collegewood
Ypsilanti, MI 48197
(313) 487-8146

Tecno Topics, Inc.
3600 Gateshane
Dongola, IL 62926
(618) 827-4912

**UCSF (University of California,
San Francisco)**
School of Nursing, N319Y
University of California
Third & Parnassus Avenues
San Francisco, CA 94143
(415) 476-4745

Williams & Wilkins (W&W)
Electronic Media Division
428 East Preston Street
Baltimore, MD 21202
(800) 527-5597 or (410) 528-4000

Name of Program	*Vendor*
SCIENCE	
Anatomy and Physiology	
Cardiac A&P	CES
Hemodynamics I: The Heart & How It Works	CES
The Engine of Life	P11 Enterprises

Medical Terminology

Elements of Medical Terminology	Applied MicroSys
Introduction to Medical Terminology	Medi-Sim/W&W

Pharmacology

Abbreviations & Equivalents—Nurse ProCalc	PDS
Clinical Simulations in Nursing Pharmacology, 2nd Edition	
A Client Using Birth Control Pills	Medi-Sim/W&W
Adjuvant Chemotherapy for Breast Cancer	Medi-Sim/W&W
Analgesia & Anesthesia for Maternity Client	Medi-Sim/W&W
Antibiotic Therapy w/Compound Fracture	Medi-Sim/W&W
A Patient Requiring Antiarrhythmic Drug Rx	Medi-Sim/W&W
Depressed Patient on Tricyclic Antidepressants	Medi-Sim/W&W
Drug Rx for Preschooler with Asthma	Medi-Sim/W&W
Immunizing Children—Communicable Disease	Medi-Sim/W&W
Iron Intoxication in a Toddler	Medi-Sim/W&W
Pharmacotherapeutics for Angina Pectoris	Medi-Sim/W&W
Pharmacotherapeutics for Gastric Pain	Medi-Sim/W&W
Psychotropic Drug Rx for Schizophrenic	Medi-Sim/W&W
Eliminating Medication Errors	CES
Eliminating Medication Errors in the Elderly	CES
Eliminating Pediatric Medication Errors	CES
Immunizations of Infants and Children	CES
Managing the Side Effects of Chemotherapy	CES
Managing the Side Effects of Chemotherapy II	CES
Potassium: A Vital Electrolyte	CES
Those Fabulous Nitrates	CES

BASIC SKILLS
CPR/ACLS

Basic Life Support	W&W
Foreign Body Airway	CES
Megacode	CES

Calculating Dosages

Calculate With Care	
Fractions	J.B. Lippincott
Ratio and Proportion	J.B. Lippincott
Drug Dosage Calculation Administration	
Symbols and Abbreviations	Medi-Sim/W&W
Systems of Measurement	Medi-Sim/W&W
Calculating Drug Dosages: Tablets & Liquids	Medi-Sim/W&W
IV Parenteral Dosages	Medi-Sim/W&W

Intravenous Calculations	W&W
Intravenous Meds: Calculation Problems	J.B. Lippincott
Math General Hospital	CES
Minims, Milliliters, and Drops: The Game	CES
Nurse ProCalc—Drugs and Solutions	PDS
The Starship Healthwise (Calculating equivalents)	CES

Communication

Effective Staff Communication	CES
The Challenge of Communication	Medi-Sim/W&W
Therapeutic Patient Communications	CES
Therapeutic Patient Communications II	CES

Computers in Nursing Practice

| Information Technology (Simulated HIS) (3.5″ disk) | Jackson & Milne |

Documentation

| Doing the "Write" Thing | CES |
| Chart Smart (demo) | College of DuPage |

General Nursing Skills

Care of the Client Receiving Internal or External Radiation Therapy	CES
Complications of IV Therapy (3.5″ disk)	CES
Death: A Personal Encounter	AJN
Ethics in Nursing Practice	
Ethical Dilemmas in Perinatal Nursing	Medi-Sim/W&W
Ethical Dilemmas in Pediatric Nursing	Medi-Sim/W&W
Everybody Needs a Nurse (Decision Making) (3.5″ disk)	CES
Fundamentally Fun Graphics (reading temp, B/P, syringes, drip rates)	PDS
Introduction of Nutritional Assessment	Medi-Sim/W&W
Legal Aspects of Nursing	CES
Potassium: A Vital Electrolyte	CES
Principles of Blood Administration	Medi-Sim/W&W
Protecting Patient's/Resident's Rights	CES
Radiation Safety: Internal and External	CES
SOS—Strategies for Problem Solving (Demo) (3.5″ disk)	C&D Enterprises
The Causes of Pressure Sores	CES

Hospital Safety
Body Mechanics	CES
Electrical Safety	CES
Fire Safety—A Hot Topic	CES
Preventing Patient Falls	CES

Infection Control
Asepsis: Principles of Nursing Practice—2nd
Edition
Introduction to Asepsis	Medi-Sim/W&W
Chain of Infection	Medi-Sim/W&W
Medical Asepsis	Medi-Sim/W&W
Surgical Asepsis	Medi-Sim/W&W
Protective Asepsis: Isolation	Medi-Sim/W&W
Handwashing	CES
Inflammation, Infection & Wound Healing: Clinical Nursing Concepts	PDS
Infection Control: Principles and Practice	CES
Universal Precautions	CES
Universal Precautions	Medware

Monitoring and Interpretation
Arterial Blood Gases
ABGee!	HSC
ABGs	CES
Acid-Base Balance: Clinical Nursing Concepts	PDS
Acid-Base Balance/Imbalance	Open Learning

EKG Interpretation
Basic Arrhythmia Teaching System	Cardionics
Basic ECG Teaching System	Cardionics
Basic Cardiac Rhythm Interpretation	
Electrical Activity of the Heart & Sinus Rhythm (3.5″ disk)	Medi-Sim/W&W
Atrial Dysrhythmias (3.5″ disk)	Medi-Sim/W&W
Junctional and Ventricular Dysrhythmias (3.5″ disk)	Medi-Sim/W&W
Heart Blocks (3.5″ disk)	Medi-Sim/W&W
C.A.R.T.A. (Cardiac Arrhythmia Recognition Training)	Techno Topics
Telemetry	CES

Fetal Monitoring
Advanced Fetal Monitor Interpretation	W&W
Antepartum Fetal Assessment	W&W
FM Tutor: Fetal Monitor Interpretation	W&W

AIDS   Medi-Sim/W&W
Lymphoma   Medi-Sim/W&W
Immunosuppression   Medi-Sim/W&W
Critical Care Series: Neonatal Nursing Series
  Neonatal Resuscitation   Medi-Sim/W&W
  Intraventricular Hemorrhage   Medi-Sim/W&W
  Respiratory Distress syndromes   Medi-Sim/W&W
  Nutrition and Fluid Management   Medi-Sim/W&W
  Meconium Aspiration   Medi-Sim/W&W
Critical Care Series: Neurological System, 2nd
  Edition
  Myasthenia Gravis   Medi-Sim/W&W
  Guillain-Barre Syndrome   Medi-Sim/W&W
  Increased Intracranial Pressure   Medi-Sim/W&W
  Intracranial Aneurysm   Medi-Sim/W&W
  Spinal Cord Injury   Medi-Sim/W&W
Critical Care Series: Pediatric
  Septic Shock   Medi-Sim/W&W
  Altered Neurological Function   Medi-Sim/W&W
  Pediatric Transport   Medi-Sim/W&W
  Low Cardiac Output   Medi-Sim/W&W
  Altered Fluid and Electrolytes   Medi-Sim/W&W
Critical Care Series: Pulmonary
  Adult Respiratory Distress Syndrome   Medi-Sim/W&W
  Pulmonary Embolus   Medi-Sim/W&W
  Acute Respiratory Failure   Medi-Sim/W&W
  COPD   Medi-Sim/W&W
  Chest Trauma   Medi-Sim/W&W
Critical Care Series: Renal System, 2nd Edition
  Altered Fluid Volume   Medi-Sim/W&W
  Electrolyte Imbalance   Medi-Sim/W&W
  Chronic Renal Failure   Medi-Sim/W&W
  Acid-Base Disturbances   Medi-Sim/W&W
  Acute Renal Failure   Medi-Sim/W&W
Critical Care Series: Response to Critical Illness
  Altered Body Image   Medi-Sim/W&W
  Pain   Medi-Sim/W&W
  Sensory Overload   Medi-Sim/W&W
  Family in Crisis   Medi-Sim/W&W
  Emotional Response/Cardiac   Medi-Sim/W&W
Death: A Personal Encounter   AJN
Meeting the Psychosocial Needs in Critical Care   CES
Meeting the Psychosocial Needs of Critically Ill
    Clients & Their Families   CES

An Adult Insulin-Dependent Diabetic	Medi-Sim/W&W
An Elderly Patient with Osteoporosis & Hip Fracture	Medi-Sim/W&W
A Patient Having Surgery for Lung Cancer	Medi-Sim/W&W
Fluids and Electrolyte Balance: Clinical Nursing Concepts	PDS
Managing the Side Effects of Chemotherapy	CES
Managing the Side Effects of Chemotherapy II	CES
Managing the Side Effects of External Radiation	CES
Nursims:	
Laura Bee: With Visual Impairment	J.B. Lippincott
Mr. Bahr: 56-year-old Diabetic with Amputation	J.B. Lippincott
Mr. Ben Lee: Undergoing Pneumonectomy	J.B. Lippincott
Mr. Carl: Undergoing Ileostomy	J.B. Lippincott
Mr. Drew: Adult Who Abuses Alcohol	J.B. Lippincott
Mr. Helm: In Cardiovascular Crisis	J.B. Lippincott
Mr. Kane: Experiencing Respiratory Distress	J.B. Lippincott
Mr. Zay: 60-year-old with Acute CVA	J.B. Lippincott
Rena Fuller in Renal Crisis	J.B. Lippincott
Nursing Care of the Cardiac Patient	
Cardiovascular Anatomy and Physiology Review (3.5″ disk)	Medi-Sim/W&W
Assessment and Diagnostic Tests (3.5″ disk)	Medi-Sim/W&W
Acute Care of the Patient after Myocardial Infarction (3.5″ disk)	Medi-Sim/W&W
Nursing Care of the Surgical Patient	
Preoperative Nursing Care	Medi-Sim/W&W
Postoperative Nursing Care	Medi-Sim/W&W
Patient Encounters—Patients Who Need Help with GI Function	
Mr. Babain: With Peptic Ulcer	J.B. Lippincott
Mr. Hansie: With Cirrhosis	J.B. Lippincott
Patient Encounters—Patients Who Need Help with Mobility	
Mrs. Peppy: With Hip Replacement	J.B. Lippincott
Mr. Ralph: With Amputation	J.B. Lippincott
Patient Encounters—Patients Who Need Help with Neurological Function	
Ms Tarbo: With Myasthenia Gravis	J.B. Lippincott
Mr. Buttons: With Alzheimers	J.B. Lippincott
Patient Encounters—Patients Who Need Help with Urinary Elimination	
Mr. Migo: With BPH	J.B. Lippincott
Mrs. Fiver: With Cystitis	J.B. Lippincott

Hypertension and Preeclampsia   W&W
Labor Management   W&W
Medical University of SC: Nurse-Midwifery
    Simulations
    Postpartum Hemorrhage   Medi-Sim/W&W
    Postpartum Complications   Medi-Sim/W&W
    Drug Therapy for Labor and Delivery   Medi-Sim/W&W
    Delivery Room Management of Newborn   Medi-Sim/W&W
    Early Labor Management   Medi-Sim/W&W
NAACOG's High Risk Maternity Nursing I
    The Pregnant Patient with Cardiac Disease   Medi-Sim/W&W
    The Pregnant Patient with Diabetes   Medi-Sim/W&W
    Sexually Transmitted Diseases in Pregnancy   Medi-Sim/W&W
NursComps:
    Pharmacological Interventions in OB   J.B. Lippincott
    12-Point Postpartum Check   J.B. Lippincott
    Interventions for Client with P.I.H.   J.B. Lippincott
    Interventions for Client with Abruptio   J.B. Lippincott
    Interventions for Pregnant Diabetic   J.B. Lippincott
Nursims:
    Mrs. West: Multip. with C-Section   J.B. Lippincott
    The Wills: Neonate & Young Mother   J.B. Lippincott
Obstetric Infections   W&W
Postpartum Care   .
    Essentials of Infant Care   Medi-Sim/W&W
    Mother Meets Baby   Medi-Sim/W&W

Pediatric Nursing
Admission of a Full Term Infant to the Nursery
    Newborn Assessment: Identification, Apgar
        Scoring, and Temp Reg.   Medi-Sim/W&W
    Maturation Assessment: Weight and Physical
        Characteristics   Medi-Sim/W&W
    Neurologic Assessment: Reflexes and Behavior
        Patterns   Medi-Sim/W&W
Clinical Simulations in Pediatric Nursing I, 2nd
    Edition
    An Infant with Vomiting   Medi-Sim/W&W
    A Toddler Hospitalized with Seizure   Medi-Sim/W&W
    A Preschooler with Meningitis   Medi-Sim/W&W
    A School Age Child with Cerebral Palsy   Medi-Sim/W&W
Clinical Simulations in Pediatric Nursing II, 2nd
    Edition
    An Infant with Congenital Heart Disease   Medi-Sim/W&W
    A Toddler with Respiratory Difficulty   Medi-Sim/W&W

A Preschooler Hospitalized with Pneumonia	Medi-Sim/W&W
A School Age Child with Leukemia	Medi-Sim/W&W
Danny Wong: In Pain	UCSF
Ellen Peterson: with Leukemia	UCSF
Eliminating Pediatric Medication Errors	CES
Ethics in Nursing Practice	
Ethical Dilemmas in Perinatal Nursing	Medi-Sim/W&W
Ethical Dilemmas in Pediatric Nursing	Medi-Sim/W&W
Immunizations of Infants and Children	CES
NursComps:	
Immediate Newborn Care	J.B. Lippincott
Continuing Newborn Care	J.B. Lippincott
Nursims:	
Ben Sims: Adolescent with Cystic Fibrosis	J.B. Lippincott
Beth Popil: Child with V.S.D.	J.B. Lippincott
Hazel: 6-year-old with Nephrosis	J.B. Lippincott
Kim Klam: With Ureteral Reimplantation	J.B. Lippincott
Lucy Webb: With Down's Syndrome	J.B. Lippincott
Sam Hill: With Tonsillectomy	J.B. Lippincott

Psychiatric Nursing

Care of the Suicidal Client	CES
Care of the Client with Borderline Personality	CES
Clinical Simulations in Psychiatric Nursing I, 2nd Edition	
A Suicidal Adolescent	Medi-Sim/W&W
A Patient with Acute Mania	Medi-Sim/W&W
A Patient with Pain and Anxiety	Medi-Sim/W&W
An Assaultive Patient	Medi-Sim/W&W
Clinical Simulations in Psychiatric Nursing II, 2nd Edition	
An Adolescent with Eating Disorder	Medi-Sim/W&W
An Adolescent with Acute Schizophrenia	Medi-Sim/W&W
Patient with History of Substance Abuse	Medi-Sim/W&W
Patient with Major Affective Disorder	Medi-Sim/W&W
Current Concepts in Mental Health Nursing	
AIDS: Psychiatric Nursing Care	Medi-Sim/W&W
The Impaired Nurse: Chemical Dependency	Medi-Sim/W&W
The Problems of Co-Dependency	Medi-Sim/W&W
The Impaired Nurse: Emotional Disturbance	Medi-Sim/W&W
NursComps:	
Bipolar Disorder	J.B. Lippincott
Anxiety Disorder	J.B. Lippincott
Anorexia Nervosa	J.B. Lippincott

Nursims:
Mr. Charles: Obsessive-Compulsive	J.B. Lippincott
Ms. Alt: Young Adult w/ Depression	J.B. Lippincott
Ms. Bale: Major Distortions in Ego Function	J.B. Lippincott
Nursing Care of Client with Bipolar Disorder	CES
Nursing Care of the Depressed Client—Mrs. Morris	CES
Nursing Care of Patients with Anxiety Disorders, 2nd Edition	Medi-Sim/W&W
The Med Clinic	CES
Therapeutic Communication with the Chemically Dependent Client	CES
Therapeutic Counseling Session	CES
Therapeutic Communications with the Chemically Dependent Client	CES

NURSING THEORY

Clinical Decision Making	ICNE
Introduction to Behavioral Objectives	J.B. Lippincott
Introduction to Nursing Diagnosis, Version 2.0	J.B. Lippincott
Introduction to Nursing Goals	J.B. Lippincott
Introduction to Nursing Orders	J.B. Lippincott
Introduction to Patient Data	J.B. Lippincott
Introduction to Patient Problems	J.B. Lippinoott
Nursing Diagnosis Vignettes in Adult Health	W&W
Nursing Diagnosis Vignettes in Child Health	W&W
Nursing Diagnosis Vignettes in Home Health	W&W
Using the Nursing Process	
Introduction to the Nursing Process	Medi-Sim/W&W
Introduction to Nursing Diagnosis	Medi-Sim/W&W
Components of Nursing Assessment	Medi-Sim/W&W
Using the Nursing Process to Establish Goals	Medi-Sim/W&W
Implementation of the Care Plan	Medi-Sim/W&W
The Importance of Evaluation	Medi-Sim/W&W

NURSING RESEARCH

Introduction to Research	
Introduction to Research (3.5" disk)	UCSF
Research Design (3.5" disk)	UCSF
Sampling (3.5" disk)	UCSF
Measurement and Instrumentation (3.5" disk)	UCSF
Data Analysis (3.5" disk)	UCSF

Appendix E
Electronic Resources

Susan K. Newbold and Miriam Jaffe

This Appendix, which is a supplement to Chapter 5, includes details on access to help nurses enter the information superhighway.

A Selection of Service Providers (phone numbers, not modem numbers)

America Online	1-800-827-6364, billing@aol.com
CompuServe	1-800-848-8199
Delphi Internet	1-800-695-4005, info@delphi.com
GEnie	1-800-638-9636
InterRamp from PSI, Inc.	1-800-PSI-0852, interramp-info@psi.com
Netcom	1-800-353-6600, info@netcom.com
PRODIGY	1-800-PRODIGY, into99a@progidy.com

To access AJNNet:

Via the Internet (telnet to ajn.org) or via modem (dial 212-582-8137). Log in as GUEST USER.

To access the Nursing Network Forum (NNF):

Via Internet, telnet delphi.com, or by modem, 1-800-695-4002
userid: JOINDELPHI
password: CUSTOM261
enter NURSE when prompted for referral name
enter GO CUS 261 at any prompt to enter the NNF
To reach JoAnn Klein, e-mail to nurse@clark.net.

A Selection of Magazines

NetGuide: The Guide to the Internet and Online Services. A CMP
  Publication.
Subscription information: 1-800-829-0421, e-mail:
  netmail@netguide.cmp.com
WWW URL: http://techweb.cmp.com

Internet World: The Magazine for Internet Users. MecklerMedia
Subscription info: 1-800-573-3062, e-mail: 74671.3430@compuserve.com
WWW URL: http://www.mecklerweb.com

Wired.
Subscription info: 1-800-SO-WIRED (1-800-769-4733),
subscriptions@wired.com

Boardwatch Magazine: Guide to Online Information Services and
  Electronic
Bulleting Boards. Jack Rickard
Subscription info: 1-800-933-6038, e-mail: subscriptions@boardwatch.com
(Good directories and ads to help you locate a BBS)

Online Access. Chicago Fine Print.
Subscription info: 1-800-36-MODEM (1-800-366-6336)
(Oriented to BBSs; a good source for locating one near you)

Computer Shopper: The Computer Magazine for Direct Buyers
Subscription info: 1-800-274-6384
(Carries an extensive BBS directory in every issue)

A Selection of Books

Engst A. *Internet Starter Kit for Macintosh (2nd ed.).* Hayden Books,
  ISBN 1-56830-111-1.
Kent P. *The Complete Idiot's Guide to the Internet.* Alpha Books, ISBN
  1-56761-414-0.
Levine JR, and Baroudi C. *The Internet for Dummies.* IDG Books, ISBN
  1-56884-024-1.
Levine JR, and Levine M. *More Internet for Dummies.* IDG Books, ISBN
  1-56884-164-7.

Nursing-Related Listservs

Many of the lists below are managed by the LISTSERV software and thus respond to a standard set of commands. To subscribe to any LISTSERV list, send a message to the administrative address (LISTSERV@place .where.list.lives) with the following line, and nothing else, in the BODY (not in the subject line) of the message:

SUB   LISTNAME   Yourfirstname Yourlastname

(substituting in the appropriate values, of course). The list name is the part before the "@" sign in the list address. To unsubscribe from any LISTSERV list, send a message to the administrative address with the following line, and nothing else, in the body of the message:

UNSUB LISTNAME

The material that follows has been excerpted from the promotional materials and welcome messages distributed by the list owners. The full text of most of these messages can be obtained from either the NURSE WWW/ Gopher sites to the NIGHTINGALE WWW/Gopher sites.

CAREPL-L

CAREPL-L is a list dedicated to the storage and retrieval of nursing care plans. Anyone can submit a care plan for review. After the care plan is approved, it will be posted to the list and archived on a monthly basis. The archives are open to retrieval and database searches via LISTSERV database commands by the public. Only care plans will be posted to the list. Discussion about care plans that are archived must take place on another forum such as SNURSE-L. The list uses LISTSERV software.

The administrative address is: listserv@ubvm.cc.buffalo.edu
The list address is: carepl-l@ubvm.cc.buffalo.edu

To submit a care plan, send a copy of your care plan to CAREPL-L@ UBVM.CC.BUFFALO.EDU. Your care plan will be forwarded to the editors of the list for review. It will then be posted to the list.

Questions should be sent to the list owner: Tim Brackett (brackett@ essex.hsc.colorado.edu).

CULTURE-AND-NURSING

CULTURE-AND-NURSING is a list for nurses and other health care professionals interested in or working in the field of cross-cultural and transcultural nursing and health care. The list allows members to discuss issues of cultural competence, theory, practice, research, and experience in an open and unmoderated forum. As of this writing, there are over 200 members from 12 different countries on the list. Recent topics have included the use of interpreters in clinical practice, teaching culturally competent care, and education aides/resources. This list uses the "majordomo" mailing list manager.

The administrative address is: majordomo@itssrvl.ucsf.edu
The list address is: culture-and-nursing@itssrv1.ucsf.edu

To subscribe to CULTURE-AND-NURSING, send the following command in the BODY of the mail message (leave the subject header blank) to the administrative address:

subscribe CULTURE-AND-NURSING

Please take note that the character after "itssrv" is the number one (1), not the letter "L." Although majordomo is similar to the LISTSERV and listproc programs, there are a few differences. To receive the command list, send a message containing the single word "help" (without the quotes) to the administrative address:

Send questions to the list manager, Chuck Pitkofsky, MS, RN, UCSF School of Nursing (chuckp@itsa.ucsf.edu).

IVTHERAPY-L

The IVTHERAPY-L list is for communication and mutual support of IV therapy nurses and other interested professionals. It uses LISTSERV software.

The administrative address is: listserv@netcom.com
The list address is: ivtherapy-l@netcom.com

Questions should be directed to the list owner, Sarah Kuykendall, RN, BS, Oregon Health Sciences University, (sarahk@netcom.com).

MIDWIFE

MIDWIFE is a list for discussion of midwifery issues. It is a semiautomated list administered by Denis Anthony at the University of Warwick.

The administrative address is: midwife-request@csv.warwick.ac.uk
The list address is   midwife@csv.warwick.ac.uk

To subscribe to the list, send a message to the administrative address asking to be added to the list. Please include your e-mail address and your name in the body of the message. The membership list for MIDWIFE is publicly available, and subscriptions from people who wish to remain anonymous are not accepted. Posts to the list are archived on the NURSE WWW/ Gopher service under the heading "Midwife List Archives." Questions should be addressed to the list owner, Denis Anthony (cudma@csv.warwick .ac.uk).

MRM

MRM is a list created to facilitate dialogue related to the nursing theory, Modeling and Role-Modeling developed by Erickson, Tomlin, and Swain. It is administered by Judy Hertz at York College of Pennsylvania (hertz@ yorkcol.edu).

The administrative address is: mrm-request@yorkcol. edu
The list address is: mrm@yorkcol.edu

NPINFO

NPINFO is a list focused on nurse practitioners of all specialties, nurse midwives, and nurse anesthetists. Sponsored by Nurse Practitioner Support Services, the list allows nurse practitioners, CNMs, and CRNAs to communicate freely across the United States and to different specialties about issues of mutual interest. The list uses the SmartList mailing list manager.

The administrative address is: npinfo-request@npl.com
The list address is: npinfo@npl.com

Address questions to the list owner, Bob Smithing, MSN, ARNP, FNP, Nurse Practitioner Support Services (nursebob@npss.win.net).

NRSING-L

NRSING-L is a list primarily for the discussion of nursing informatics topics. It uses the "listproc" mailing list manager, which is similar to LISTSERV but has several major differences in syntax.

The administrative address is: listproc@lists.umass.edu
The list address is: nrsing-l@lists.umass.edu

To subscribe to NRSING-L, send a message to the administrative address with a blank subject line and the single line

sub nrsing-l Yourfirstname Yourlastname

in the body of the message. Questions should be directed to the list owner, Gordon Larrivee, M.S., R.N. (larrivee@umassmed.ummed.edu).

NRSINGED

NRSINGED provides a forum for the discussion of topics and issues in nursing education. Discussion is meant to be wide ranging, from teaching methodologies to philosophical issues, to meet the diverse needs of nurse educators. It uses the LISTSERV mailing list manager.

The administrative address is: listserv@ulkyvm.louisville.edu
The list address is: nrsinged@ulkyvm.louisville.edu

The list is not "moderated," but you must be subscribed to the list before LISTSERV will let you post to it. Address questions to the list owner, Patricia K. Lacefield EdD, RN (pklace01@ulkyvm.louisville.edu or pklace 01@ulkyvm.bitnet)

NURCENS

NURCENS is a forum for issues related to nurse management centers. It uses the LISTSERV mailing list manager.

The administrative address is: listserv@gibbs.oit.unc.edu
The list address is: nurcens@gibbs.oit.unc.edu

Direct questions to the list owner, Dr. P. Allen Gray (gray@vxc.ocis .uncwil.edu).

NURSENET

NURSENET is an international conference for discourse about diverse nursing issues in the areas of nursing administration, nursing education, nursing practice, and nursing research. It is open and unmoderated and uses the LISTSERV mailing list manager.

The administrative address is: listserv@vm.utcc.utoronto.ca
The list address is: nursenet@vm.utcc.utoronto.ca

As of this writing, NURSENET is the largest and the most prolific of the nursing lists, with 1347 members in 23 countries as of January 31, 1995. List volume can top 50 messages a day, so if you are new to e-mail, be sure you know whether you will be incurring per-message charges with your service provider before you subscribe. The NURSENET archives are available from the University of Toronto gopher and can be viewed and retrieved from that site (gopher.vm.utcc.utotonto.ca).

Questions should be directed to the list owner, Judy Norris (jnorris@ oise.on.ca).

NURSERES

As mentioned in the text, NURSERES focuses on nursing research and nursing practice. The list underwent a merger with the list GRADNRSE, a list devoted to nursing practice issues, and that list no longer exists. NURSERES uses the LISTSERV software.

The administrative address is: listserv@kentvm.kent.edu
The list address is: nurseres@kentvm.kent.edu

Address questions to the list owner, Linda Q. Thede, RN (Ithede@kentvm.kent.edu).

NURSE-UK

NURSE-UK is a list for discussion of nursing issues in the United Kingdom. It is a semiautomated list administered by Denis Anthony at the University of Warwick.

The administrative address is: nurse-uk-request@csv.warwick.ac.uk
The list address is: nurse-uk@csv.warwick.ac.uk

To subscribe to the list, send a message to the administrative address asking to be added to the list. Please include your e-mail address and your name in the body of the message. The membership list for NURSE-UK is publicly available, and subscriptions from people who wish to remain anonymous are not accepted. Posts to the list are archived on the NURSE WWW/ Gopher service under the heading "NURSE-UK Archives." Questions should be addressed to the list owner, Mr. Denis Anthony (cudma@csv.warwick.ac.uk).

PNN-L

PNN-L, the Parish Nursing Network, exists to facilitate dialogue and resource sharing among persons of all faith traditions regarding the professional practice of health promotion, prevention, and education integrated with the spirituality of the particular faith community within which that practice is exercised. This list welcomes both RN and non-RN practitioners, physicians, health ministers, clergy and nonordained, experts and beginners, and all others interested in religion and health. It uses the majordomo mailing list manager.

The administrative address is: majordomo@interaccess.com
The list address is: pnn-l@interaccess.com

To subscribe, send a message to the administrative address, with this and only this statement in the message body:

subscribe PNN-L <your Internet e-mail address>

Please note that majordomo wants to see your Internet e-mail address, not your name, in the command line.

PSYCHIATRIC-NURSING

PSYCHIATRIC-NURSING is a list that is part of InterPsych, an international, multidisciplinary organization of people interested in mental health issues. It uses the mailbase mailing list manager.

The administrative address is: mailbase@mailbase.ac.uk
The list address is: psychiatric-nursing@mailbase.ac.uk

To subscribe, send a message to the administrative address with the following in the body:

join psychiatric-nursing firstname lastname
stop

SCHLRN-L

SCHLRN-L, the School Nurse Network, is a forum for school nurses, school nurse practitioners, school nurse teachers, and school nurse managers. The list encourages networking; helps spread information about research and technological advances, educational and funding opportunities, advanced practice, and professional organizations; and supports those nurses working in isolated educational settings. It uses the LISTSERV software.

The administrative address is: listserv@ubvm.cc.buffalo.edu
The list address is: schlrn-l@ubvm.cc.buffalo.edu

Address questions to the list owner, Martha Dewey Bergren, RN (C179gu7r@ubvm.cc.buffalo.edu).

SNURSE-L

SNURSE-L is a global electronic forum for nursing students. This list is open to anyone who would like to join. The topics include nursing issues, student issues, electronic databases and libraries useful to nursing students, and National Student Nursing Association issues and events. It uses the LISTSERV software.

The administrative address is: listserv@ubvm.cc.buffalo.edu
The list address is: snurse-l@ubvm.cc.buffalo.edu

Direct questions to the list owner, Tim Brackett (brackett@essex.hsc.colorado.edu).

A Selection of Usenet Newsgroups of Potential Interest to Nurses

Nursing Newsgroups

sci.med.nursing	A general forum for nursing
alt.npractitioners	Nurse practitioners
bit.listserv.snurse-l	Student nurses; the Usenet gateway for the mailing list

Medical/Health-Related Usenet Newsgroups

sci.med	Medicine & related products and regulations
sci.cognitive	Perception, memory, judgment, & reasoning
sci.med.aids (moderated)	Medical discussion of AIDS/HIV virus
sci.med.diseases.cancer	Medical discussion of cancer
sci.med.immunology	Immunology
sci.med.nutrition	Nutrition & diet
sci.med.occupational	Occupational medicine & therapy
sci.med.pharmacy	Pharmacy
sci.med.psychobiology	Psychiatry & psychobiology
sci.med.radiology	Radiology and imaging
sci.med.telemedicine	Telemedicine and related applications
sci.med.transcription	Medical transcription issues
sci.med.vision	Vision, ophthalmology, eye care
sci.psychology	General psychology
sci.psychology.digest	Psychology electronic journal
sci.psychology.research (moderated)	Research issues in psychology
misc.education.medical	Medical education
misc.health.aids	General discussions about AIDS
misc.health.alternative	Alternative health
misc.health.arthritis	Arthritis
misc.health.diabetes	Diabetes, hypoglycemia
misc.kids.health	Children's health issues
bit.listserv.c+health	Usenet gateway for C+HEALTH (computers and health) mailing list
bit.listserv.tbi-support	Usenet gateway for TBI-SPRT (traumatic brain injury support) mailing list
bit.med.resp-care.world	Usenet gateway for RC_WORLD (respiratory care) mailing list
alt.infertility	Causes & treatment of infertility

alt.med.allergy	Allergy
alt.med.cfs	Chronic fatigue syndrome
alt.med.fibromyalgia	Fibromyalgia
alt.psychology.help	General help with psychological problems
alt.psychology.personality	Personality taxonomies/assessment/models
alt.abuse.offender.recovery	Recovery for abuse offenders/perpetrators
alt.abuse.recovery	Recovering from all types of abuse
alt.abuse.transcendence	Alternate models of dealing with abuse
alt.abuse-recovery (m)	Moderated version of alt.sexual.abuse.recovery
alt.recovery	General topics in recovery
alt.recovery.addiction. sexual	Recovering from sexual addictions
alt.recovery.codependency	Codependency
alt.recovery.religion	Recovering from the effects of religion
alt.sexual.abuse.recovery	Recovering from sexual abuse
alt.support.abuse-partners	Partners of childhood sexual abuse survivors
alt.support.anxiety-panic	Anxiety and panic disorders
alt.support.arthritis	Arthritis
alt.support.asthma	Asthma
alt.support.attn-deficit	Attention-deficit disorders
alt.support.big-folks	Fat acceptance with no dieting talk
alt.support.cancer	Cancer
alt.support.cerebral-palsy	Cerebral palsy
alt.support.crohns-colitis	Crohn's disease & ulcerative colitis
alt.support.depression	Depression & mood disorders
alt.support.dev-delays	Developmental delay
alt.support.diabetes.kids	Parents & family of children with diabetes
alt.support.diet	Dieting/losing weight/nutrition
alt.support.dissociation	Persons w/ dissociative disorders (e.g., MPD)
alt.support.divorce	Divorce/marital breakups
alt.support.eating-disord	Eating disorders (anorexia, bulimia, etc.)
alt.support.epilepsy	Epilepsy
alt.support.grief	Grief and loss
alt.support.headaches. migraine	Migraine and headache ailments
alt.support.loneliness	Loneliness
alt.support.mult-sclerosis	Multiple sclerosis
alt.support.musc-dystrophy	Muscular dystrophy
alt.support.non-smokers	Effects of second-hand smoke
alt.support.obesity	Obesity
alt.support.ocd	Obsessive-compulsive disorder
alt.support.short	Issues of interest to short people

alt.support.shyness	Shyness
alt.support.single-parents	Single parents
alt.support.sleep-disorder	Sleep disorders
alt.support.spina-bifida	Spina-bifida
alt.support.step-parents	Help being a stepparent
alt.support.stop-smoking	Stopping or quitting smoking
alt.support.stuttering	Stuttering & other speaking difficulties
alt.support.tall	Issues of interest to tall people
alt.support.tinnitus	Tinnitus/ringing ears/other head noises
alt.transgendered	Transgendered, transsexual, intersexed persons
alt.support	Other support topics & questions not covered by existing groups
alt.sigma2.height	People far from average height
soc.support.youth.gay-lesbian-bi	Gay, lesbian, and bisexual youth
soc.support.transgendered	Transgendered & intersexed persons

A Selection of Nursing Related Gopher and World-Wide Web Sites

Clearinghouse of Subject-Oriented Resource Guides
gopher to una.hh.lib.umich.edu choose inetdirs
Gopher URL: gopher://una.hh.lib.umich.edu:70/11/inetdirs

HIV/AIDS Nursing from the National Institutes of Health
gopher to odie.niaid.nih.gov choose AIDS/Nursing
Gopher URL: gopher://odie.niaid.nih.gov:70/11/aids/nursing

Idea Nurse
WWW URL: http://www.silcom.com/~peter/nurse.html

Galaxy Nursing section
WWW URL: http://galaxy.einet.net/galaxy/Medicine/Nursing.html

NIGHTINGALE, at the College of Nursing, University of Tennessee, U.S.A.
NIGHTINGALE exists in both gopher and WWW formats
gopher to nightingale.con.utk.edu
Gopher URL: gopher://nightingale.con.utk.edu:70
WWW URL: http://nightingale.con.utk.edu:70/0/homepage.html

NURSE, at the School of Nursing, Warwick University, England
NURSE exists in both gopher and WWW formats
gopher to nurse.csv.warwick.ac.uk
Gopher URL: gopher://nurse.csv.warwick.ac.uk:70/11/
WWW URL: http://www.csv.warwick.ac.uk:8000

Nursing Services at Duke University Medical Center
WWW URL: http://nursing-www.mc.duke.edu/nursing/nshomepg.html

Ohio State University College of Nursing
WWW URL: http://www.con.ohio-state.edu:80/

University of California, San Francisco School of Nursing
WWW URL: http://nurseweb.ucsf.edu/www/ucsfson.html/

University of Delaware College of Nursing
WWW URL: http://www.udel.edu/brentt/UD_Nursing.html

University of Iowa Nursing Page
WWW URL: http://indy.radiology.uiowa.edu/Nursing/
    ColOfNurseHP.html

University of Maryland at Baltimore School of Nursing
gopher to umabnet.ab.umd.edu choose Schools/Nursing
Gopher URL: gopher://umabnet.ab.umd.edu:70/11/.schools/.nursing
WWW URL: http://www.nursing.ab.umd.edu/

University of Washington School of Nursing
WWW URL: http://www_son.hs.washington.edu/

University of Michigan, Ann Arbor
gopher to gopher.itd.umich.edu choose University of Michigan/Schools/
    Nursing
Gopher URL: gopher://gopher.itd.umich.edu/11/presoff/nursing/gopher

Yahoo—A Guide to WWW
WWW URL: http://akebono.stanford.edu/yahoo/

Nursing Organizations and Nursing Publications With Electronic Mail Access

American Journal of Nursing
555 W. 57th Street, New York, NY 10019
1-800-CALL-AJN

ajn.editorial@ajn.org (Editor, American Journal of Nursing)
circulation@ajn.org (Circulation Department)
mcn.editorial@ajn.org (Editor, Maternal Child Nursing)
nr.editorial@ajn.org (Editor, Nursing Research)
telnet: ajn.org or WWW URL: http://www.ajn.org

American Nurses Association
600 Maryland Avenue, Suite 100 West, SW
Washington, DC 20024-2571 U.S.A.
202-651-7000, taneditor@ana.org (Editor, The American Nurse)

Computers in Nursing
University of Southern Maine
96 Falmouth Street, Portland, ME 04103 U.S.A.
lnicoll@maine.maine.edu (Editor-in-Chief, Dr. Leslie Nicoll)

National League for Nursing
350 Hudson Street, New York, NY 10014 U.S.A.
1-800-669-1656, 212-989-9393, nlninform@nln.org

Nursing
Springhouse Corporation
215-646-8700
73751.42@compuserve.com

Sigma Theta Tau International Honor Society of Nursing
550 West North Street, Indianapolis, IN 46202
317-634-8171
member address changes: dtownsenestti_sun.iupui.edu
Online Journal of Knowledge Synthesis for Nursing
barnstnr@son.nursing.upenn.edu (Editor, Dr. Jane Barnsteiner)

Sigma Theta Tau International Honor Society of Nursing
Virginia Henderson International Library
telnet: stti-sun.iupui.edu (password is visitor)

Springer-Verlag New York, Inc.
175 Fifth Avenue
New York, NY 10010 U.S.A.
1-800-777-4643
custserv@spint.compuserve.com (Customer Service)
bookorders@spint.compuserve.com (Orders)

Nursing Informatics Special Interest Groups

Name: American Medical Informatics Association, Nursing
                Informatics
            Working Group and Student Working Group
Area: United States
Contact: American Medical Informatics Association
            4915 St Elmo Avenue, Suite 401, Bethesda, MD 20814
                U.S.A.
            301-657-1291, mail@amia2.amia.org

Name   American Nurses Association Council on Nursing Services
                and Informatics
Area: United States
Contact: American Nurses Association
            600 Maryland Avenue, Suite 100 West, SW
            Washington, DC 20024-2571 U.S.A., taneditor.ana.org

Name: American Nursing Informatics Association
Area: Southern California, U.S.A.
Contact: Ms. Melodie Kaltenbaugh
            21710 Clearwater Dr, Yorba Linda, CA 92687 U.S.A.
            melodiekrn@aol.com,bob@kaiwan.com, or
                pwetsch@delphi.com

Name: Australian Nursing Informatics Council (ANIC)
Area: Australia
Contact: Health Informatics Society Australia, Inc.
            Suite G1, 63 Stead Street, South Melbourne VIC 3205
                Australia
            61-3-690-5388, 61-3-690-5488 (f), hisa@vaxc.cc.monash.edu.au

Name: Boston Area Nursing Informatics Consortium (BANIC)
Area: Boston and Vicinity, U.S.A.
Contact: Alice Siders   617-632-8806

Name: Canadian Health Informatics Association (COACH) Nursing
            Informatics Special Interest Group,
            Suite 216, 10458-Mayfield Road,
            Edmonton, Alberta, Canada T5P 4P4
Area: Canada
Contact: Carol Robinson   75051.2272@compuserve.com
            Pat Jeselon   pjeselon@gvhs.gov.bc.ca

Name: Capital Area Roundtable on Informatics in NursinG
             (CARING)
Area: Maryland, Virginia, Washington, DC, U.S.A.
Contact: Marina Douglas   703-709-2363
             Susan K. Newbold   410-531-9244
             snewbold@umabnet.ab.umd.edu
             Chris Wierz   703-698-3677

Name: Computers in Healthcare Interfacing with Nursing (CHIN)
Area: Connecticut, U.S.A.
Contact: Laurel Perry   203-650-8069
             Ann Bello   nk_bello@apollo.commnet.edu

Name: Delaware Valley Nursing Computer Network (DVNCN)
Area: Delaware, New Jersey, and Pennsylvania, U.S.A.
Contact: Mary Ellen Sweeney   302-633-5545
             James Cannon   cannon2@aol.com

Name: International Medical Informatics Association, Special
             Interest Group on Nursing Informatics (SIGNI)
Area: The World
Contact: Ulla Gerdin Jelger, Sweden
             Evelyn Hovenga, Australia, e.hovenga@ucq.edu.au
             Virginia Saba, U.S.A.,
             vsaba01@gumedlib.dml.georgetown.edu

Name: Michigan Nursing Informatics Group (MINIG)
Area: Michigan, U.S.A.
Contact: Donna Hoff-Grambau MS, RN, C
             Mid Michigan Community College, Health Education
             1375 South Clare Avenue, Harrison, Michigan 48625
             1-517-386-6648, dhoffgr@edcen.ehhs.cmich.edu

Name: Midwest Alliance for Nursing Informatics (MANI)
             PO Box 9313, Downers Grove, IL 60515 U.S.A.
Area: Midwest United States
Contact: Joyce Sensmeier   708-923-4531

Name: Midwest Nursing Research Society (MNRS), Nursing
             Informatics Research Section
Area: Midwest United States
Contact: Connie Delaney   319-541-3600,
             connie-delaney@uiowa.edu
             MNRS Office   317-541-3600

Name: National League for Nursing, Council on Nursing Informatics
Area: United States
Contact: National League for Nursing
          350 Hudson Street, New York, NY 10014 U.S.A.
          1-800-669-1656, 212-989-9393, nlninform@nln.org

Name: North Carolina State Nurses Association Council on Nursing
            Informatics (CONI)
Area: North Carolina, U.S.A.
Contact: Dr. Mary Curran   704-547-3355,
            macurran@unccvm.uncc.edu

Name: Northern California Nursing Informatics Association
            (NCNIA)
Area: Northern California, U.S.A.
Contact: Michael Moore   mmoore@nbn.com
          Kathy Douglas   415-812-7418, kathy@oceania.com

Name: Nursing Informatics Systems Discussion Group (NISDG)
Area: Minneapolis and St. Paul, Minnesota, and vicinity, U.S.A.
Contact: Florence C. Marks, 617-347-3366,
          Hennepin County Medical Center
          flossy.marks@co.hennepin.us or
            marke003@maroon.tc.umn.edu

Name: Nursing Informatics New Zealand (NINZ)
Area: New Zealand
Contact: exe@ninz.gen.nz or
          Robyn Carr   rlc@ninz.gen.nz

Name: Ontario Nursing Informatics Group (ONIG)
Area: Canada
Contact: Rose Dzugan, 905-521-2100 x
            5471   dzugan@ihis.cmb.on.ca

Name: Tri-State Nursing Computer Network (TNCN)
Area: Pennsylvania, Ohio, West Virginia, U.S.A.
Contact: Dr. Ramona Nelson   412-738-2325, ren@sruvm.sru.edu

Name: Western New York Nursing Informatics Group (WNYNIG)
Area: Buffalo, NY, U.S.A.
Contact: Kathleen Plowcha
          Nursing Systems Coordinator, Buffalo General Hospital
          100 High Street, Buffalo, NY 14203 U.S.A. 716-845-2908
          ned001@po1.bgh.edu
          Martha Dewey Bergren, c179gu7r@ubvm.cc.buffalo.edu

Name: Wisconsin Computers in Nursing (WICAN)
Area: Wisconsin, U.S.A.
Contact: Judy Murphy   414-541-1589

Index

Contributors

Patricia A. Abbott, M.S., R.N.
Clinical Specialist for Information Systems, GRECC, Baltimore VA
Medical Center, Baltimore, MD, USA (abbott@umbc2.umbc.edu)

Kathleen C. Allan, M.H.A., R.N.
Product Manager, SMS, Malvern, PA, USA

Betty J. Anderson, R.N., B.Sc.N., M.N.
Clinical Nurse Specialist, Royal Alexandra Hospital, Edmonton, Alberta,
Canada

John Anderson
Technical Systems, SMS, Malvern, PA, USA

Kathleen M. Andolina, R.N., M.S., C.S.
Consultant, The Center for Case Management, Inc., South Natick, MA,
USA

Marion J. Ball, Ed.D.
Vice President Information Services, University of Maryland, Baltimore,
MD, USA (mjb@umabnet.ab.umd.edu)

Christine Bolwell, M.S.N., R.N.
President, Diskovery, San Jose, CA, USA

Patricia Flatley Brennan, R.N., Ph.D., F.A.A.N., F.A.C.M.I.
Associate Professor, Frances Payne Bolton School of Nursing, Case
Western Reserve University, Cleveland, OH, USA (pfb@po.cwru.edu)

Gail R. Casper, M.S., R.N.
Project Director, Frances Payne Bolton School of Nursing, Case Western Reserve University, Cleveland, OH, USA (grc2@po.cwru.edu)

Elizabeth B. Concordia, M.A.S.
Senior Director Clinical Services, Johns Hopkins Bayview Medical Center, Baltimore, MD, USA

Christine R. Curran, M.S.N., R.N., C.N.A.
Director, Division of Surgical Nursing, Penn State's University Hospital at the Milton S. Hershey Medical Center, Hershey, PA, USA (ccurran@nursing.hmc.psu.edu)

Marguerite A. Daniels, M.A., C.C.C.
Manager, Strategic Products, SMS, Malvern, PA, USA

Judith V. Douglas, M.H.S.
Director, Information Services, University of Maryland, Baltimore, MD, USA (judy@umabnet.ab.umd.edu)

Marina Douglas, M.S., R.N.
Manager, Patient Care Systems, The Compucare Company, Reston, VA, USA

Linda Edmunds, M.S., R.N.
Director of Design, Highland Reserves, Inc., Atlanta, GA, USA (linda edmds@aol.com)

Margaret J.A. Edwards, Ph.D., R.N.
Margaret JA Edwards & Associates, Inc., Calgary, Alberta, Canada (marge@cs.athabascau.ca)

Marjorie H. Farver, M.S.N., R.N.
Director of Information Systems, Visiting Nurse Association of Washington, DC and Suburban Maryland, Washington, DC, USA (mhfl@mhg.edu)

James M. Gabler, M.S.
Gabler Consulting, Phoenix, AZ, USA (jmgabler@aol.com)

Carole A. Gassert, Ph.D., R.N.
Assistant Professor, Coordinator of Nursing Informatics, University of Maryland at Baltimore, Baltimore, MD, USA (cgassert@umabnet.ab.umd.edu)

Gary D. Hales, Ph.D.
Founding Editor-in-Chief, Computers in Nursing

Gary L. Hammon, B.S.B.A.
Manager, Superior Consultant Company, Inc., San Antonio, TX, USA
(gary_hammon@super.#u#dtw.ccmail.compuserve.com)

Kathryn J. Hannah, Ph.D., R.N.
Professor, Department of Community Health Sciences, Faculty of Medicine, The University of Calgary, Calgary, Alberta, Canada (khannah@acs
.ucalgary.ca)

Barbara A. Happ, Ph.D., R.N.
Senior Consultant, Hamilton/KSA, Fairfax, VA, USA (72123.2333@compu
serv.com)

Bennie E. Harsanyi, Ed.D., R.N.
Nursing Consultant, SMS, Malvern, PA, USA

Margaret M. Hassett, M.S., R.N.
Nursing MIS Coordinator, St. Elizabeth's Medical Center, Boston, MA,
USA (mhassett@world.std.com)

Detsy S. Hersher, B.S.
President, Hersher Associates, Ltd., Northbrook, IL, USA

Shirley J. Hughes, R.N.
President, SJ Hughes Consulting, Chandler, AZ, USA

Miriam Jaffe, B.A.
Information Services, University of Maryland at Baltimore, Baltimore, MD,
USA (mjaffe@umabnet.ab.umd.edu)

Suzanne Jenkins, B.S.N., R.N.
Account Executive, The Compucare Company, Reston, VA, USA

Nancy M. Lorenzi, Ph.D.
Associate Senior Vice President, University of Cincinnati Medical Center,
Cincinnati, OH, USA (lorenzi@uc.edu)

Kathleen A. McCormick, Ph.D., R.N., F.A.A.N.
Senior Science Advisor, Agency for Health Care Policy and Research,
Rockville, MD, USA

Salah H. Mandil, Ph.D.
Director-Advisor on Informatics, World Health Organization, Geneva, Switzerland (mandilsewho.ch)

Kerry E. Meyer, Ph.D., A.R.N.P., R.N.
(formerly Kerry E. Meyer-Petrucci), Assistant Professor, University of Washington, Seattle, WA, USA (petrucci@carson.u.washington.edu)

Mary Etta Mills, Sc.D., C.N.A.A., R.N.
Associate Professor and Chair, University of Maryland at Baltimore School of Nursing, Baltimore, MD, USA (mmills@umabnet.ab.umd.edu)

Susan K. Newbold, M.S., R.N.
University of Maryland at Baltimore, Baltimore, MD, USA (snewbold@umabnet.ab.umd.edu)

Robert T. Riley, Ph.D.
President, Riley Associates, Cincinnati, OH, USA (rileyrt@uc.edu)

Judith Shamian, Ph.D., R.N.
Vice-President, Nursing, Mount Sinai Hospital, Toronto, Ontario, Canada (jshamian@gpu.utcc.utoronto.ca)

Diane J. Skiba, Ph.D.
Associate Professor and Director of Informatics, University of Colorado Health Sciences Center, School of Nursing, Denver, CO, USA (dskiba@freenet.hsc.colorado.edu)

Nancy Staggers, Ph.D., R.N.
Deputy Director, Corporate Informatics, OASD (HA), HSO&R—Health Affairs, Washington, DC, USA (nstagger@ha.osd.mil)

James P. Turley, Ph.D., R.N.
Associate Professor, The University of Texas—Houston, Health Science Center School of Nursing, Houston, TX, USA (jturley@sonl.nur.uth.tmc.edu)

Ann Warnock-Matheron, M.N., R.N.
Patient Care Information Systems Specialist, Calgary General Hospital, Calgary, Alberta Canada (warnock@acs.ucalgary.ca)

David Williams, M.S., R.N.
Nursing Informatics Manager, U.S. Army, Madigan Army Hospital, Tacoma, WA, USA

David H. Wilson, M.D.
Physician Consultant, SMS, Malvern, PA, USA

Karen Lafferty Zimmerman, B.S.N., R.N.
Consultant, Information Services, Carilion Health System, Roanoke, VA, USA

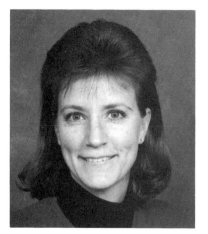

PATRICIA A. ABBOTT

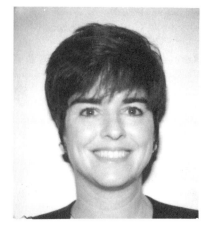

KATHLEEN C. ALLAN

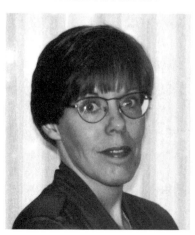

BETTY J. ANDERSON

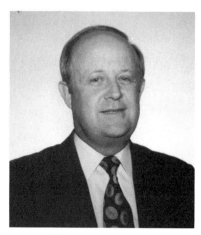

JOHN ANDERSON

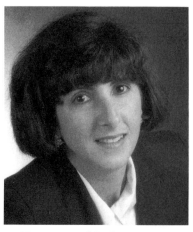

KATHLEEN M. ANDOLINA

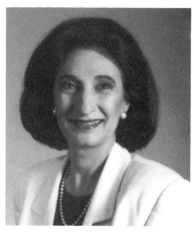

MARION J. BALL

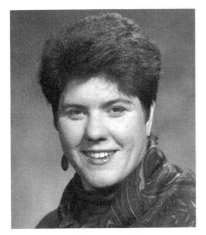

PATRICIA FLATLEY BRENNAN

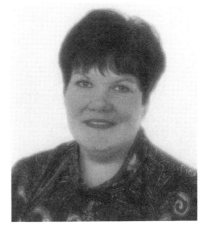

GAIL R. CASPER

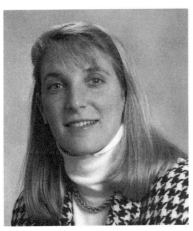

ELIZABETH B. CONCORDIA

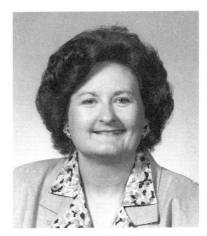

CHRISTINE R. CURRAN

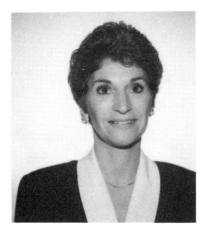

MARGUERITE A. DANIELS

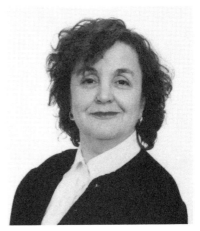

JUDITH V. DOUGLAS

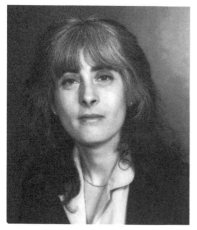

LINDA EDMUNDS

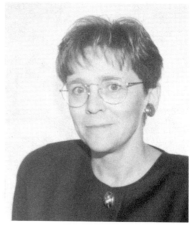

MARGARET J. A. EDWARDS

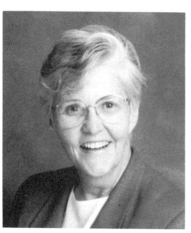

MARJORIE H. FARVER

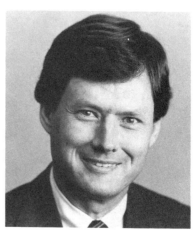

JAMES M. GABLER

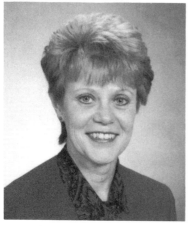

CAROLE A. GASSERT

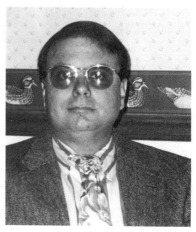

GARY D. HALES

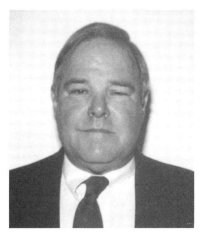

Gary L. Hammon

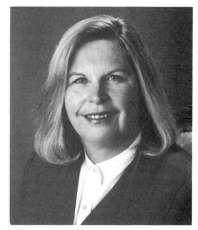

Kathryn J. Hannah

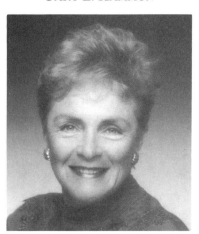

Barbara A. Happ

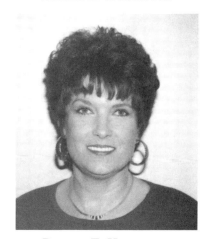

Bennie E. Harsanyi

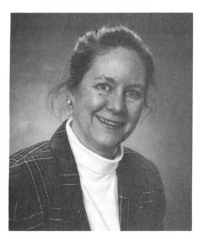

Margaret M. Hassett

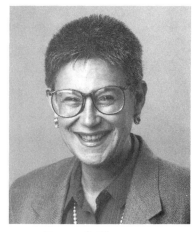

Betsy S. Hersher

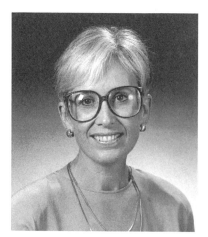

SHIRLEY J. HUGHES

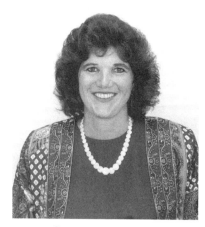

SUZANNE JENKINS

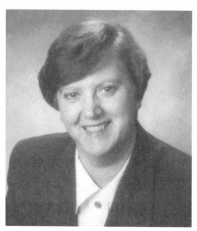

NANCY M. LORENZI

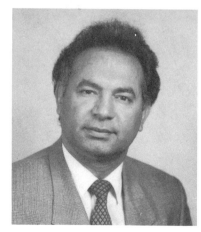

SALAH H. MANDIL

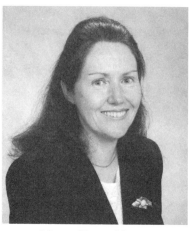

MARY ETTA MILLS

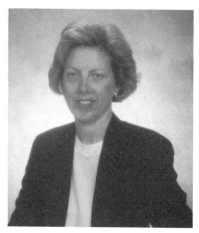

SUSAN K. NEWBOLD

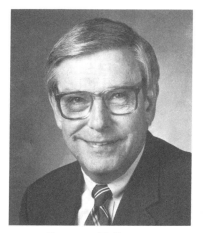

ROBERT T. RILEY

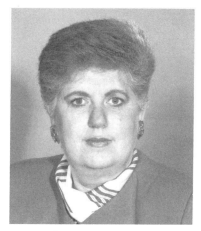

JUDITH SHAMIAN

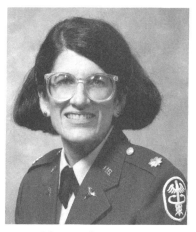

NANCY STAGGERS

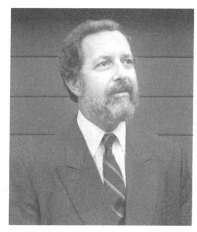

JAMES P. TURLEY

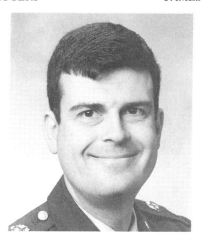

DAVID WILLIAMS

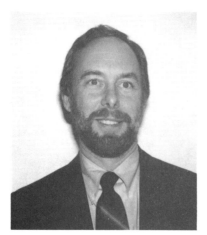

DAVID H. WILSON

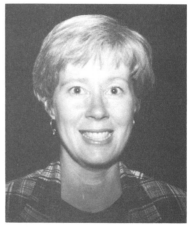

KAREN LAFFERTY ZIMMERMAN